Small Animal Anesthesia and Analgesia

Small Animal Anesthesia and Analgesia

Edited by Gwendolyn L. Carroll

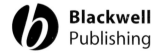

Blackwell
Publishing

GWENDOLYN LIGHT CARROLL, MS, DVM, DACVA, CVA is a Professor of Anesthesiology at Texas A&M University College of Veterinary Medicine and Biomedical Sciences, Department of Small Animal Clincal Sciences. Dr. Carroll received an AB in biopsychology from Vassar College. She was a small animal practitioner for several years before completing a residency in anesthesiology. The common thread in her education, training, practice, and research is a persistent interest in animal behavior and well-being. She currently lives with her husband Tim and three red tabbies: DJ, Felix, and Oscar.

Blackwell Publishing Professional
2121 State Avenue, Ames, Iowa 50014, USA

Orders: 1-800-862-6657
Office: 1-515-292-0140
Fax: 1-515-292-3348
Web site: www.blackwellprofessional.com

Blackwell Publishing Ltd
9600 Garsington Road, Oxford OX4 2DQ, UK
Tel.: +44 (0)1865 776868

Blackwell Publishing Asia
550 Swanston Street, Carlton, Victoria 3053, Australia
Tel.: +61 (0)3 8359 1011

Authorization to photocopy items for internal or personal use, or the internal or personal use of specific clients, is granted by Blackwell Publishing, provided that the base fee is paid directly to the Copyright Clearance Center, 222 Rosewood Drive, Danvers, MA 01923. For those organizations that have been granted a photocopy license by CCC, a separate system of payments has been arranged. The fee codes for users of the Transactional Reporting Service are ISBN-13: 978-0-8138-0230-5/2008.

First edition, 2008

Library of Congress Cataloging-in-Publication Data
Carroll, Gwendolyn L.
    Small animal anesthesia and analgesia / Gwendolyn L. Carroll. – 1st ed.
        p.   ;   cm.
    Includes bibliographical references and index.
    ISBN-13: 978-0-8138-0230-5 (alk. paper)
    ISBN-10: 0-8138-0230-X (alk. paper)
    1. Veterinary anesthesia.   2. Analgesia.
3. Pets–Surgery.   I. Title.
    [DNLM: 1. Dogs–surgery.   2. Analgesia–methods.   3. Analgesia–veterinary.
4. Anesthesia–methods.   5. Anesthesia–veterinary.   6. Cats–surgery. SF 991 C319s 2008]

    SF914.C37 2008
    636.089'796–dc22
                                        2007028217

Disclaimer
The contents of this work are intended to further general scientific research, understanding, and discussion only and are not intended and should not be relied upon as recommending or promoting a specific method, diagnosis, or treatment by practitioners for any particular patient. The publisher and the author make no representations or warranties with respect to the accuracy or completeness of the contents of this work and specifically disclaim all warranties, including without limitation any implied warranties of fitness for a particular purpose. In view of ongoing research, equipment modifications, changes in governmental regulations, and the constant flow of information relating to the use of medicines, equipment, and devices, the reader is urged to review and evaluate the information provided in the package insert or instructions for each medicine, equipment, or device for, among other things, any changes in the instructions or indication of usage and for added warnings and precautions. Readers should consult with a specialist where appropriate. The fact that an organization or Website is referred to in this work as a citation and/or a potential source of further information does not mean that the author or the publisher endorses the information the organization or Website may provide or recommendations it may make. Further, readers should be aware that Internet Websites listed in this work may have changed or disappeared between when this work was written and when it is read. No warranty may be created or extended by any promotional statements for this work. Neither the publisher nor the author shall be liable for any damages arising herefrom.

The last digit is the print number: 9 8 7 6 5 4 3 2 1

Dedication

This book is dedicated to my mother and mentor, Frances Light Currie, to my husband and captain, Tim Carroll, and to my sister and hero, Dr. Jennifer Light. This book would not be possible without my pets and patients whose fear and pain sadden me and whose spirit and humor make me laugh.

Table of Contents

Foreword

If there were not a *reason* to anesthetize an animal, you would not bother doing so. General anesthesia has, since its inception, been a means to an end—to enable the surgeon to operate on a still patient and so that the patient does not experience potentially severe pain during an operation. This facilitative nature of anesthesia may be responsible for the fact that, in veterinary medicine and laboratory animal research, the individual who administers and monitors general anesthesia is most often *not* a veterinarian. However, because it is facilitative, it has been said that there is zero tolerance for anesthetic-related complications. Safety is paramount, for not only does the anesthetist largely take over control of the patient's circulatory, respiratory, and neurologic systems, she or he also bears the responsibility for inadvertent injury due to handling and positioning during general anesthesia.

Meanwhile, a quiet revolution in the veterinary care of small animals has been occurring. To paraphrase an observation from Chapter 13 of this textbook, the nature of our patients, goals, and responsibilities has changed so much over the past decade that anesthesia of the elderly, or morbidly ill, or systemically or genetically impaired dog or cat is often proposed with little second thought. Surgical and diagnostic procedures of increasing sophistication are performed, necessitating long or specialized anesthesia management. Veterinarians are also recognizing the importance of perioperative management of pain and fear or anxiety in their patients. In short, veterinary anesthesia is no longer simple, if it ever was! When one considers that nearly all small-animal veterinarians must also be the experts who oversee sedation and anesthesia of their patients, it seems obvious that this expertise must grow with every new expectation of the profession. For this reason, a crucial role is played by the board-certified veterinary anesthesiologist in advancing knowledge, setting standards, and training of each veterinarian who graduates.

Yet, so much of what we do as veterinary anesthesiologists, our "best practice," is still not completely based on rigorous data and clinical trial outcomes, as is that of our medical doctor counterparts. Rather it is based on the body of human medical and basic physiology literature and supported by "nodes" of veterinary basic and applied research elucidating some of the things we need to know. A skilled anesthesiologist is therefore responsible for interpretation of fact, experience, and lore, crafting them into the coherent discipline of veterinary anesthesiology. In this textbook, the author has made available a career's worth of experience and knowledge specifically about dog and cat anesthesia. She has managed to distill an enormous amount of information about general anesthesia, from taking a history to recovery. Information for troubleshooting problems is included along with discussions of equipment and physiology. The commonsense approach to patient workup prior to anesthesia presented in Chapter 4 thoroughly discusses factors to consider and probably is the best real-life description I have seen. There is a marvelously successful chapter on pain, which includes a review of the pain physiology, as well as treatment strategies. And a unique feature is a chapter on some physical medicine techniques that can be used to complement standard pain medicine therapy.

For those who learn best when presented with a reason "why" a fact is important, this text will be an excellent resource. Although pharmacologic and physiologic information is cited to support concepts, it spares the reader from having to interpret a litany of published findings—in other words, it is not overreferenced, and the interpretation is there for you. As I read through it, I found myself nodding in appreciation of how seamlessly the author has blended descriptions of techniques into the contextual supporting information that help justify an idea. "Pearls" of wisdom are offered at times to highlight or reinforce a concept. There is an almost "stream of consciousness" quality to the writing that makes it easy to read.

The book will effectively dispel the notion that "one size fits all" anesthetic regimens or techniques can be used on every patient and will enhance the reader's knowledge and thus ability to safely anesthetize animals, while also providing for their comfort. If I did not also have to teach veterinary students about horses, farm animals, and exotics, I would make this book THE reference for their anesthesiology and pain medicine course. However, the book is invaluable, not only for veterinary students but also for veterinary technician students, anesthesiology residents, practicing small-animal veterinarians, and especially any nonveterinarian who will be administering anesthesia for any purpose (e.g., researchers).

—Alicia Z. Karas MS, DVM, Dipl. ACVA
Assistant Professor, Department of Clinical
Sciences Cummings School of Veterinary
Medicine at Tufts University North Grafton,
MA Member, Board of Directors, International
Veterinary Academy of Pain Management

Preface

Small Animal Anesthesia and Analgesia was written with the student needing a quick review and the busy practitioner in mind. The intent of this text is to provide protocols and monitoring techniques such that "survival" is not the yardstick by which we measure outcomes in patients undergoing anesthesia and surgery. For practitioners that currently use limited analgesics and analgesic techniques in their practice, I have provided basic information that will be easy to follow, useful, and reliable. The information provided can be used the first day. For practitioners that currently rely heavily on advanced anesthetic and analgesic techniques in their practice, there is information that complements the drugs and techniques already employed. The text necessarily reflects my bias. As in any case management, clinical judgment must be used to individualize treatment for any given patient.

The references cited have been limited to those that are particularly helpful, those that provide specific drug dosages or techniques that I do not normally employ, and those that provide recent new evidence of efficacy of analgesics or analgesic techniques.

This text is intended to be a quick reference and is not intended to replace chapters and journal articles or more complete previously published texts. The interested reader should consult these references for further information.

Acknowledgements

I would like to acknowledge the Herculean contribution of my coauthors, all of whom are experts in their fields. Their gift of time can never be repaid.

The photographer at Texas A&M, Larry Wadsworth, who helped me with photographs and the artist, Mark M. Miller of Miller Medical Illustration & Design who provided fantastic illustrations with little direction, were excellent collaborators, often with little notice.

Ms. Elaine Lippard is a word processing genius for whom I am daily grateful.

As regards to Blackwell, I have had enormous support. There are several individuals in particular whom have had a helpful hand in this endeavor: Erin Gardner was the Commissioning Editor for whom I am very grateful. Dede Anderson picked up as the Managing Editor. Even though I was a bit of an onus, she never complained. Erin Magnani is the Production Editor and again is a patient soul. I am also grateful for the hard work of Allison Esposito, the copy editor, Tad Ringo, the proofreader, and Robert and Cynthia Swanson, the indexers.

A special thanks to Drs. Hartsfield, Matthews, Crist, Baetge, Guedes, Lepiz, and Martinez for their clinical service during this endeavor.

List of Contributors

M.A. Crist, DVM, CVA, CCH
College of Veterinary Medicine and Biomedical
  Sciences
Texas A&M University

Steven M. Fox, MS, DVM, MBA, PhD
Director of Pain Management
Novartis Animal Health

Tamara L. Grubb, DVM, MS, DACVA
Pfizer

Alonso G.P. Guedes, DVM, PhD, DACVA
College of Veterinary Medicine and Biomedical
  Sciences
Texas A&M University

Sandee M. Hartsfield, DVM, MS, DACVA
Department of Small Animal Clinical Sciences
College of Veterinary Medicine and Biomedical
  Sciences
Texas A&M University

Kris T. Kruse-Elliott, DVM, PhD, DACVA
Medical Director
San Francisco Iams Pet Imaging Center

Phillip Lerche, BVSc, PhD, DACVA
Ohio

Nora S. Matthews, DVM, DACVA
Department of Small Animal Clinical Sciences
College of Veterinary Medicine and Biomedical
  Sciences
Texas A&M University

Maureen McMichael, DVM, DACVECC
Illinois

William Muir, DVM, PhD, ACVA, ACVECC
Professor
Department of Veterinary Clinical Sciences
Ohio State University

Carin A. Ponder, RVT
College of Veterinary Medicine and Biomedical
  Sciences
Texas A&M University

Katy W. Waddle, RVT, VTS (ECC/Anesthesia)
College of Veterinary Medicine and Biomedical
  Sciences
Texas A&M University

Small Animal Anesthesia and Analgesia

Chapter 1
Anesthesia Equipment

Sandee M. Hartsfield

Various pieces of medical equipment are necessary for the proper conduct of general anesthesia in veterinary patients. Endotracheal tubes are vital for security of the airway. Anesthesia machines, vaporizers, and breathing systems facilitate the administration of oxygen alone or an oxygen and anesthetic mixture. Furthermore, facemasks, anesthetic chambers, laryngoscopes, and ventilators often play vital roles in the management of anesthesia.

The purpose of this chapter is to provide an overview of equipment that is commonly used in anesthetic management of veterinary patients. Detailed descriptions of these and other pieces of anesthetic equipment are available in textbooks intended as relatively exhaustive references to support both human and veterinary anesthesia (Dorsch and Dorsch 1984, 1994, 1999; Ehrenwerth and Eisenkraft 1993; Hartsfield 1987, 1996, 1999).

> Equipment malfunctions and improper use of equipment are common causes of anesthetic complications.

ENDOTRACHEAL TUBES, MASKS, ANESTHETIC CHAMBERS, AND LARYNGOSCOPES

Endotracheal Tubes

Endotracheal (ET) tubes are required for most patients anesthetized with inhalant anesthetics in oxygen. A properly placed ET tube with a correctly inflated cuff establishes a patent airway, allows effective spontaneous and controlled ventilation, protects the respiratory system from entry of foreign material, and assists in prevention of contamination of the workplace with waste anesthetic gases. ET tubes should be clean, dry, and preferably sterile when placed into a patient's respiratory system.

A common ET tube is depicted in Figure 1.1. The parts of a cuffed ET tube include the tube itself, the adapter-connector (15-mm outside diameter [O.D.] for connection to the anesthesia breathing system), and the cuff, pilot balloon, pilot line, and inflation-deflation valve complex. For orientation, the patient end of an ET tube is equivalent to the distal end (beveled end), and the machine end is synonymous with the proximal end.

Commercial ET tubes for humans and animals have various markings and abbreviations that describe each tube, and markings may include the manufacturer, internal and external diameters (in millimeters or French units), length (in centimeters), and codes indicating tissue toxicity or implantation testing (e.g., I.T., F29, Z79). For application in human patients, a radiopaque marker is required near the distal end of the ET tube or along the entire length of the tube.

In sizing ET tubes, it is common to refer to the internal diameter (I.D.) of the tube measured in millimeters. The I.D. of a tube may be referred to as the oral size, and the O.D. as the nasal size. A larger I.D. reduces resistance to ventilation, but the O.D. limits the tube to a specific size of patient. Generally, the length of the ET tube should be selected to allow the distal end of the tube to be located at the level of the mid-cervical trachea (distal to the larynx and near the thoracic inlet) when the proximal end of the tube is located at the level of the patient's incisor teeth.

The safest cuffs for ET tubes appear to be of the high-volume, low-pressure design, which allows the airway to be sealed between the external wall of the ET tube and the trachea without putting undue pressure on the tracheal mucosa. Excessive pressure

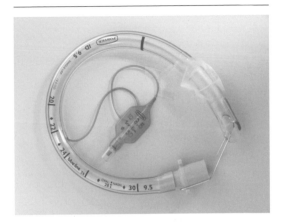

Figure 1.1. A Murphy-style endotracheal tube showing the parts of the tube (connector, inflation apparatus, cuff, Murphy eye or side hole, end hole, and bevel) and the common markings (manufacturer = Portex, internal diameter in millimeters = 9.5, outside diameter in millimeters = 13, length markings in centimeters from the distal end of the tube = 20, 22 . . . 30, indication that the tube can be used orally or nasally, indication that the tube is for single use).

(30 cm H_2O or greater) can limit blood supply to the mucosa (Dorsch and Dorsch 1999) and lead to sloughing of tissue, scarring, and constriction of the tracheal lumen. Overinflation of the cuff should be avoided. A common practice is to inflate the cuff with only enough air to prevent leakage of gases past the cuff when pressures of 20 to 25 cm H_2O are applied to the respiratory system.

The kinds of ET tubes that have been available for small animal anesthesia include Murphy, Magill, and Cole styles; Murphy-type tubes are used most commonly. A Murphy tube (Fig. 1.1) has the same internal and external diameters throughout its length and has a side hole (Murphy eye) near the distal end opposite the bevel. The side hole facilitates gas flow if the end hole should become occluded. Tubes designed for human use may be curved slightly to facilitate placement, while some tubes designed for veterinary patients are straight. Magill tubes are similar to Murphy tubes but do not have a side hole. A Cole tube has larger internal and external diameters at the proximal end and smaller diameters at the distal end. The distal end of the tube fits into the larynx and trachea, and the point at which the diameters gradually change (shoulder) allows a seal between the tube and the airway, if the correct size of tube has been selected and the tube has been properly placed and secured. It is possible for pressure from the shoulder of the tube to damage laryngeal tissues. In practice, Cole tubes do not produce the same degree of airway security and protection as cuffed tubes.

Commercial ET tubes for small animal use are usually made from polyvinyl chloride or silicone rubber. Materials used for the manufacture of ET tubes and cuffs should have been shown to be nontoxic to tissues. Silicone tubes appear to be minimally traumatic to tissues if they are placed carefully and are well secured. ET tubes are usually clear, rather than opaque, so that the lumen can be inspected to ensure that the tube remains unobstructed.

Specially designed ET tubes are available for certain purposes. Armored or spiral embedded ET tubes contain helical wire or nylon to retard collapse of the tube and obstruction of the lumen when the patient's neck is flexed. A double-lumen ET tube may be used to allow one-lung ventilation for certain kinds of thoracic and pulmonary surgery.

Tracheostomy tubes are used to maintain a patent and protected airway in unanesthetized patients with upper airway obstruction. They are designed with a removable liner that can be changed and cleaned to prevent the buildup of dried secretions within the lumen of the tube. Standard ET tubes can be placed through a tracheostomy site for maintenance of anesthesia (e.g., laryngeal surgery), but they are usually replaced with tracheostomy tubes before the patient recovers from anesthesia.

Manual resuscitators allow controlled ventilation in patients with ET tubes or tracheostomy tubes in place. A manual resuscitator (Fig. 1.2) is a compressible, self-reinflating bag equipped with a nonrebreathing valve that attaches to the ET tube connector. "Ambu (Army Manual Breathing Unit) bag" is a common term used to refer to these types of resuscitators. A manual resuscitator can function with ambient air or can be supplied with a source of oxygen to enrich inspired gases. Unless an additional reservoir is added to the resuscitator bag, inspired gases will usually contain less than 100% oxygen because air will be entrained as the bag self-inflates (Dorsch and Dorsch 1999).

Masks

Masks (Fig. 1.3) can be used to facilitate delivery of oxygen to patients before induction of anesthesia

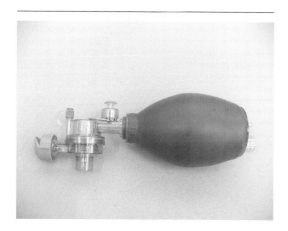

Figure 1.2. A self-inflating manual resuscitator showing the nonrebreathing valve, the reservoir bag, a port for attaching an oxygen source, and a valve for entraining room air.

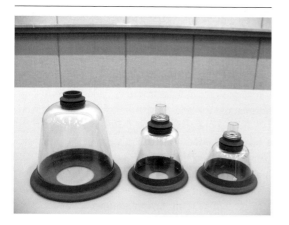

Figure 1.3. Three sizes of clear veterinary masks, each with a diaphragm to create a seal around the patient's mouth and nose.

and placement of an ET tube and during recovery from anesthesia after the ET tube has been removed. Masks are also used for induction of anesthesia with oxygen and inhalant anesthetics. Masks should fit snugly over the nose and mouth to speed induction and prevent leakage and dilution of anesthetic gases with air. A clear mask with a diaphragm allows for a good seal and an unimpaired view of the nose and mouth during the masking process.

Masks should be attached to an anesthesia breathing system (e.g., circle system) that supplies oxygen and anesthetic gases, has a reservoir (e.g., bag) of gases to meet the patient's inspiratory demand for tidal volume, and provides for elimination of excess gases via a scavenging system. The best practice is to use masks for induction of anesthesia only when necessary and to use them in well-ventilated induction and surgery rooms (preferably in a fume hood).

Generally, induction of anesthesia with a mask is faster if relatively high fresh gas flow rates are supplied to the breathing system. In most small-animal patients, fresh gas flow rates should be between 2 L/min and 5 L/min. Mask induction can be advantageous in selected cases, but disadvantages include an unprotected airway, potentially prolonged induction times if patients do not breathe deeply, and contamination of the workplace with waste gases.

Closed Containers

Closed containers (anesthetic chambers) can be used for oxygenation and delivery of inhalant anesthetics. Induction chambers should be made of clear plastic to facilitate a good view of the patient at all times. If the patient is easily excited, the container can be partially covered with a towel to decrease visual stimuli while the animal is in the container. The container should be near the size of the patient that is being anesthetized. Excessively large containers will lead to long induction times. The container and lid should fit and be almost air-tight, and there should be an entry port for fresh gases and an exit port for waste gases; waste gases should be delivered to a scavenging system. Ideally, closed container inductions should be done under a fume hood.

Generally, induction of anesthesia in a closed container is faster if relatively high fresh gas flow rates are supplied to the container. In most small animal patients, fresh gas flow rates should be between 2 L/min and 5 L/min. After allowing the patient to breathe oxygen for about 5 minutes, a gradual increase in the concentration of inhalant anesthetic (approximately 0.5% every 10 to 15 seconds until the desired maximum is reached) may reduce the tendency for some patients to become excited during the induction.

Advantages of closed container inductions include the delivery of anesthetic with minimal restraint, which can be of significant value in certain kinds of patients (e.g., the aggressive cat). Cats, small laboratory animals, and some exotic and wild species may be candidates for induction in a closed container. The disadvantages are the same as those

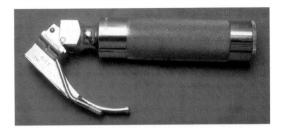

Figure 1.4. A laryngoscope showing the handle (batteries inside), a MacIntosh laryngoscope blade, and the light bulb to serve as a source of illumination.

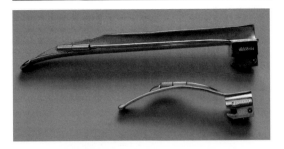

Figure 1.5. Miller (longer blade) and Bizarri-Guiffrida (shorter blade) laryngoscope blades.

listed above for mask induction. In addition, some animals become excited in the container and may hit their head against the wall of the container, and there is less control over the airway in a closed container compared with using a mask. If a question arises about whether the patient's airway is patent during induction, the animal should be removed from the container and induction completed with a mask or intravenous anesthetic.

Laryngoscopes

Laryngoscopes can be vital in the performance of rapid intubation of the trachea in small animals. They are useful for completing a good examination of the mouth, pharynx, and larynx. A laryngoscope has a handle (with batteries) and a blade with a light near the distal end (Fig. 1.4). Both disposable and permanent laryngoscopes are available, and laryngoscopes may be powered by various sizes of batteries (commonly, C cells). In preparation for anesthesia, laryngoscopes should be checked for proper function before induction.

Many types of blades are available for laryngoscopes. The Miller blade (Fig. 1.5) is very common and comes in a wide variety of sizes. Other useful blades include the MacIntosh (Fig. 1.4) and the Bizarri-Guiffrida (Fig. 1.5). A good practice is to have several blades of varying sizes (e.g., 0, 2, and 4) available. A blade length of 205 mm is a good size to use with a large dog.

For small animals, a laryngoscope is most useful to the anesthetist if an assistant grasps the patient's muzzle and retracts the lips with one hand and extends the tongue with the other. This allows the anesthetist to manipulate the laryngoscope with one hand and to pass the ET tube or guide tube with the

other. The blade should be placed flat on the tongue with the tip of the blade just rostral to the base of the epiglottis. Gentle pressure on the tip of the blade allows the epiglottis to move ventrally and rostrally to expose the glottis. Improper use of the laryngoscope can impair visualization of the airway and/or passage of the ET tube.

ANESTHESIA MACHINES

An anesthesia machine creates a precise, but variable, combination of anesthetic gases (a volatile liquid halogenated hydrocarbon anesthetic and/or nitrous oxide) and oxygen (Dorsch and Dorsch 1984). The gas mixture is delivered to a patient via a breathing system (e.g., circle system). The basic components of an anesthesia machine (Fig. 1.6) include the following:

- Source of oxygen (compressed gas cylinders)
- Regulator for oxygen
- Flowmeter for oxygen
- Vaporizer for a volatile liquid anesthetic (e.g., sevoflurane or isoflurane)

If the anesthesia machine is fitted for delivery of nitrous oxide, the basic components (source of nitrous oxide, regulator for nitrous oxide, and flowmeter for nitrous oxide) will run in parallel with the components for delivery of oxygen. The two gases mix before they reach the inlet to the vaporizer.

BREATHING SYSTEMS

A breathing system is attached to an anesthesia machine for the following purposes:

- Delivery of oxygen to the patient
- Delivery of anesthetic gas(es) to the patient

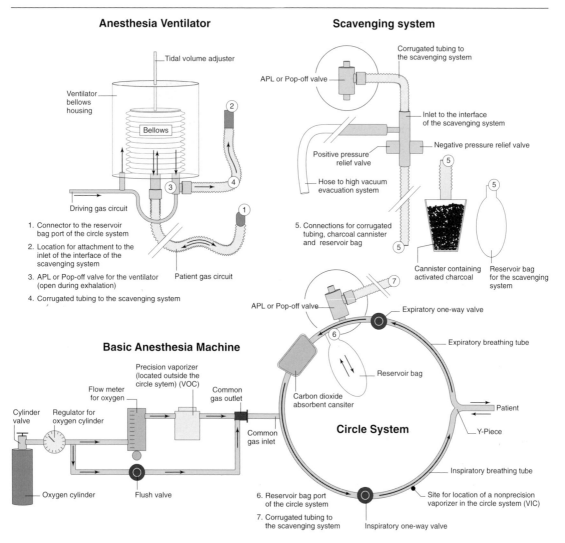

Figure 1.6. Diagrams of a basic anesthesia machine, a circle breathing system, an anesthesia ventilator, and a scavenging system. (Illustration by Mark M. Miller, Miller Medical Illustration & Design.)

- Removal of carbon dioxide from exhaled gases
- Provision of a method for controlled ventilation

Breathing systems have been classified in numerous schemes (Dorsch and Dorsch 1999). For the purpose of this chapter, breathing systems will be discussed in two groups: *circle systems* and *non-rebreathing (NRB) systems*. Depending on the design of the NRB system and the flow rate of fresh gas into a NRB system, some exhaled gases may be inspired during inspiration; thus, the term "non-rebreathing" could be a misnomer under certain conditions (e.g., inadequate fresh gas inflow).

Perhaps the best way to describe the use of a breathing system for any patient is to provide the following information (Hamilton 1964):
- Name and describe the breathing system (e.g., circle system)
- Define the patient by its body weight and/or metabolic rate
- State the flow rate of each medical gas into the breathing system

Circle Systems

Circle systems retain all or part of the patient's expired gases, after the removal of carbon dioxide, and some of the retained gases are inspired during the patient's next breath. The amount of expired gas that is retained depends entirely on the fresh gas flow rate into the circle system. Very little expired gas is retained if the fresh gas flow rate into the circle is very high; most of the expired gas exits at the pop-off valve. Conversely, most of the expired gas (except for carbon dioxide) is retained if the fresh gas flow rate approximates the patient's rate of consumption of oxygen. The following terms have been used to describe circle systems according to fresh gas flow into the system:

Closed circle system: Fresh gas flow equals the patient's oxygen consumption.

Low-flow circle system: Fresh gas flow is greater than the patient's oxygen consumption, but less than the fresh gas flow in a semi-closed circle.

Semiclosed circle system: Fresh gas flow rate is much greater than the patient's oxygen consumption. Traditionally, an oxygen flow rate of 22 to 44 ml/kg per minute has been used for semiclosed circles. A guideline for oxygen flow for maintenance in semiclosed circles is three times the patient's oxygen consumption.

The consumption of oxygen by anesthetized dogs has been reviewed and reported to range from 3 ml/kg per minute to 14 ml/kg per minute (Hartsfield 1996). This variability depends on the anesthetic used, the patient's body weight and surface area or metabolic rate, and the patient's body temperature.

The prime advantage of higher fresh gas flow rates to the breathing system is stability of concentration in the circle and thus stability of anesthetic depth. With use of a higher fresh gas flow, a change in the vaporizer concentration is reflected in the patient's inspired anesthetic concentration very quickly. This enables the anesthetist to effect changes in anesthetic depth as fast as possible, given the limitations of the particular inhalant anesthetic (e.g., the blood-gas partition coefficient). Advantages of lower fresh gas flow rates include production of less waste anesthetic gas, potentially less exposure of personnel to waste gases, better economy, and less effect on the patient's body temperature. Higher fresh gas flow rates promote hypothermia. Nitrous oxide should not be used in low flow or closed systems without continuous instrumental monitoring of the inspired oxygen concentration.

Basic components of a circle system are diagrammed in Figure 1.6. Gases move in one direction around a circle breathing system. Fresh gases enter the circle at the fresh gas inlet which is commonly located near the inspiratory one-way valve. On inspiration, gases move from the reservoir bag through the carbon dioxide absorbent canister, through the inspiratory one-way valve, through the inspiratory breathing hose, through the Y-piece, through the endotracheal tube, and into the patient's lungs. On expiration, gases move from the lungs through the trachea, ET tube, Y-piece, expiratory breathing hose, expiratory one-way valve, and into the reservoir bag. At any time during the respiratory cycle, excess gases in the circle system are "popped off" through the overflow (pop-off) valve to the hoses of the scavenging system and are either absorbed by activated charcoal or vented outside the workplace through a negative pressure exhaust system.

Some of the details about the function of the various components of circle breathing systems are listed next. These components are diagrammed in Figure 1.6, and some are illustrated in Figure 1.7:

Fresh Gas Inlet

The fresh gas inlet is the source of oxygen to the circle system. If the anesthesia machine is configured with a vaporizer outside the breathing system (VOC), oxygen and inhalant anesthetic enter the circle at the fresh gas inlet. If the anesthesia machine is configured with a vaporizer inside the circle (VIC), only oxygen enters at the fresh gas inlet. If nitrous oxide is used, it travels in parallel and mixes with oxygen and enters the breathing system at the fresh gas inlet. The fresh gas inlet is the portal for delivery of oxygen to the circle if the flush valve is activated.

Reservoir Bag

The reservoir bag attaches to a 22-mm bag port on the circle system and serves to provide gases to meet the peak flow demand during inspiration. Peak flow during the short period of inspiration exceeds the maintenance flow of oxygen into the breathing system. Some general and traditional guidelines are

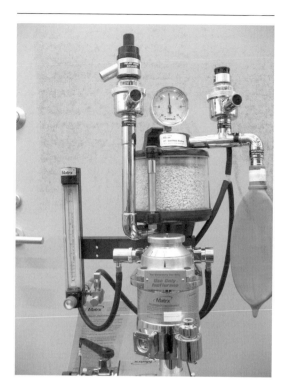

Figure 1.7. Matrx VMS anesthesia machine showing the reservoir bag, unidirectional valves, carbon dioxide absorbent canister with a manometer on top, pop-off valve atop the expiratory one-way valve, negative-pressure relief valve atop the inspiratory one-way valve, a vaporizer (inlet on the left and outlet on the right), flowmeter, and flush valve.

that the bag's minimum volume should be about six times the patient's tidal volume (an estimate of tidal volume is 11 ml/kg) and that the bag should remain about three-quarters full during maintenance of anesthesia. Bags of different sizes can be used, but excessively large bags add volume to the system, make monitoring of ventilation more difficult (movement of the bag is harder to assess), and slow equilibration of gas concentration when vaporizer settings are changed. Small bags are more easily overfilled, which can lead to overpressurization and damage to the lung.

CARBON DIOXIDE ABSORBENT CANISTER

The absorbent canister contains the chemical absorbent (Fig. 1.7) for exhaled carbon dioxide. A general formula (Dorsch and Dorsch 1999) that depicts the chemical absorption of CO_2 by soda lime is:

$$2NaOH + 2H_2CO_3 + Ca(OH)_2 \rightarrow CaCO_3 + Na_2CO_3 + 4H_2O + heat \quad (1.1)$$

The volume of the canister should be at least twice the patient's tidal volume, because approximately half the gas volume of the canister is occupied by the absorbent itself. The presence of an effective chemical absorbent for carbon dioxide allows only exhaled oxygen and anesthetic to be rebreathed by the patient on the next inspiration. Canisters are designed with screens and baffles, the former to prevent absorbent granules from moving into other parts of the breathing system and the latter to reduce channeling of gases along the side of the canister. Channeling of gases in the canister reduces the effectiveness of carbon dioxide absorption.

CHEMICAL CARBON DIOXIDE ABSORBENTS

Two products are commonly used in circle systems as chemical carbon dioxide absorbents: soda lime and baralyme. In both, calcium hydroxide is the primary component of the granular material. Absorbent granules should be added to completely fill the canister leaving only a small space at the top (Fig. 1.8). The canister should be tapped gently during filling to settle the granules, but granules should not be packed tightly. Fresh absorbent is white in color and is easily crumbled under pressure. Expended absorbent undergoes a pH sensitive color change (white to violet or white to pink) and becomes hard (calcium carbonate = limestone). The reaction involved with carbon dioxide absorption is exothermic, and a "heat line" is produced which usually can be identified on the side of the canister during active use of a circle system. The absorbent in the canister should be changed regularly to ensure effective absorption of carbon dioxide. Water is a component of the carbon dioxide absorbents, and absorbents should not remain exposed to air and allowed to dry. Dry absorbents may not function properly.

Some degradation of the inhalant anesthetics occurs with their exposure to carbon dioxide absorbents (Dorsch and Dorsch 1999); sevoflurane has the greatest potential for degradation, producing Compound A. Factors associated with an increase

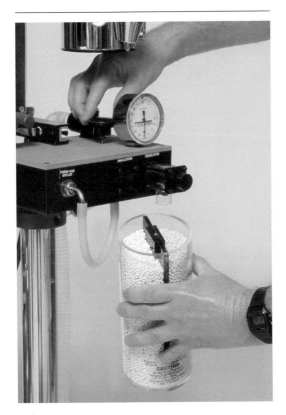

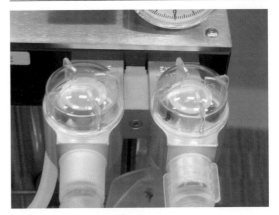

Figure 1.9. Unidirectional (one-way) valves on a SurgiVet anesthesia machine with the expiratory valve on the *right* and the inspiratory valve on the *left*.

Figure 1.8. Changing soda lime in a circle system on an Anesco anesthesia machine illustrating the small open space at the top of the canister after filling the canister with soda lime; the fresh gas or common gas outlet is shown on the left side of the unit with tubing leading to the fresh gas inlet of the circle system.

in the concentration of Compound A in the breathing system include dry absorbent, high concentration of sevoflurane, high temperature of absorbent, low fresh gas inflow, and use of baralyme instead of soda lime. While renal effects due to exposure to Compound A have been suggested, the clinical significance of Compound A in routine anesthesia for small animals has not been determined.

Carbon monoxide (CO) may be produced when inhalant anesthetics are delivered using absorbers that have been idle for at least 24 hours (Dorsch and Dorsch 1999). Carbon monoxide production is greatest with desflurane (desflurane > enflurane > isoflurane > halothane = sevoflurane). Similar factors as listed for Compound A tend to increase production of CO. Increased time of exposure also increases production of CO. Use of soda lime rather than baralyme, using fresh absorbent, and using semiclosed rather than closed or low-flow circle systems should minimize the potential for detrimental effects of either Compound A or CO.

INSPIRATORY ONE-WAY (UNIDIRECTIONAL) VALVE

During inspiration, the inspiratory one-way valve opens to allow gases from the reservoir bag to move into the patient's respiratory system. This valve works in unison with the expiratory one-way valve which closes during inspiration (Fig. 1.9).

INSPIRATORY BREATHING TUBE

The inspiratory breathing tube connects the Y-piece to the inspiratory one-way valve. It connects to the 22-mm O.D. inspiratory port of the circle system and to the 22-mm male port of the Y-piece. The tube is made of plastic or rubber and is corrugated to be flexible without kinking.

Y-PIECE

The Y-piece (22 mm O.D.) connects the inspiratory and expiratory breathing hoses (22 mm I.D.), and the Y-piece (15 mm I.D.) attaches to the ET tube connector (15 mm O.D.). The Y-piece will connect to a standard face mask.

EXPIRATORY BREATHING TUBE

The expiratory breathing tube connects the Y-piece to the expiratory one-way valve. It connects to the

22-mm O.D. expiratory port of the circle system and to the 22-mm male port of the Y-piece. The tube is made of plastic or rubber and is corrugated to be flexible without kinking.

Expiratory One-Way (Unidirectional) Valve

During expiration, the expiratory one-way valve opens to allow exhaled gases to move from the patient's respiratory system into the reservoir bag. This valve works in unison with the inspiratory one-way valve which closes during expiration (Fig. 1.9).

Overflow Valve

Synonyms include pop-off valve, pressure relief valve, and adjustable pressure limiting (APL) valve (Dorsch and Dorsch 1999). The overflow valve allows escape of excess gases from the circle system. If the valve is functioning properly, gases should escape into the scavenging system if pressure in the circle exceeds 1 to 3 cm H_2O. The overflow valve is a safety valve and should remain fully open during spontaneous ventilation. It may be closed slightly if the reservoir bag collapses when the overflow valve is fully open, but the pressure required for release of gases should remain at 1 to 3 cm H_2O. The valve may be closed temporarily if the operator is applying manually assisted or controlled ventilation (Fig. 1.10).

Scavenging System

The scavenging system includes the overflow valve, an interface, and a waste gas elimination system. The scavenging system is diagrammed in Figure 1.6. The waste gas eliminating system can be one of the following: a high negative pressure system, a low negative pressure system, or an activated charcoal system. Activated charcoal canisters are available from multiple manufacturers, and they are not effective for scavenging nitrous oxide. One manufacturer provides a detection system (Fig. 1.11) that alerts the operator if halogenated hydrocarbon anesthetic gases are not being absorbed completely.

The most important method for prevention of contamination of the workplace with waste anesthetic gases is a properly functioning scavenging system. Other procedures should be used as well,

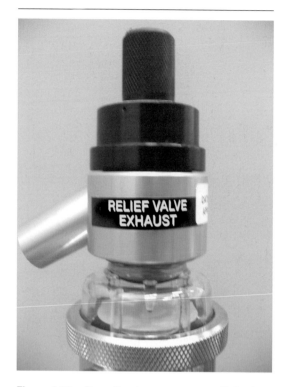

Figure 1.10. Pop-off valve or pressure relief valve atop the expiratory one-way valve on the circle system of a Matrx anesthesia machine; the angled tube to the left leads to the scavenging system.

including care in filling vaporizers, proper maintenance of all anesthetic equipment, minimizing the use of mask and closed container inductions, evacuating breathing systems into scavenging systems before patients are disconnected from the systems, and use of a monitoring program to ensure that concentrations of waste gases in the workplace do not exceed standard minimums (Hartsfield et al. 1996).

Coaxial Breathing Tubes

The Universal F system can be used to replace the standard breathing tubes and Y-piece. An F system is designed as a tube within a tube—the inspiratory tube (15 mm) located on the inside of the expiratory tube (25 mm). The patient end of the F system adapts to an ET tube connector due to its 15 mm I.D. dimension and to a face mask due to its 22 mm O.D. external diameter. An F system is compact and

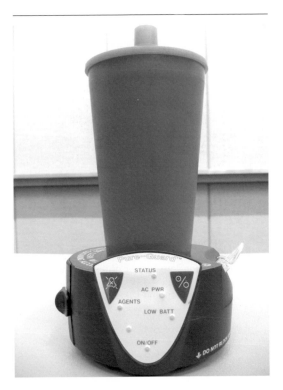

Figure 1.11. SurgiVet activated charcoal canister with a detection system for unabsorbed halogenated hydrocarbon anesthetic gases.

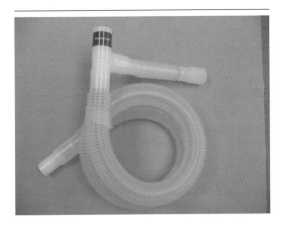

Figure 1.12. A set of coaxial breathing tubes (F circuit) that can be used to replace the traditional hoses and Y-piece on a circle system.

lightweight and is easy to manipulate when it is attached to a patient. The coaxial arrangement may provide a mechanism for heat exchange between expired and inspired gases (Fig. 1.12).

MANOMETER

Modern circle breathing systems have a pressure gauge (manometer) attached to the absorbent canister (Fig. 1.7). This allows the anesthetist to check the approximate pressure being applied to the patient's respiratory system during assisted or controlled ventilation and the pressure applied to the equipment during preanesthetic checkout procedures for machines and breathing systems. Typically, the scale for the manometer is graduated in units of kilopascals (kPa) or centimeters of water (cm H_2O).

NEGATIVE PRESSURE RELIEF VALVE

This is an intake valve designed to allow fresh air to enter the circle system if the oxygen supply to the circle system should fail. Currently, this component of the circle is commonly present on only one brand of veterinary anesthesia machines, and it is located atop the expiratory one-way valve (Fig. 1.7).

NONREBREATHING SYSTEMS

Bain, Magill, Ayre's T-piece, and Norman Elbow breathing systems are examples of nonrebreathing (NRB) systems. They have been applied in human pediatric anesthesia and have been popular for inhalant anesthesia in small veterinary patients. The most common pediatric systems in veterinary anesthesia today are the Bain and various modifications of the Ayre's T-piece system (e.g., Jackson-Rees system). A NRB system replaces the circle system; it receives fresh gases that come directly from the common gas outlet (or the outlet from the vaporizer) of the anesthesia machine.

Selection of patients for maintenance with NRB systems is a matter of personal preference. For example, some anesthesiologists use pediatric systems for patients weighing less than 7 kg, while others continue to use circle systems for patients weighing more than 3 kg (Dunlop 1992). A pediatric system is most important if the patient is expected to breathe spontaneously; the arguments for pediatric systems include lower resistance during breathing, less mechanical dead space, less total volume in the system, and reduced effort by the patient on inspiration. If ventilation is controlled and effective flow rates are used, the breathing system selected, whether a circle or NRB system, may be immaterial.

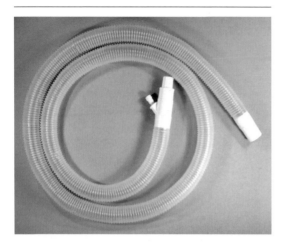

Figure 1.13. An adult Bain breathing circuit; the endotracheal tube joins the connector at the right side of the picture, and the reservoir bag with its attachment to the scavenging system and the fresh gas delivery hose attach to the plastic apparatus in the center of the picture.

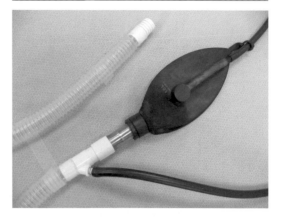

Figure 1.14. A pediatric Bain system showing the fresh gas delivery hose (black) and the reservoir bag with the overflow (center of the bag near the 1-liter mark indicating the volume of the bag) leading to the scavenging system.

While NRB systems are relatively inexpensive to purchase compared to circle systems, they are more costly to use because high fresh gas flow rates are necessary to prevent rebreathing of carbon dioxide. Consequences of higher flows include greater loss of body heat and humidity and more waste anesthetic gases. Because of the large amount of waste gas, the operator should ensure that the scavenging system functions properly. The primary advantage of NRB systems is rapid control of the anesthetic concentration in the breathing system, which translates into rapid control of depth of anesthesia.

A Bain breathing circuit (modified Mapleson D system) (Fig. 1.13) is a coaxial (tube within a tube) system without valves. The inner tube delivers fresh gases to the system, and the outer corrugated tube conducts gases to the reservoir. Excess gases exit the Bain circuit and enter the scavenging system (Fig. 1.14).

Because there is no chemical absorbent for carbon dioxide in a Bain system, the fresh gas flow rate must be relatively high. Between breaths (end of exhalation to the beginning of the next inspiration), the high fresh gas flow (oxygen and anesthetic) into the Bain circuit flushes carbon dioxide from the outer tube of the Bain circuit toward the reservoir bag. Because of the high rate of gas flow

on inspiration that is required to deliver the patient's tidal volume, the patient inhales gases provided from both the fresh gas source (flow from the inner tube) and the corrugated outer tube. When the patient exhales, expired gases flow into the outer corrugated tube and are directed toward the reservoir bag. Simultaneously, the high fresh gas flow from the inner tube dilutes carbon dioxide and flushes expired gases toward the reservoir (and ultimately into the scavenging system). This purging of carbon dioxide continues as described above until the patient starts its next inspiration. If the fresh gas flow rate is adequate, the patient rebreathes no carbon dioxide, even though a portion of the tidal volume arises from the outer corrugated tube. However, multiple recommendations exist for fresh gas flow rates during clinical use of the Bain system.

Fresh gas flow rates of two to three times the patient's minute volume are expected to ensure essentially no rebreathing of carbon dioxide. One reference recommended a flow rate of 100 to 130 ml/kg/min for spontaneously breathing patients and 100 ml/kg/min during controlled ventilation (Manley and McDonnell 1979). Others have recommended higher flows such as 200 ml/kg/min (Hodgeson 1992). Flow rates of 440 to 660 ml/kg/min prevent rebreathing of carbon dioxide in essentially all patients. The increased availability of monitors for measuring inhaled and exhaled carbon dioxide concentrations provides a means for ensuring that carbon dioxide is not rebreathed. Without instrumental monitoring of carbon dioxide tensions, the best practice is to err on the side of higher fresh gas flow rates.

Ayre's T-piece, Norman-elbow, and Jackson-Rees systems are options for pediatric breathing systems. They can be used in a manner similar to that for Bain systems. Generally, two to three times the patient's minute volume is recommended for these systems. As described above, monitoring of inspired and expired carbon dioxide concentrations can be used to ensure that fresh gas flow is adequate to prevent rebreathing of carbon dioxide.

ANESTHESIA VENTILATORS

An anesthesia ventilator is designed to be used with an anesthesia machine, and it provides the mechanism for artificial ventilation during inhalant anesthesia. The ventilator's bellows (reservoir bag) replaces the reservoir bag of the breathing circuit (e.g., circle system). Automatically controlled intermittent positive pressure applied to the outside of the ventilator's reservoir drives inspiration at an established rate and a predetermined tidal volume or inspired pressure.

The purpose of intermittent positive-pressure ventilation (IPPV) or intermittent positive-pressure breathing (IPPB) is to ensure adequate minute ventilation in anesthetized patients. A high percentage of anesthetized spontaneously breathing patients do not maintain normal minute ventilation and develop respiratory acidemia during anesthesia. In addition, patients anesthetized for thoracic surgery or repair of diaphragmatic hernias cannot generate the negative intrathoracic pressure required for normal inspiration, and artificial ventilation (mechanical or manual) is necessary. An anesthesia ventilator can be used to free the anesthetist from the laborious task of manually breathing for an anesthetized patient.

Double-circuit ventilators (Fig. 1.6) are commonly used with anesthesia machines. *Double-circuit* refers to the driving gas circuit and the patient circuit (Hartsfield 1996). The driving gas circuit is supplied by gas (often oxygen) under moderate pressure (e.g., 50 psig) delivered directly to the bellows housing of the ventilator; this circuit functions to compress the bellows, which forces gas

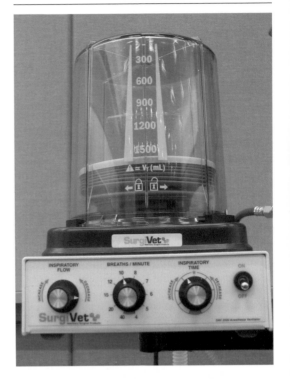

Figure 1.15. SurgiVet anesthesia ventilator showing the bellows, bellows housing, and controls (inspiratory flow, respiratory rate, inspiratory time, and power switch).

within the patient circuit into the patient's lungs on inspiration. The gases in the patient circuit are supplied from the anesthesia machine (oxygen from the machine's flowmeter and anesthetic agent from the vaporizer). An anesthesia ventilator is fitted with an automatic overflow (pop-off) valve that closes during inspiration to allow positive pressure to develop, leading to inflation of the lungs; the ventilator's automatic pop-off valve opens during expiration to allow escape of excess gases from the patient circuit.

Anesthesia ventilators may be configured with an ascending or a descending bellows, the definition being dependent on whether the bellows rises or falls during expiration. An ascending bellows rises on expiration, and is compressed toward the bottom of the bellows housing on inspiration (Figs. 1.15 and 1.16). A significant advantage of ascending bellows is that the bellows will collapse if there is an inadvertent disconnection (e.g., a loose fitting

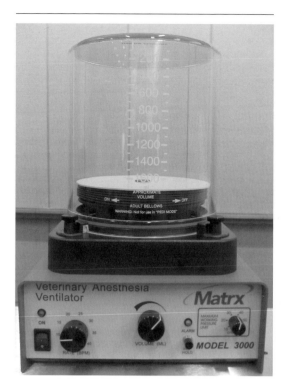

Figure 1.16. Matrx anesthesia ventilator showing the bellows, bellows housing, and controls (power switch, respiratory rate, inspiratory flow, and maximum working pressure).

thoracic or pulmonary compliance. Pressure preset describes a mode of ventilation in which the ventilator's bellow's delivers gases into the patient's lungs until a specific pressure is reached, at which point the expiratory phase of ventilation begins. The practical concern with a pressure preset mode is that tidal volume may vary with changes in thoracic or pulmonary compliance, potentially leading to inadequate minute ventilation. Most anesthesiologists prefer to operate anesthesia ventilators for small animals in a tidal volume preset mode. It is common for anesthesia ventilators to be time-cycled as the primary way of controlling respiratory rate, and most anesthesia ventilators have a maximum pressure limit to prevent overpressurizing the lung during inspiration.

Most anesthesia ventilators have controls (Figs. 1.15 and 1.16) that allow the operator to adjust most or all of the respiratory variables listed below. The usual guidelines for application of IPPB in small animals include the following:

- Respiratory rate (RPM or f) = 8 to 12 breaths/min
- Tidal volume (V_T) = 10 to 20 ml/kg of body weight
- Inspiratory pressure (P_I) = 15 to 20 cm H_2O
- Inspiratory time = 1 to 1.5 seconds
- Inspiratory time to expiratory time (I : E) ratio = 1 : 2 or less (e.g., 1 : 3, 1 : 4, . . .)

An anesthesia ventilator should be operated in accordance with the instructions that are supplied by the manufacturer. Some preparatory considerations in the setup of an anesthesia machine and anesthesia ventilator include the following:

- The patient should have a correctly sized ET tube in place with the cuff properly inflated to prevent leakage of gas around the cuff when positive pressure is applied to the airway.
- The anesthesia machine and breathing system should have no leaks when the overflow valve is closed, the Y-piece is occluded, and positive pressure of approximately 30 cm H_2O is applied (see the checkout procedures for anesthesia machines and breathing systems near the end of this chapter).
- The anesthesia machine should be properly connected to adequate sources of oxygen and

between the ET tube connector and the Y-piece of the circle breathing system) between the ventilator and the patient. A collapsed bellows is easily noticed as a malfunction by the operator. In contrast, a descending bellows can appear to be functioning normally during such a disconnection.

Anesthesia ventilators may be powered electrically, by compressed gas, or, more commonly, by a combination of the two. Typically, the bellows is compressed during inspiration by pressurized gas. *Tidal volume preset* and *pressure preset* are terms that are used to describe the way that an anesthesia ventilator functions. Generally and simplistically, tidal volume preset refers to a mode of mechanical ventilation in which the ventilator's bellows delivers a specific tidal volume to the patient with each breath. With some exceptions, this ensures that tidal volume is maintained consistently throughout the period of IPPB, but the pressure generated on inspiration may vary with changes in the patient's correctly fitted with a vaporizer for delivery of inhalant anesthetic.

- The patient's ET tube should be attached to the breathing system, and proper function of the anesthesia machine and breathing system should be ensured before the ventilator is connected to the breathing system.
- The ventilator should be checked for proper connections to electrical and pressurized gas sources, and its reservoir bag and connecting gas hose should be ensured to be free from leaks. The operator should follow the pre-use checkout procedures provided by the manufacturer of the ventilator.
- The ventilator should be connected by a corrugated breathing hose to the port for the anesthesia breathing system's reservoir bag after the breathing system's reservoir bag has been removed and the overflow valve on the breathing system has been closed.
- The ventilator's controls should be set to ensure correct values for f, V_T, P_I, inspiratory time, and I:E ratio.
- The anesthetist should ensure by auscultation and observation that air flows into both lungs during inspiration and that there is no impairment to expiration. The anesthetist should evaluate f, V_T, P_I, inspiratory time, and I:E ratio regularly throughout the period of IPPB to ascertain continued and correct function of the ventilator. Monitoring of arterial blood gases and end-tidal carbon dioxide data is an excellent approach to ensuring proper function of the ventilator and appropriate application of IPPB.

At the end of a period of anesthesia with IPPB, the patient must regain its ability to breathe spontaneously. The procedure involved in changing from controlled to spontaneous ventilation is commonly called "weaning the patient from a ventilator." This is accomplished by some combination of decreasing the depth of anesthesia and increasing the patient's Pa_{CO_2}. The inspired concentration of inhalant anesthetic will be reduced, often to zero, and respiratory rate will be decreased (e.g., from 8 breaths/min to 4 breaths/min), effectively lowering minute ventilation and allowing Pa_{CO_2} to increase slightly and stimulate spontaneous breathing. While it is generally acceptable to allow Pa_{CO_2} to increase to 45 to 50 mm Hg, it is not appropriate to allow development of a significant respiratory acidosis. Other options to promote spontaneous ventilation include stimulation of the patient (e.g., turning the patient) and reversing the effects of drugs used during anesthesia that might be causing respiratory depression (e.g., antagonism of an opioid). Hypothermia may contribute to postanesthetic respiratory depression, and cold patients should be actively warmed toward normal body temperature. The use of respiratory stimulants (e.g., doxapram) is not recommended. During the transition to spontaneous ventilation and continuing throughout the recovery period, the Sp_{O_2} should be monitored with a pulse oximeter, and the patient should be supported with supplemental oxygen if necessary.

Demand valves and manual resuscitators (Hartsfield 1996) can be used in the recovery period to control or assist ventilation until spontaneous ventilation becomes adequate in both rate and tidal volume to ensure appropriate ventilation and oxygenation. Demand valves are attached to a source of compressed oxygen. The valve can be attached to the ET tube connector (15 mm O.D.), and it forces inspiration and delivers oxygen until the patient begins to exhale or until a preset inspiratory pressure is reached. The demand valve can be triggered manually (operator sets the respiratory rate) or by the patient creating a negative pressure as it begins inspiration (patient sets the respiratory rate). Oxygen flow during inspiration varies with the pressure of the oxygen source. Demand valves should be used cautiously to ensure that excessive pressure is not applied to the lungs during inspiration.

As with most mechanical devices, hazards, malfunctions, and mishaps are possible with the use of anesthesia ventilators (Dorsch and Dorsch 1994; Hartsfield 1996). Therefore, monitoring is important during IPPB. Some of the common problems that can occur include the following:

- Loss of a seal due to leakage of the ET tube cuff
- Leaks in the bellows or other rubber or plastic components
- Anesthesia machine's overflow valve opened inadvertently
- Disconnection at the ET tube–breathing system interface

- Loss of electrical power to the ventilator
- Loss of gas supply from central gas source to the driving gas circuit
- Inadequate supply of gases to the patient circuit
- Inadvertent changes in settings on the ventilator
- Failure to inflate the lungs adequately
- Excessive depth of anesthesia
- Animal becomes too light
- Excessive pressure on inspiration
- Hypoventilation and respiratory acidosis
- Hyperventilation and respiratory alkalosis
- Obstruction of flow
- Hypoxemia
- Bucking the ventilator (patient attempts to exhale during the ventilator's inspiratory phase)

> As with most mechanical devices, hazards, malfunctions, and mishaps are possible with the use of anesthesia ventilators.

MEDICAL GASES

Oxygen and nitrous oxide are two medical gases that are commonly available for veterinary anesthesia, and anesthesia machines are often designed for the delivery of both gases (Fig. 1.17). Oxygen is essential and nitrous oxide is optional. The use of nitrous oxide has diminished in veterinary anesthesia to the point that the drug is of minimal importance. Equipment for delivery of medical gases incorporates a number of engineering mechanisms to prevent the inadvertent interchange of these two medical gases.

Medical gases may be supplied from bulk sources (e.g., liquid oxygen tanks), oxygen-generating systems, and central source manifold systems (oxygen and nitrous oxide) fitted for large gas cylinders (e.g., H cylinders). These sources connect to distribution systems (pipelines) to deliver gases to station outlets in appropriate locations in the hospital. High-pressure hoses connect anesthesia machines to the station outlets. Attachments to station outlets and to the pipeline inlets on anesthesia machines are made with fittings that have specific diameters and thread types (diameter-indexed safety system [DISS]) to prevent the inadvertent interchange of gases. Alternately, proprietary quick connections may be used; these systems have specific connectors that prevent interchange of oxygen and nitrous oxide, and they can be easily and rapidly

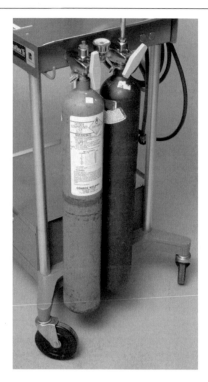

Figure 1.17. E cylinders of oxygen and nitrous oxide attached to hanger yokes on a veterinary anesthesia machine. Cylinders are color-coded; the oxygen cylinder is green and the nitrous oxide cylinder is blue. Inadvertent interchange of these cylinders is presented by the pin-index safety system.

connected and disconnected if movement of the anesthesia machine is required.

Small gas cylinders (E cylinders) attach to the hanger yokes (Fig. 1.18) of anesthesia machines and serve as portable and emergency gas supplies. Gas from the cylinder is delivered through a regulator, which reduces the pressure and supplies a constant pressure (usually 50 psi) to the flowmeter on the anesthesia machine. Inadvertent interchange of gases is prevented by the pin index safety system, which uses pins and a nipple on the hanger yoke (Fig. 1.19) that correspond to pin holes and the gas inlet on the cylinder's valve body. The alignment of the pins is different for each medical gas.

Gas cylinders are color coded; nitrous oxide cylinders are blue and oxygen cylinders are green in the United States. Each cylinder must have a label that includes the color code, the hazards associated with the gas and the cylinder, and the name and

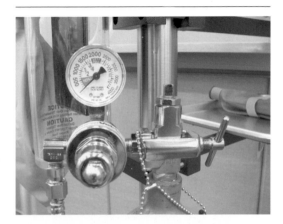

Figure 1.18. Hanger yoke with the retaining screw *(right)*, regulator *(center)*, and pressure gauge *(atop* the regulator) on a SurgiVet anesthesia machine.

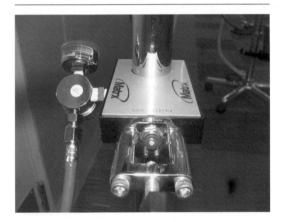

Figure 1.19. Hanger yoke on a Matrx anesthesia machine illustrating the pin-index safety system; the regulator and pressure gauge are shown from the rear.

address of the manufacturer or distributor. Hazards for oxygen and nitrous oxide cylinders relate to the high pressure and the presence of oxidizing agents and include explosion and fire.

Gas cylinders are made of steel, steel alloy, or aluminum, the latter being necessary if a portable oxygen source is needed for patients undergoing magnetic resonance imaging. Aluminum cylinders are not as heavy as steel cylinders. Large cylinders (e.g., H cylinders) generally supply gases more economically that small cylinders (e.g., E cylinders).

The service pressure (maximum filling pressure at 70°F) for oxygen cylinders is about 2000 psi; a full H cylinder contains approximately 7000 L of oxygen gas and a full E cylinder contains about 700 L of oxygen gas. The content of an oxygen cylinder is proportional to the pressure. If a full E cylinder contains 700 L at a pressure of 2000 psi, then the E cylinder contains about 175 L at a pressure of 500 psi.

REGULATORS AND PRESSURE GAUGES

Gases from the primary source pass through a regulator (Fig. 1.18) in route to a flowmeter in route to the vaporizer. If an anesthesia machine is fitted for both oxygen and nitrous oxide, each must have its own regulator and pressure gauge. A regulator reduces the high pressure of gas from the primary source to about 50 psi in veterinary anesthesia machines and maintains a constant pressure downstream from the regulator. This allows the flowmeter to function accurately as the medical gas cylinder empties and the pressure decreases. The lower, constant pressure allows manual adjustment of the flowmeter control without undue sensitivity. A pressure gauge is often located on or near the regulator (Fig. 1.18); the gauge reflects the pressure in the cylinder. Small cylinders attached to anesthesia machines are usually changed when the pressure drops below 500 psi.

FLOWMETERS

Flowmeters are located downstream from regulators (Figs. 1.6 and 1.7). Separate flowmeters are used for oxygen and nitrous oxide; that is, oxygen and nitrous oxide run in parallel until the gases mix just before they enter the vaporizer of the anesthesia machine. Flowmeters allow delivery of a quantity of oxygen that will meet or exceed the patient's metabolic oxygen demands. If nitrous oxide is used, flowmeters are set to ensure that the concentration (greater than 30% oxygen in the gases delivered to the breathing system) of oxygen is sufficient for the patient to saturate its hemoglobin.

Gas flow through a flowmeter is from the bottom to the top of the glass tube. Flow is controlled by a needle valve and is adjusted as the indicator (float) rises in the glass tube using a scale indicating rate of flow (Fig. 1.7). Needle valves are easily damaged and should not be overtightened. Flowmeter control valves should be in the off position before exposing the flowmeter to pressure from a gas cylinder and regulator; this will prevent sudden application of pressure from slamming the indicator into the stop at the top of the glass tube, which could damage the indicator. Flow rates less than that lowest mark on the scale should not be extrapolated. The indicator is read at the center if it is in the shape of a ball; all other indicators are read at the top of the indicator. Gases that exit the flowmeter move to the vaporizer.

VAPORIZERS

Vaporizers change liquid anesthetic into vapor and add a controlled amount of vapor to the other gases flowing to the patient (Dorsch and Dorsch 1999). With the potent, highly volatile inhalant anesthetics that are common in veterinary anesthesia today, the best practice is the use of modern, concentration-calibrated, accurate vaporizers.

Precision, concentration-calibrated vaporizers are classified as variable-bypass (method of output regulation), flow-over with a wick (method of vaporization), out-of-the-circle (VOC; location; Figure 1.6), thermo-compensated, and agent-specific (a different vaporizer specifically calibrated for each anesthetic agent). Modern vaporizers are temperature, flow, and back-pressure compensated. Precision vaporizers maintain consistent output during spontaneous ventilation or controlled ventilation, and output is maintained with reasonable changes in liquid anesthetic temperature and fresh gas flow. The degree of flow compensation varies with the model of vaporizer, but most will compensate between 0.5 L/min and 10 L/min. Likewise, temperature compensation varies with the model of vaporizer, but is usually effective in the range of 15° to 35°C.

A nonprecision, low-resistance, in-the-circle (VIC; Figure 1.6) vaporizer continues to be available for veterinary use. Without instrumental monitoring of the inspired anesthetic concentration, use of nonprecision vaporizers would appear to add unnecessary risk during the administration of potent, volatile drugs like isoflurane and sevoflurane.

Specific vaporizers available for use in veterinary anesthesia include Tec-type vaporizers, Ohio-calibrated-type vaporizers, and Penlon-type vaporizers. Tec 3 (Fig. 1.7), Tec 4 (Fig. 1.20), Tec 5 (Fig. 1.21), and Tec 6 vaporizers are common. The Tec 6 is designed specifically for desflurane, an agent that

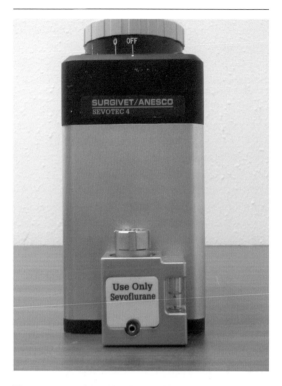

Figure 1.20. SurgiVet/Anesco Sevotec 4 vaporizer with a standard filling mechanism.

is not in common use in veterinary anesthesia due to the cost of the drug, the cost of the vaporizer, and the cost of maintenance of the vaporizer. Tec 3 vaporizers work well for small animal anesthesia, but Tec 4 and Tec 5 vaporizers offer some advantages. The Tec 5 has a larger capacity for liquid anesthetic (300 ml), allowing it to be used longer without a refill; the Tec 3 and 4 vaporizers hold approximately 125 ml of liquid. Both the Tec 4 and Tec 5 are less vulnerable to uncontrolled changes in output if they are tipped. Penlon-type vaporizers (liquid capacity = 250 ml) and Ohio-calibrated vaporizers (liquid capacity = 225 ml) have similar characteristics to the Tec-type vaporizers.

Vaporizers can have standard filler ports (Figs. 1.7 and 1.20) or keyed filler ports (Fig. 1.21), the latter intended to prevent inadvertently filling a vaporizer with the wrong anesthetic agent and to reduce contamination of the workplace with anesthetic gases. When filling a vaporizer with a standard filler port, a spout should be used on the bottle to reduce spillage. If a vaporizer is to be removed

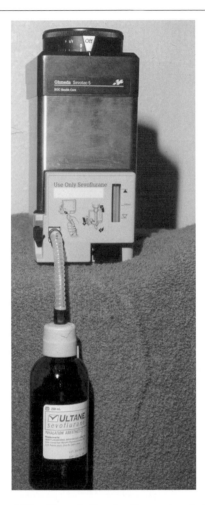

Figure 1.21. Ohmeda Sevotec 5 vaporizer being emptied with a keyed filler apparatus.

from a machine or if the machine and vaporizer are to be transported, the vaporizer should be emptied (Figs. 1.21 and 1.22).

Maintenance and recalibration of vaporizers should be done according to the recommendations of the manufacturers. Anesthetic agent monitors have become more prevalent in veterinary medicine in recent years and can be used to measure anesthetic output from vaporizers. Significant deviations from the setting on the vaporizer's control dial provide a reason for immediately seeking service and recalibration from a qualified vaporizer technician. A proper recalibration of a vaporizer should include evaluation of the vaporizer's output at multiple flow rates and temperatures.

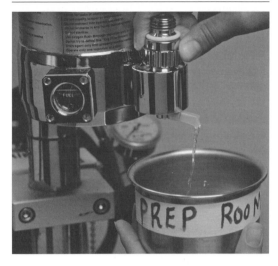

Figure 1.22. Tec 3 vaporizer being emptied with a standard filler port system; note that the inverted cap for the filler port serves as a wrench to open and close the drain for the vaporizer. Emptying and filling a vaporizer with a standard filler port system should be done in a well-ventilated location.

COMMON GAS OUTLET

Medical gases originating in compressed gas cylinders flow through the cylinder valve, regulator, flowmeter, and vaporizer to reach the common gas outlet (Fig. 1.8). If the flush valve is activated, oxygen immediately downstream from the regulator is diverted, bypasses the flowmeter and vaporizer, and reaches the common gas outlet. Some veterinary anesthesia machines are designed very simply and have the gas hose from the flush valve and the gas hose from the outlet of the vaporizer join immediately upstream from the inlet to the breathing system (Fig. 1.7); that is, there is no identifiable common gas outlet as a separate component.

FLUSH VALVES

Flush valves are optional components of anesthesia machines, but most veterinary machines are fitted with flush valves (Fig. 1.7). Flush valves may deliver oxygen to the common gas outlet at a rate of 35 to 75 L/min. The flow originates downstream from the regulator (oxygen pressure of about 50 psi) and bypasses the flowmeter and vaporizer (VOC). The flush valve is intended to rapidly fill the circle breathing system with oxygen in emergencies. To avoid overpressurization of the breathing system, the flush valve should not be activated when a pediatric breathing system is in use. The best design for a flush valve is to have a guard around the valve to prevent inadvertent activation.

DEVICES FOR MAINTAINING BODY TEMPERATURE IN THE ANESTHETIZED PATIENT

Hypothermia develops in most anesthetized small animal patients unless active warming techniques are used. Monitoring of body temperature is essential during anesthesia. Forced warm air (Fig. 1.23) is an effective way to prevent hypothermia. Warm water–circulating blankets (Fig. 1.24) placed under the anesthetized patient may be helpful but normally will not prevent hypothermia unless the patient is wrapped with the blanket. Fluid warmers, especially those that warm fluids in the intravenous infusion line near the point that fluid enters the vein, can be used to control the patient's temperature. In general, electric heating pads are considered dangerous due to the variations in temperature produced and multiple incidences of severe burns in anesthetized patients.

Forced air warmers (Fig. 1.23) make use of "blankets" with small holes for escape of warm air. The blanket may even surround the patient and delivers warm air to areas of the body that do not include the surgical site. These warmers may have multiple temperature settings and rates of air flow. Patients can become overheated if forced air warmers are misused. Monitoring of body temperature is important whenever external sources of heat are used.

ROUTINE FOR CHECKOUT AND MAINTENANCE OF ANESTHESIA EQUIPMENT

Consistent evaluation of anesthesia equipment should be part of standard operating procedures (SOP) and should be used to prevent malfunctions and hazards associated with inhalant anesthesia (Dorsch and Dorsch 1999; Hartsfield 1996; Mason 1993). Malfunction of equipment can cause injury to a patient or even death and can contribute to an unsafe working environment if there is leakage of medical gases and/or anesthetics. Routine maintenance and checkout procedures are typically recommended by the manufacturers and/or distributors of anesthesia machines, breathing systems, and ventilators; the user should become familiar with the operations manual for each piece of equipment. Some checkout procedures should be done daily, and some should be done before each anesthetic episode. It is good practice to maintain a log that documents maintenance and checkout procedures for each anesthesia machine and its associated components and each ventilator. Although not intended to be inclusive, some common checkout procedures

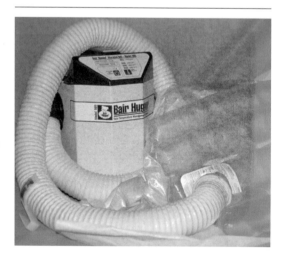

Figure 1.23. Bair Hugger forced warm air system for controlling body temperature in anesthetized patients; the plastic blanket has small holes to allow warm air to move next to the patient to control body temperature.

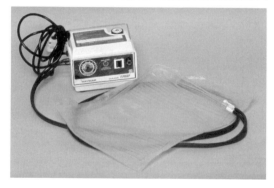

Figure 1.24. A warm water-circulating blanket for supporting body temperature in anesthetized patients; water-circulating blankets are inefficient unless the patient is wrapped in the blanket.

are listed below for anesthesia machines, circle breathing systems, and NRB systems. More detailed descriptions of checkout and maintenance procedures have been published elsewhere.

EVALUATION OF THE ANESTHESIA MACHINE AND BREATHING SYSTEMS

The first step in checkout of anesthesia machines and breathing systems is to assess the overall condition the equipment. A knowledgeable operator should ensure that all parts of the machine and breathing system are present, properly maintained, not defective, and correctly connected. The following suggestions should help to prevent complications due to equipment malfunction:

- Central gas supplies (oxygen and nitrous oxide) should be adequate in quantity and pressure. The line pressures should not fluctuate and should remain at about 50 psi when flowmeters on the anesthesia machine are adjusted to a mid range of flow rates.
- Portable gas supplies (small oxygen and nitrous oxide cylinders on the anesthesia machine) should be adequate in quantity and pressure.
- Small cylinders attached to the anesthesia machine should be evaluated for leaks. With the flowmeter control "off" and the cylinder valve open, there should be no decrease in cylinder pressure over time (e.g., 10 minutes).
- With the cylinder valves open, flowmeters should be assessed through a complete range of flow rates from zero to the maximum setting on the scale. The indicator should not stick or move erratically.
- Vaporizers should be filled with liquid anesthetic, the control dial should be in the "off" position, the inlet and outlet connections should be secure, and the filler cap should be sealed. With the vaporizer control dial in the "off" position, no odor of anesthetic should be detected when the oxygen flowmeter is turned on.
- If the scavenging system involves a charcoal canister, the quality of the charcoal absorbent should be ensured.

EVALUATION OF A CIRCLE BREATHING SYSTEM

Circle breathing systems should be inspected and evaluated before being used on each patient.

All parts of the circle should be present, not defective, and properly connected.

The fresh gas inlet to the circle should be correctly connected to the common gas outlet of the anesthesia machine or, alternately, to the outlet of the vaporizer in simple anesthesia machines.

The absorbent for carbon dioxide should be evaluated; ineffective absorbent should be changed before the breathing system is used.

The integrity and function of the one-way valves should be ensured. Exhaling through the Y-piece should produce movement of the disc of the expiratory valve. Closing the pop-off valve and compressing the reservoir bag should cause movement of the disc in the inspiratory one-way valve.

Leak tests are important in preparing for use of circle systems. Several kinds of tests can be done. The primary purposes are to ensure delivery of anesthetic and oxygen to the patient and the ability to use the system to apply positive pressure ventilation. Secondarily, leak tests are used to ensure no obvious source of waste gases to contaminate the working environment. The following procedures have been useful:

- With the pop-off valve closed, the Y-piece occluded, and the system filled to a pressure of 30 cm H_2O, the pressure in the system should

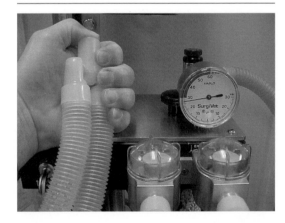

Figure 1.25. A pressure check being conducted on a circle breathing system; the pop-off valve is closed, the Y-piece is occluded, and the pressure in the circle system has been raised to near 30 cm H_2O. A system without significant leaks should hold without any reduction in pressure for at least 10 seconds.

remain at 30 cm H$_2$O for at least 10 seconds (Fig. 1.25). Alternately, the leak rate at 30 cm H$_2$O should be less than 250 ml/min.

- The pressure in the system should be raised to about 50 cm H$_2$O by squeezing the bag to ensure the integrity of the system during the short period of higher pressure.
- With the pop-off valve open and the Y-piece occluded, changes in pressure (either positive or negative) should be negligible at flow rates of oxygen between 0 and 5 L/min.
- With the pop-off valve open, pressure relief should be obvious if the flush valve is activated.

EVALUATION OF NONREBREATHING SYSTEMS

Bain systems and other NRB systems should be inspected and evaluated before use on each patient. A complete system check should be done with the NRB system attached to the common gas outlet of the anesthesia machine (or the outlet of the vaporizer)—the patient port should be occluded, the overflow blocked, and the bag distended. With the flowmeters set at zero, there should be no loss of pressure; the reservoir bag should remain distended.

For Bain systems, an additional test has been recommended for the inner tube. With the Bain system properly connected to the anesthesia machine and the oxygen flowmeter set at 1 L/min, the inner tube is occluded briefly using the plunger from a small syringe. If there are no leaks, the indicator in the glass tube of the flowmeter should fall to zero.

REFERENCES

Dorsch, J.A., and Dorsch, S.E. 1999. *Understanding Anesthesia Equipment*, 4th ed. Baltimore: Williams and Wilkins.

Dorsch, J.A., and Dorsch, S.E. 1994. *Understanding Anesthesia Equipment*, 3rd ed. Baltimore: Williams and Wilkins.

Dorsch, J.A., and Dorsch, S.E. 1984. *Understanding Anesthesia Equipment*, 2nd ed. Baltimore: Williams and Wilkins.

Dunlop, C.I. 1992. The case for rebreathing circuit for very small animals. *Vet Clin North Am Small Anim Prac* 22:400–403.

Ehrenwerth, J., and Eisenkraft, J.B. 1993. *Anesthesia Equipment: Principles and Application*. St. Louis: C.V. Mosby.

Hamilton, W.K. 1964. Nomenclature of inhalation anesthetic systems. *Anesthesiology* 25:3–5.

Hartsfield, S.M. 1987. Machines and breathing systems for administration of inhalation anesthetics. In *Principles and Practice of Veterinary Anesthesia*, edited by Charles E. Short, pp. 395–418. Baltimore: Williams & Wilkins.

Hartsfield, S.M. 1996. Anesthesia machines and breathing systems. In *Lumb and Jones' Veterinary Anesthesia*, 3rd ed., edited by J.C. Thurmon, W.J. Tranquilli, and G.J. Benson, pp. 366–408. Baltimore: Williams & Wilkins.

Hartsfield, S.M. 1996. Airway management and ventilation. In *Lumb and Jones' Veterinary Anesthesia*, 3rd ed., edited by J.C. Thurmon, W.J. Tranquilli, and G.J. Benson, pp. 515–556. Baltimore: Williams & Wilkins.

Hartsfield, S.M., Cornick-Seahorn, J., Cuvelliez, S., Gaynor, J. and McGrath, C. 1996. Commentary and recommendations on control of waste anesthetic gases in the workplace. *J Am Vet Med Assoc* 209: 75–77.

Hartsfield, S.M. 1999. Anesthetic equipment. In *Manual of Small Animal Anesthesia*, 2nd ed., edited by Robert R. Paddleford, pp. 89–109. Philadelphia: W.B. Saunders Company.

Hodgson, D.S. 1992. The case for nonrebreathing systems in very small patients. *Vet Clin North Am Small Anim Prac* 22:397–399.

Manley, S.V., and McDonnell, W.N. 1979. Clinical evaluation of the Bain breathing circuit in small animal anesthesia. *J Am Anin Hosp Assoc* 15:67–72.

Mason, D.E. 1993. Anesthesia machine checkout and troubleshooting. *Semin Vet Med Surg* 8:104–108.

Chapter 2
Monitoring

Nora S. Matthews

There are no safe anesthetics, only safe anesthetists.

Anesthesia should be a totally reversible process.

All anesthetics are dangerous. The most important way to ensure "safe anesthesia" is vigilant monitoring. Conscientious monitoring not only ensures that anesthesia is reversible but also that the patient will be adequately anesthetized with a rapid recovery and no permanent damage to vital organs. Patient drug requirements vary widely depending on physical status, previous drug administration, and individual differences; monitoring is the best way to "customize" the anesthetic experience. No single method of monitoring is guaranteed to keep a patient safe.

The patient should be monitored with as many different techniques as possible; both physical methods (e.g., palpating pulse, observing respiration and mucous membrane color) and mechanical methods (e.g., pulse oximetry, electrocardiogram) should be used. To some extent, even duplication of monitoring may provide supplemental information because different monitors may give slightly different information or artifacts observed by one monitor may be refuted by another method. If the heart rate from the pulse oximeter does not match the heart rate from the blood pressure machine or neither matches the ausculted heart rate, the other information provided by the monitors is suspect. A more emergent situation is the loss of a pulse oximetry reading. The loss of a pulse oximetry reading warrants immediate palpation of a pulse or auscultation of heartbeat to determine whether the probe has simply fallen off or cardiac arrest has just occurred! If all the monitoring equipment fails at the same time, look to a patient factor.

Knowledge of normal values for many variables is essential for monitoring the anesthetized patient. Normal awake values for dogs and cats (Table 2.1) for heart and respiratory rates, temperature, arterial blood pressure, pain score (see Chapter 9), hemoglobin saturation, and other important variables should be examined and recorded before and at the conclusion of anesthesia. Depending on the physical status (see Chapter 4) of the patient, additional information should be garnered. Values for many blood parameters (hematologic and biochemical) vary with the laboratory used and are not included. Normal values from your laboratory should be available to facilitate interpretation of lab work. The variables included here represent those that are routinely evaluated for all preoperative patients (vicious dogs and cats excepted).

ANESTHESIA RECORDS

The anesthetic record is a legal document and should be completed in blue or black ink (Fig. 2.1). Information contained in the anesthetic record should include patient identification and signalment, date, accurate weight (indicate if estimated), procedure to be performed, and, if appropriate, the correct limb. At regular intervals, vital signs should be recorded; drugs (in milligrams, not milliliters), time, and route of administration, type of monitoring, and values obtained should be recorded at regular intervals. Observed problems and measures taken to correct them should be recorded throughout anesthesia and during recovery. Problems experienced in recovery and intervention required should

Table 2.1. Normal values for conscious dogs and cats on room air (21% oxygen).

Variable (units)	Dog	Cat
Heart rate (beats/min)	60–120	100–200
Respiratory rate (breaths/min)	10–20	15–25
Temperature (°C)	37.0–39.2	37.5–39.5
Arterial blood pressure (mm Hg)		
Systolic	100–150	100–150
Diastolic	60–90	60–90
Mean	80–100	80–100
Central venous pressure (cm H_2O)	<5	<5
Urine production (ml/hr)	1	1
Pain score[1] (visual analogue score [VAS] interactive)	0	0

[1]Regardless of the method used to evaluate pain, a pain score should be assigned each time a physical exam is conducted. If analgesic treatment is indicated, the intervention and response should be recorded.

also be recorded. The completed anesthetic record should not contain empty spaces. If information is not available, a single line should be drawn through the space. If an erroneous entry is made, a single line drawn through the entry, initials, and date of the correction should be noted on the record.

Rather than viewing the record as a necessary evil, it should be viewed as providing useful information about the patient—both during the procedure and for subsequent anesthetic episodes. Complete anesthetic records allow troubleshooting within the clinic and provide information about the incidence of preventable problems. Information required on anesthetic records may vary from state to state but is generally minimal. The veterinarian should consult the state veterinary medical practice act for local requirements.

NEUROLOGIC MONITORING

Reflexes

Monitoring various reflexes, such as swallowing, corneal and palpebral reflexes, pupil size, and jaw and anal tone, provides valuable information about the patient's depth of anesthesia. It is important to be aware of which anesthetic drugs have been used

because some reflexes will vary with the drug used. For example, when ketamine is used for anesthetic maintenance, eye signs will remain brisk and the eyeball will remain centrally located, unlike what is seen when an inhalant is used for maintenance. Rather than dividing anesthesia into stages and planes of anesthesia which were originally developed for ether anesthesia, the current planes of anesthesia are based on expected reflexes at light, surgical, and deep planes of anesthesia.

Planes of Anesthesia

Not all animals "read the book;" some individual variation is always seen:

- **Light plane of anesthesia:** Muscle relaxation is present (only barely), swallowing, nystagmus, corneal, and palpebral reflexes are present, and tearing may occur. The eyeball is centrally positioned, pupils may be dilated, and anal tone is strong.
- **Surgical plane of anesthesia:** Muscle relaxation is good, swallowing, nystagmus and palpebral reflex are absent, although corneal reflex should be maintained. The eye is usually rotated ventrally, and anal tone is relaxed.

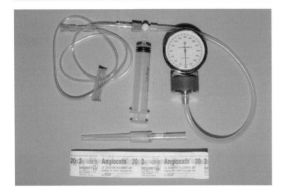

Figure 2.5. An aneroid manometer is an inexpensive method for measuring direct arterial blood pressure.

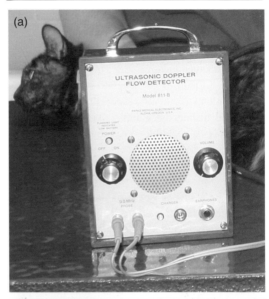

(a)

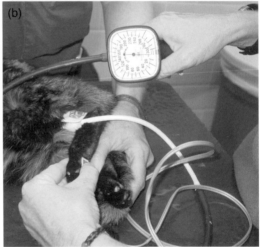

(b)

Figure 2.6. A Doppler (*A*) involves placement of the piezoelectric crystal (*B*) over a peripheral artery distal to a cuff used to occlude the artery.

is also not practical in very small patients, where catheterizing an artery is technically very difficult. Therefore, indirect methods are widely used and the equipment has become more accurate as veterinary monitors (instead of human monitors redirected to veterinary medicine) have been developed.

The simplest and least expensive way to measure blood pressure directly is with an aneroid manometer connected to the arterial catheter via tubing filled with heparinized saline (Fig. 2.5). This allows measurement of mean arterial blood pressure only, but is very useful for ensuring that mean arterial pressure is maintained over 60 to 70 mm Hg (to protect renal function) and to allow trending of the depth of anesthesia. Use of a transducer connected to an arterial catheter allows measurement of systolic, diastolic, and mean blood pressures and evaluation of the pulse pressure wave. Several manufacturers make multiparameter monitors with the capability of invasive blood pressure (IBP). For best accuracy, the stopcock, which is opened to the air during zeroing of the manometer or transducer, needs to be placed at the level of the patient's heart. The stopcock is often connected to the manometer or transducer, and placing the manometer or transducer at the level of the heart is equivalent.

Noninvasive blood pressure measurement (NIBP) may use the Doppler method (which gives systolic pressures only) or an oscillometric technique. The Doppler unit is inexpensive but involves placement of the piezoelectric crystal over a peripheral artery, with manual inflation of the cuff (which is posi-

tioned proximal to the crystal) until blood flow through the artery is occluded (Fig. 2.6). Careful deflation of the cuff until blood flow is heard via the crystal (as blood flow is allowed through the artery again) gives the systolic blood pressure reading.

The oscillometric method is automated (allowing readings at variable intervals) and gives systolic, diastolic, and mean blood pressures as well as heart rate. With all NIBP monitors, the best accuracy is obtained with a correctly sized cuff (width should equal 40% to 60% of circumference of the tail or limb) and readings must be adjusted for distance of the cuff above or below the heart (correction factor varies with manufacturer, so see the manual). It may be more difficult to get accurate readings on very small patients (i.e., cats), especially when the cuff is placed distally on a limb; placing the cuff as proximally as possible (i.e., above the hock or carpus) may be helpful.

Human NIBP monitors may have difficulty in measuring blood pressures in very small patients if inflation pressure is not variable. Some monitors detect the cuff size connected to the monitor and automatically set inflation pressures accordingly. So when a "neonatal" cuff is selected (as would be used for a small dog or cat), the monitor will not measure a systolic pressure above 120 mm Hg (refer to the manual for specific model), which may not be high enough to get a reading. Newer monitors such as the Cardell (MINRAD Inc., Orchard Park, New York 14127; Fig. 2.7) have been shown to produce accurate readings in cats (Pedersen 2002) and dogs (Sawyer 2004), although some underestimation of systolic pressure is seen with hypertension.

> Some older human noninvasive blood pressure monitors are inaccurate if the heart rate is slow or irregular (e.g., sinus bradycardia, cardiac dysrhythmia) or the patient is small.

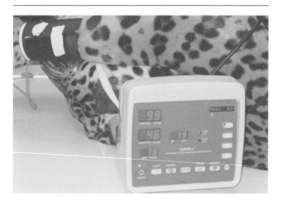

Figure 2.7. A Cardell oscillometric blood pressure monitor measures indirect blood pressure; the Cardell is particularly useful for small dogs and cats.

Urine Output

Urine output (1 ml/kg/hr; Table 2.1) should be monitored in patients with renal compromise and in patients at risk for hypovolemia or hypotension. Placing a urinary catheter and closed collection system is described in Chapter 15.

Central Venous Pressure

The central venous pressure (CVP) is a reflection of the right atrial pressure in the absence of confounding factors (e.g., a clot on the end of the catheter or the catheter wedged up against the wall). The CVP is used to estimate blood volume and to guide fluid administration in hypovolemia. Typically, increased venous return (preload) results in an improved cardiac output. If patients are not responding to treatment for hypotension, CVP may offer helpful information (e.g., inotropes do not function in the absence of volume). CVP may also be used to document ongoing blood loss or continuing hypovolemia secondary to major fluid shifts or loss. In many cases, CVP may be measured with a jugular catheter.

Pulse Oximetry

The pulse oximeter noninvasively measures hemoglobin saturation of blood with oxygen (Sao_2) and measures peripheral pulse through plethysmography. It uses red and infrared light to measure the relative absorption of oxygenated versus reduced hemoglobin to calculate Sao_2. Because only two wavelengths are used, the pulse oximeter cannot differentiate other types of hemoglobin (i.e., methemoglobin and carboxyhemoglobin), which can lead to errors in Sao_2 when these forms of hemoglobin are present. Carboxyhemoglobin will falsely elevate Sao_2, whereas methemoglobin will cause Spo_2 readings trending toward 85%.

Patient oxygenation can be estimated from the Spo_2 based on the relationship of the oxyhemoglobin-dissociation curve; an Spo_2 of 90% equals a Pao_2 of approximately 60 mm Hg. If the patient's Pao_2 is greater than 100 mm Hg (as is the normal patient's Pao_2 on supplemental oxygen), the Spo_2 will be 98% to 100%. In this case, Spo_2 does not accurately reflect Pao_2 (which might range from 100 to 400 mm Hg). The Spo_2 is evidence that the patient is at least well oxygenated. When Pao_2 drops below 60 mm Hg, Spo_2 tends to follow it very quickly and so is accurate in predicting Pa_{O_2} and detecting hypoxemia in the patient.

Numerous factors impact on accuracy of the pulse oximeter: motion, pigmentation, hair, vasoconstriction, hypothermia, ambient light, probe type and position, and accuracy of the nomogram used to calculate Sp_{O_2} by the manufacturer. Some of these factors have been improved with newer technology; motion and pigmentation are less of a problem than in older models (Barker 2002). Not all companies have tested the accuracy of their pulse oximeters in veterinary species, nor have all companies developed probe types that are versatile for veterinary use. The tongue is the most consistent site for probe placement on most animals. For procedures in the mouth, other sites that often work well include the toe, lip, prepuce, vulva, and ear (Fig. 2.8). Rectal sensors are reflectance (or transflectance) probes that send the light beam through vascular tissue, bounce it against bone, and receive it back at the probe. Unless positioned close to a pelvic bone, rectal sensors may not work well; reflectance probes may sometimes be successfully placed on the gum or hard palate. Vasoconstriction, usually induced by anesthetic drugs (e.g., ketamine, medetomidine), is a major cause of poor signal strength and inability to obtain readings. The hypothermic patient is usually also vasoconstricted; therefore, readings may not be obtainable.

The pulse oximeter will not provide useful information about blood pressure! Especially in the presence of inhalant agents, which are potent vasodilators, profound hypotension may occur before Sp_{O_2} readings are lost. The pulse oximeter also does not provide information about how well the patient is ventilating; Sp_{O_2} may be completely normal in the face of significant respiratory hypercapnia and acidosis. Use of a capnograph or blood gas analysis is required to confirm hypoventilation.

The pulse oximeter is very useful in providing dynamic information about the patient's oxygenation, pulse rate, and peripheral perfusion. Low Sp_{O_2} values indicate the need for oxygen therapy in patients anesthetized with injectable anesthetics, during recovery, or after extubation. Sp_{O_2} readings in the range of 92% to 94% may indicate hypoventilation ($F_{IO_2} = 0.21$) or accidental endobronchial intubation ($F_{IO_2} > 0.21$) (see Chapter 3 for differentials for low Pa_{O_2}). Decreasing Sp_{O_2} values may

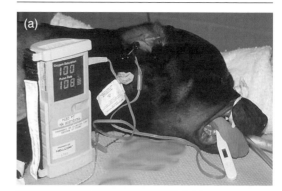

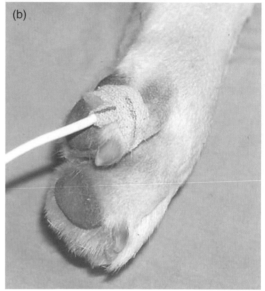

Figure 2.8. A pulse oximeter with probe attached to the (*A*) ear and (*B*) toe; there must be pulsatile flow for the pulse oximeter to provide a reading. The displayed heart rate should match a manual count.

indicate the presence of pneumothorax or other thoracic pathology that affects oxygenation. A sudden loss of Sp_{O_2} reading requires immediate palpation of pulses or auscultation of the heart, because it may indicate cardiac arrest.

Troubleshooting a pulse oximeter which does not seem to be giving accurate readings, may include checking the probe on your own finger to make sure it is working. Comparing the pulse rate displayed by the oximeter against palpable pulse rate is another way to make sure it is finding a good reading (i.e., perfused capillary bed). Comparing the SaO$_2$ from a blood gas sample to the SpO$_2$ will also ensure accuracy of the reading.

Capnography

Capnography noninvasively measures expired carbon dioxide (ETCO$_2$), which is an estimate of arterial carbon dioxide (PaCO$_2$) and provides information about adequacy of ventilation. The capnograph also provides information about metabolism (a high ETCO$_2$ would be expected in a hypermetabolic patient) and circulation (ETCO$_2$ drops to zero almost instantly during cardiac arrest). Anesthetized patients often hypoventilate in a dose-dependent manner; the deeper the plane of anesthesia, the more hypoventilation that occurs. Therefore, the capnograph provides guidance for evaluating the depth of anesthesia (i.e., can you lighten the plane of anesthesia?) and for assessing the adequacy of ventilation (i.e., does the patient need assisted ventilation?). In normal small animals, the difference between ETCO$_2$ and PaCO$_2$ (alveolar − arterial gradient or A-a gradient) is 3 to 5 mm Hg. An ETCO$_2$ of 30 to 40 mm Hg indicates that the patient is ventilating normally; the PaCO$_2$ is expected to equal 35 to 45 mm Hg). An anesthetized patient with an ETCO$_2$ equal 65 mm Hg is hypoventilating (i.e., the PaCO$_2$ is expected to equal 70 mm Hg). Blood gas analysis would show a respiratory acidosis, which may be very detrimental to the patient.

Thoracic pathology or abnormal lung function (e.g., collapsed lung, pneumonia) will cause the A-a gradient to be increased such that the capnograph reading no longer accurately reflects ventilation status. In this case, a blood gas sample is necessary to measure PaCO$_2$. Evaluation of the waveform of the capnograph may also be helpful in detecting exhausted sodasorb, faulty flutter valves (seen as an inspired carbon dioxide [FICO$_2$] greater than zero or elevation of the waveform from baseline), leaks in the circuit, apnea, esophageal intubation, and other abnormal conditions. The normal waveform should rise sharply with exhalation, peak at the end of expiration, and return to zero just before the beginning of the next inspiratory cycle (Fig. 2.9). Most capnographs use infrared analysis to measure carbon dioxide and may sample expired gases remotely (side-stream analysis) by removing gas from the circuit or directly (sensor is between the patient and anesthetic circuit (mainstream analysis). Mainstream analysis has a more rapid response to

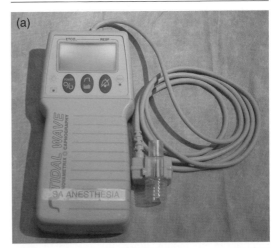

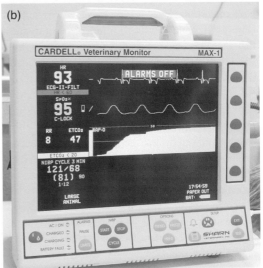

Figure 2.9. A capnograph is used to measure end-tidal carbon dioxide (ETCO$_2$). (*A*) Hand-held ETCO$_2$ monitor Tidal Wave displays a wave form. (*B*) Multiparameter monitors (e.g., Cardell) may incorporate many parameters, including the presence of a ETCO$_2$ wave form, which allows the anesthetist to make assumptions about the breathing pattern.

each breath, but the sensor is more vulnerable to damage or contamination with mucous or water. Side-stream analysis has a longer response; the time required to get the sample to the analyzer depends on the sampling rate of the unit, which may be variable. Accurate readings in small patients are difficult to obtain due to small tidal volumes and the large oxygen flow rates used with nonrebreathing systems, which tend to dilute out the carbon dioxide in each breath.

Qualitative carbon dioxide monitors are also available (e.g., Easy CapII; Mallinckrodt Corporate Headquarters, Hazelwood, MO 63042); these are designed to distinguish esophageal intubation from endotracheal intubation and are not designed to quantitate $ETCO_2$.

Respirometer

The respirometer, or volumeter, measures the volume of air moved with each breath (tidal volume [V_T]) and minute ventilation (amount of volume moved over a minute [MV]). This monitor is very useful for determining if the patient is breathing adequately to prevent hypercapnia and respiratory acidosis. For example, in an anesthetized patient that has received a neuromuscular blocking drug (to facilitate cataract removal), the anesthetist needs to know if the neuromuscular junction has recovered sufficiently to allow adequate ventilation before the patient is awakened. Attaching a respirometer into the system allows quantitation of V_T and MV. Normal V_T is approximately 10 to 15 ml/kg body weight and respiratory rate is 10 to 13 breaths/minute; MV is about 150 to 200 ml/kg/min. The most commonly used respirometer is the Wright respirometer (Grace Medical, Inc., Memphis, TN 38133; Fig. 2.10), which costs less than $1000. While capnography or blood gas analysis is a more accurate assessment of ventilation, the respirometer can help to determine when assisted or controlled ventilation is indicated.

Agent Analyzer

Agent analyzers (Fig. 2.11) measure anesthetic gases (halothane, isoflurane, sevoflurane, nitrous oxide) in the circuit and usually quantitate oxygen concentration. Newer monitors use infrared analysis, mass spectrometry, or Ramen spectrometry. Piezoelectric analysis can be used if the agent to be measured is selected; however, it is more affected by water vapor in the circuit. Accuracy of the various monitors varies with the methodology and all but the Ramen spectrometer may misidentify gases that could exist within the breathing circuit (e.g., methane gas may be identified as halothane). The reader interested in more specific information is referred to a detailed reference (Dorsch and Dorsch 1999). Older infrared analyzers were unable to differentiate between methane and halothane and so were very inaccurate when used with ruminants and horses.

Use of an agent analyzer allows the anesthetist to measure expired inhalant concentration; initially, this concentration will be significantly less than the concentration coming directly out of the vaporizer.

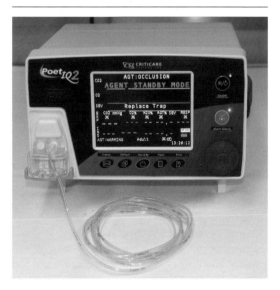

Figure 2.11. The Poet IQ2 measures $ETCO_2$ and inhalant agent.

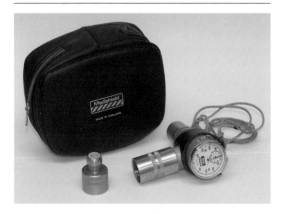

Figure 2.10. A respirometer measures tidal volume (V_T) and may be used to measure minute ventilation.

The initial expired inhalant ($ET_{INHALANT}$) is determined by the breathing circuit volume, the carrier gas flow rate, the gases present in the circuit, and the inhalant uptake by the patient. Over time, as the circuit and patient become saturated with inhalant and uptake by tissues is minimal, inspired inhalant ($FI_{INHALANT}$) and $ET_{INHALANT}$ concentration come closer together and can provide useful information about depth of anesthesia. Patient anesthetic depth can be "fine-tuned" by monitoring $ET_{INHALANT}$ concentration; surgical conditions usually require 1.25 to 1.5 × the minimum alveolar concentration (MAC) for the agent being used (e.g., if isoflurane is being used, the desired $ET_{INHALANT}$ concentration should be approximately 1.6% to 1.9%).

Agent monitors usually also measure oxygen, carbon dioxide, and nitrous oxide (if used) in the anesthetic circuit, thereby providing much useful information about the patient. Unfortunately, these monitors have remained expensive, so they are not frequently used by practitioners.

pH and Blood Gas Analysis With Electrolytes

Until recently, most veterinarians were unable to measure pH and blood gases because analyzers were very expensive and required extensive up-keep and calibration. However, a new generation of inexpensive, portable blood gas analyzers that use disposable microelectrodes have made it practical to obtain this information very rapidly. Because pH and blood gas values are very dynamic and represent the summation of respiration and metabolism, the veterinarian must be able to interpret the values and understand how they may be changed.

Blood gas and pH interpretation is discussed in Chapter 3. Whether the patient is acidotic, normal, or alkalotic (see Table 3.1) is represented by pH. These abnormal states may be caused by aberrations in respiration, metabolism, or both. Arterial blood carbon dioxide ($PaCO_2$) represents how well the patient is ventilating; a high $PaCO_2$ reflects hypoventilation (which will produce acidosis), while a low $PaCO_2$ reflects hyperventilation. Depending on the information needed, an arterial or a venous sample may be collected. Both arterial and venous blood (as long as it is sampled from freely flowing, large veins) samples are adequate to evaluate pH and PCO_2. If the veterinarian is interested in assessing respiratory efficiency (i.e., PaO_2), an arterial blood sample is necessary because oxygen has normally been extracted from venous blood.

SAMPLING FOR BLOOD GAS ANALYSIS

Arterial blood samples can be collected from several sites; femoral and dorsal metatarsal arteries are most commonly used, although the lingual artery can be used in the anesthetized patient. The site should always be thoroughly cleaned, a small-gauge needle should be used and the puncture site should be held off with firm pressure for 5 minutes to prevent hematoma formation. Once drawn, any air in the syringe should be expelled, because this will falsely decrease oxygen content. Venous samples should be taken from the largest, most rapidly flowing vein possible (e.g., jugular vein). In general, samples should be drawn into heparinized syringes (lithium heparin is preferred if electrolytes are to be determined) and the volume of anticoagulant should be small compared with the blood volume (to prevent dilutional errors). Samples should be immediately analyzed or stored in ice water slush and completely mixed before analysis (because cells rapidly settle).

Examples of the newer, point-of-care monitors that analyze pH, blood gases, and electrolytes (Fig. 2.12) include the IRMA TRUpoint Blood Analysis System (ITC Corp., Edison, NJ 08820), I-Stat Portable Clinical Analyzer (Heska Corp., Loveland, CO 80538), and Vet-Stat (Idexx, Inc., Westbrook, MA 04092). All are fairly similarly priced and can

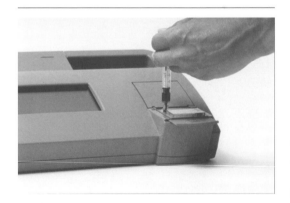

Figure 2.12. The IRMA pH and blood gas analyzer is one of many "bedside" monitors that allow anesthetists to make real-time decision about the ventilatory status of a patient.

of hyperventilation interspersed between periods of apnea. During hyperventilation, the V_T increases and decreases, and then respiration stops.

Dyspnea is difficult breathing and is subjectively associated with patient distress.

A *gasp* is a brief spasmodic inspiratory effort, usually maximal, that ends abruptly. A gasp may occur as a terminal event or during severe hypoxia.

Kussmaul respiration is deep and rapid ventilation seen in patients that have a metabolic acidosis and is observed in diabetic acidosis. See *air hunger*.

Panting is a rapid movement of dead space ventilation. Panting typically results in hypoventilation (CO_2 retention) rather than hyperventilation. Panting may be seen in response to opioid administration, which resets the hypothalamic thermoregulatory center. Cats rarely open mouth breathe. The flehmen (or grimace) that may be confused with open mouth breathing in the cat results from sampling air using the vomeronasal organ in the roof of the mouth.

Intermittent Positive-Pressure Ventilation

IPPV may be used to assist or control ventilation. During assisted ventilation, the anesthetist may offer two or three additional breaths per minute or may augment V_T to assist the patient's own ventilation. In controlled ventilation, the patient is not allowed to ventilate spontaneously and all ventilation is controlled by the anesthetist. Typically, 8 to 12 respirations per minute are used in controlled ventilation. The goals of IPPV are to maintain $Paco_2$ and Pao_2, speed induction, maintain a stable anesthetic plane, and control respiratory movements. A "sigh" (e.g., a larger than normal breath administered to an inspiratory pressure of approximately 30 mm Hg) may be offered periodically to renew surfactant. It is difficult to overcome the closing pressure of the alveoli and reexpand collapsed alveoli by IPPV. In anesthetized patients, it is only possible to temporarily recruit alveoli that are atelectic. In dogs, lateral recumbency is more important in the development of atelectasis than is the Fio_2 (Morandi et al. 2003).

Keeping your patient in sternal recumbency after premedicants and throughout anesthesia will prevent atelectasis. In dogs, the Fio_2 is a trivial source of atelectasis.

There are disadvantages to IPPV. IPPV may increase anesthetic depth, particularly with in-circle vaporizers (VICs). With most inhalants, respiration stops as the patient becomes too deep, but during IPPV, respiration is lost as an indicator of anesthetic depth. Other complications of IPPV may include hyperventilation and alkalosis, barotrauma, and impaired cardiovascular function. When positive pressure is introduced into the lung, thoracic pressure is increased which causes decreased venous return, decreased cardiac output, decreased arterial blood pressure, impairment of tissue perfusion, and increased resistance to pulmonary blood flow. The clinical impact of IPPV on cardiovascular function is greater in patients with inadequate blood volume.

A mechanical ventilator may be used as an "extra pair of hands" during IPPV (see Chapter 1), or the anesthetist may manually provide IPPV. Guidelines for IPPV in dogs and cats are similar. Tidal volume should be about 15 ml/kg and the respiratory rate should be 8 to 12 respirations/min. When providing IPPV, the inspiratory time should be about 1.5 seconds and the ratio of inspiratory time to expiratory time should be 1 : 2 or less (e.g., 1 : 3, 1 : 4). The inspiratory pressure should be 12 to 25 cm H_2O. In young patients with healthy lungs and in patients with thoracic disease or trauma, such as bulla or pneumothorax, lower inspiratory pressures should be used. In patients with thoracic trauma, manual ventilation is preferred over mechanical ventilation so that the anesthetist may appreciate a change in lung compliance. In patients with thoracic disease or abdominal distension, higher inspiratory pressure may be needed to deliver adequate V_T. With IPPV, MV should be adjusted according to blood-gas and pH analyses.

A mechanical ventilator acts as "an extra pair of hands" to squeeze the bag during IPPV.

If a patient continues to breathe during IPPV (i.e., "bucks" ventilation), an equipment problem (e.g., sticky valves, leak in system) should be ruled out (see Chapter 1). If there is no equipment problem, the patient may be inadequately anesthetized (i.e., "too light"), inadequately ventilated (i.e., $Paco_2$ greater than 45 mm Hg), or hypoxemic (i.e., Pao_2

less than 60 mm Hg). In order for a patient to resume spontaneous ventilation after IPPV, the respiratory rate should be briefly decreased so that the $Paco_2$ increases and stimulates ventilation. If the patient does not begin spontaneous ventilation after decreasing MV, the patient should be reevaluated. Do not to allow the $Paco_2$ to increase to a concentration that is depressing to the central nervous system (e.g., 30% CO_2 produces anesthesia, 90 to 120 mm Hg produces narcosis, greater than 100 to 150 mm Hg results in cessation of breathing). Decreasing anesthetic depth will also facilitate spontaneous ventilation. Hypoxemia should not be used to drive ventilation.

DERANGEMENTS IN VENTILATION

Hypoventilation is, by definition, arterial retention of CO_2 ($Paco_2$ greater than 45 mm Hg). Carbon dioxide retention results from an imbalance of production and elimination. Increased production can result from shivering, hyperthermia (e.g., septicemia, malignant hyperthermia), or inotrope (e.g., dobutamine, dopamine) administration. In the presence of increased production, MV should be increased and any underlying pathology addressed.

Inadequate CO_2 elimination occurs with decreased MV, ventilation-perfusion ($\dot{V}/\dot{Q}$) mismatch, or rebreathing. Decreased MV may result from anesthesia, as described earlier. Other differentials for reduced MV include positioning (i.e., head down surgical position), obesity (i.e., "Pickwickian"[2]), central nervous system derangements, and thoracic pathology. MV should be increased if hypoventilation causes an excessively high $Paco_2$.

Ventilation-perfusion mismatch may occur as a result of venous admixture (i.e., physiologic shunt) or dead space ventilation. A large physiologic shunt affects Pao_2 more than $Paco_2$ because the difference in arterial and venous O_2 is greater than the difference in arterial and venous CO_2. If equal parts of venous and arterial blood are mixed, the effect on oxygen will be greater than on carbon dioxide. Ventilation-perfusion mismatch is discussed at greater length in the section on hypoxemia.

Rebreathing of CO_2 may occur with exhausted CO_2 absorbent in a circle breathing system, inadequate fresh gas flow rate in a nonrebreathing anesthesia circuit, or incompetent one-way valves in a circle system. If malfunction of the breathing system is the cause for inadequate elimination of CO_2, the problem should be identified and corrected. Rebreathing is easily identified with an end-tidal CO_2 ($ETCO_2$) monitor (see Chapter 2).

There are a few potentially beneficial effects of hypoventilation, but far more untoward effects. Carbon dioxide retention shifts the oxyhemoglobin dissociation curve to the right, facilitating oxygen offloading in the tissues (see p. 46, the discussion of hypoxemia). Permissive hypoventilation may be used to support cardiac output. Carbon dioxide retention results in a sympathetically mediated maintenance of arterial blood pressure and cardiac output. However, the catecholamine release may also result in cardiac arrhythmias.

The negative effects of hypoventilation may be dangerous. In room air ($Fio_2 = 0.21$), hypoxemia may result from hypoventilation. In anesthetized patients breathing 100% O_2, hypoventilation has minimal impact on Pao_2. However, after premedication with respiratory depressants (e.g., opioids, α_2-agonists) or during anesthetic recovery, hypoventilation in a patient breathing air may have clinically significant consequences. An increase in $Paco_2$ produces a similar decrease in Pao_2 (e.g., if $Paco_2$ increases by 40 mm Hg to 80 mm Hg, Pao_2 will decrease by about 40 mm Hg to 60 mm Hg). Hypoxemia and its treatment are discussed after hypoventilation.

> Hypoventilation is not an important differential for hypoxemic patients inspiring a high concentration of oxygen.

As stated, the cardiovascular effects of an elevated $Paco_2$ result from sympathetic stimulation. However, in isolated heart preparations, myocardial depression (decreases in both contractility and rate) occurs. This may be important in traumatized or chronically ill patients that are unable to increase the concentration of circulating catecholamines.

Cerebral blood flow increases with increasing CO_2 as a result of extracellular pH changes around the arterioles. The calvarium is essentially a closed cavity that houses brain, cerebrospinal fluid (CSF), and blood. The volume of brain tissue and CSF cannot be changed, but the amount of blood in the

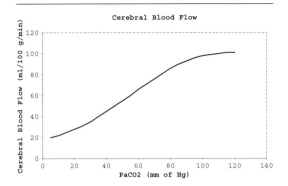

Figure 3.2. An approximation of the relationship between $Paco_2$ and cerebral blood flow.

calvarium can be altered. Figure 3.2 illustrates the relationship between $Paco_2$ and cerebral blood flow.

Premedication with drugs that cause hypoventilation (e.g., opioids, α_2-agonists) should be avoided in patients with increased intracranial pressure (ICP). "Permissive" hyperventilation of patients with increased ICP is controversial. Previously, patients with increased ICP were hyperventilated in an attempt to vasoconstrict the cerebral vasculature prior to exposure to the vasodilatory effects of inhalants. Profound hyperventilation ($Paco_2$ less than 25 mm Hg) should be avoided since brain ischemia may result. Conservative IPPV to an ETCO$_2$ of 27 to 32 mm Hg ($Paco_2$ = 32 to 37 mm Hg) seems prudent. Ideally, a $Paco_2$ should be compared to a simultaneous ETCO$_2$ to determine the gradient between $Paco_2$ and ETCO$_2$ (e.g., dead space); that difference should be used to determine the appropriate beginning ETCO$_2$. For example, if the $Paco_2$ = 45 mm Hg and the ETCO$_2$ = 40 mm Hg, the gradient is 5 mm Hg. If the desired $Paco_2$ = 35 mm Hg, ventilation should be increased to result in an ETCO$_2$ = 30 mm Hg. During a prolonged procedure, periodic arterial blood gas may be examined to see if ventilation should be changed to account for changes in dead space (i.e., changes in the difference between $Paco_2$ and ETCO$_2$).

Central nervous system depression may occur as $Paco_2$ increases. Thirty percent CO$_2$ in inhaled gases is sufficient to produce anesthesia at high partial pressures ($Paco_2$ greater than 100 to 150 mm Hg) but causes frequent seizures. Carbon dioxide narcosis occurs with $Paco_2$ in the range of 90 to 120 mm Hg. Even though CO$_2$ stimulates ventilation at lower partial pressures, ventilation is depressed at high partial pressures ($Paco_2$ greater than 100 to 150 mm Hg) and apnea occurs at $Paco_2$ greater than 150 mm Hg.

Catecholamine release and arrhythmia formation as a result of increased $Paco_2$ were discussed earlier. Bradycardia may occur as a consequence of increased vagal tone resulting from reduced acetylcholine hydrolysis in an acidic environment. However, the most common consequence of hypoventilation in anesthetized patients breathing 100% oxygen is respiratory acidosis.

Arterial Acid-Base Derangements

In order to interpret and treat arterial blood gas derangements, the relationship between $Paco_2$ and bicarbonate ion (HCO$_3^-$) must be understood. The carbonic acid equilibrium equation (Equation 3.2) reveals the relationship. In the presence of carbonic anhydrase (CA), carbon dioxide (CO$_2$) and water (H$_2$O) combine to produce carbonic acid (H$_2$CO$_3$) which dissociates to produce hydrogen ion (H$^+$) and bicarbonate ion (HCO$_3^-$).

$$CO_2 + H_2O \xleftarrow{\;CA\;} H_2CO_3 \leftrightarrow H^+ + HCO_3^- \quad (3.2)$$

This buffering occurs at the level of the red blood cell and is not the result of compensation by the kidneys, which takes days. Dissolved CO$_2$ exerts a pressure according to Henry's law[3] and can be measured as the partial pressure of carbon dioxide in the plasma ($Paco_2$). The dissolved CO$_2$ determines the gradient responsible for CO$_2$ entering or leaving the blood.

Determination of $Paco_2$ in an anesthetized patient may not accurately reflect the ventilatory status of an awake patient, especially if the patient has been heavily premedicated. As indicated earlier, anesthetics depress ventilation, the patient's ability to increase MV in response to increased $Paco_2$ is shifted, and ventilatory status in an anesthetized patient is not reflective of the conscious patient. Obviously, $Paco_2$ measured in patients whose ventilation is being assisted or controlled is being artificially adjusted.

Metabolic status is also changed by anesthesia. Diagnosis of a metabolic acidosis in an anesthetized patient may reflect lactic acidosis that results from poor circulation. The blood gas and pH changes

Table 3.1. Normal values for arterial blood gases ($F_{IO_2} = 0.21$).

Variable	Normal Values at 37°C
pHa	7.35 to 7.45
Pa_{O_2} (mm Hg)	80 to 100
Pa_{CO_2} (mm Hg)	35 to 45
HCO_3^- (mEq/L)	22 to 27
Base excess (BE) (mEq/L)	−4 to +4

in an anesthetized patient reflect the adequacy of ventilation (removing too much CO_2 or not enough) and the adequacy of circulation (presence of a lactic acidosis). In an anesthetized patient with normal circulation, a preexisting metabolic derangement may be discovered. Shapiro et al. (1994) provides an extensive review of the clinical application of blood gases.

Evaluating Blood Gas Results

The advent of point of care blood gas and pH analyzers (e.g., IRMA) makes it possible and economically feasible to evaluate blood gases and acid-base balance in practice. The normal values for arterial blood gases appear in Table 3.1.

Interpreting arterial blood gases is best accomplished by establishing a routine. The following sequence may be used to interpret the data in the anesthetized patient.

1. Examine the pH to diagnose status, either acidotic or alkalotic.
2. Evaluate the Pa_{O_2} to determine oxygenation.
3. Evaluate the Pa_{CO_2} to determine ventilatory status. The Pa_{CO_2} is the only objective determinant of ventilation.
4. Determine if the HCO_3^- is reflective of metabolic status or should be adjusted for ventilatory status. The HCO_3^- reflects metabolic status but is influenced by ventilation as a result of the carbonic acid equilibrium. Bicarbonate concentration increases with increases in Pa_{CO_2} and vice versa.
5. Adjust HCO_3^- for acute changes in Pa_{CO_2} according to rules of thumb:

   a. HCO_3^- increases by 1 to 2 mEq/L for each acute 10–mm Hg increase in Pa_{CO_2} above 40 mm Hg.
   b. HCO_3^- decreases by 1 to 2 mEq/L for each acute 10–mm Hg decrease in Pa_{CO_2} below 40 mm Hg.

   or

   c. Use base excess (+BE) or base deficit (−BE) to simplify blood gas interpretation. Base excess/deficit is a mathematically generated number that reflects the metabolic status of a normally ventilated patient. It reflects how much acid or base per liter should be added to normalize the pH in a normally ventilated patient (Pa_{CO_2} 40 mm Hg).

6. Match changes in Pa_{CO_2} and HCO_3^- or both with pH.
7. Determine presence of compensation if pH is normal. If the arterial blood gas sample was not taken shortly after induction or if the patient is heavily premedicated, the result of the blood gas may not be reflective of the patient's conscious status. If available, the total CO_2 (T_{CO_2}) on the venous preoperative screening blood work may indicate the need for a blood-gas immediately after induction. This may not true for dogs that are excited and panting (dead space ventilation) for an extended time. The T_{CO_2} may be lowered to about 20 mEq/L by panting. If the T_{CO_2} is less than 20 mEq/L, it is unlikely due to panting alone.

Because pH and blood gas data are affected by body temperature, the patient's temperature may be considered during evaluation of the measurements. Most point-of-care blood gas machines are set to reflect normal human body temperature and may be changed to species variation in body temperatures. The value of correcting blood gas data for body temperature is debated. Consistency in interpretation is probably more important than correcting data for small changes in body temperature.

Treatment of Blood Gas Derangements

Once the data from the blood gas analysis have been interpreted, the treatment should be determined. A respiratory acidosis (Pa_{CO_2} 45 mm Hg or greater) or alkalosis (Pa_{CO_2} 35 mm Hg or less) is easily remedied by increasing or decreasing ventilation, respectively. When changing the MV, either the RR or V_T

may be changed. If possible, the V_T rather than RR should be increased in hemodynamically unstable patients. During IPPV, venous return is decreased during inspiration. Decreasing venous return decreases preload to the heart. The fewer times per minute venous return is decreased, the better. Whether the V_T may be increased is determined by thoracic compliance and the inspiratory pressure generated during IPPV. In most instances, inspiratory pressure should not exceed 20 cm H_2O. In young patients, lower inspiratory pressures provide adequate ventilation; in older patients, higher inspiratory pressures may be required. For patients with thoracic trauma (e.g., pneumothorax, bulla), which may be worsened by high inspiratory pressures, 12 to 15 cm H_2O should not be exceeded and the patient should be hand-ventilated. In a normal chest, barotrauma does not occur until the inspiratory pressure is greater than 60 cm H_2O. The RR may be increased if the V_T cannot be altered.

If respiratory acidosis ($Paco_2$ greater than 45 mm Hg) and metabolic acidosis (BE less than −4 mEq/L) require treatment, the respiratory component should be treated first because the administration of sodium bicarbonate produces more arterial CO_2. If artificial ventilation will not be possible after bicarbonate administration (e.g., surgery or diagnostics are almost completed and recovery from anesthesia is imminent), it is better to reevaluate the pH and blood gases after the patient awakens.

The guidelines for treatment of metabolic acidosis are changing. Generally, in an anesthetized patient, pH 7.2 or less (due solely to metabolic acidosis) warrants treatment with sodium bicarbonate or another alkalinizing drug (see Chapter 12). The amount of HCO_3^- replacement is easily determined. In most patients, the extracellular fluid volume is 30% of the body weight (BW; in kg). Base deficit (BE) units are given in mEq/L. Equation 3.3 is used to calculate the total milliequivalents of sodium bicarbonate for intravenous administration.

$$\text{Deficit mEq } HCO_3^-$$
$$= \text{BW (kg)} \times 0.3 \times \text{BE mEq/L} \quad (3.3)$$

One half to one third of the calculated deficit should be administered slowly (over 20 minutes) intravenously and the pH and blood gas data reevaluated 30 minutes after the bicarbonate administra-tion has ended.[4] The important concept is to avoid overcorrection.

> Bicarbonate therapy is not without risk!

The administration of sodium bicarbonate is not necessarily benign. There may be untoward effects of bicarbonate administration. An alkalosis may be created, especially with overdosage or rapid intravenous administration. There may be decreased oxygen delivery to tissue due to increased affinity of hemoglobin for oxygen (i.e., alkalosis shifts the oxyhemoglobin curve to the left). There may be negative inotropy, hyperosmolarity (increased sodium concentration), hypokalemia, or hypocalcemia. Vasodilation may occur. The additional sodium may lead to volume overload. Due to differences in solubilities of CO_2 and H^+ across the blood-brain barrier, a paradoxical CSF acidosis may occur. The administration of sodium bicarbonate results in the production of CO_2. The CO_2 easily crosses the blood-brain barrier, hydrates to carbonic acid, and liberates hydrogen ions to which the blood-brain barrier is not permeable. Other non–CO_2-generating buffers are discussed later (see Chapter 12).

Although quite rare in small animals, a metabolic alkalosis may be treated by changing from an alkalinizing fluid (e.g., lactated Ringer's solution) to an acidifying fluid such as normal saline (0.9% NaCl). Most instances of metabolic alkalosis are associated with significant derangements in blood concentrations of sodium, chloride, and potassium. Properly addressing electrolyte imbalances usually leads to correction of the metabolic alkalosis.

Clinical Signs of Hypoventilation

The least reliable method of evaluating the adequacy of ventilation is comparing the expected MV of a patient with the apparent MV. There should be an obvious thoracic excursion with each breath and the respiratory rate should be adequate. A respirometer may be used on the inspiratory arm of the breathing circuit or between the breathing system and endotracheal to determine V_T and/or MV (see Chapter 2).

Hypoventilation may be diagnosed by monitoring ETCO$_2$, which is discussed in Chapter 2. End-tidal CO_2 will be about 2 to 10 mm Hg lower than the $Paco_2$. If the $Paco_2$ value is compared to a simultaneous ETCO$_2$ value and the patient's positioning does not change, the difference between the Paco$_2$ and the ETCO$_2$ should remain relatively constant during anesthesia.

Clinically, the mucous membranes may become brick red due to vasodilation during hypoventilation. The patient may "buck" the ventilator during inspiration, as previously discussed. Tachycardia and arrhythmias may occur due to the sympathetic stimulation associated with an increased Paco$_2$.

HYPOXEMIA

Inadequate oxygen in the blood causes hypoxemia. Hypoxemia is the most common final event in an anesthetic-related death. Hypoxemia may be absolute (Pao$_2$ equals 60 mm Hg or less) or relative. If the Pao$_2$ is adequate (Pao$_2$ equals 80 mm Hg or greater) but less than expected, hypoxemia is relative. The expected Pao$_2$ can be calculated for a given FIO$_2$ and level of ventilation using the ideal alveolar gas (Pao$_2$) equation (Equation 3.4).

$$P_{AO_2} = F_{IO_2} \times (P_B - P_{A_{H_2O}}) - (P_{aco_2}/RQ)$$
$$P_B = \text{barometric pressure,}$$
$$P_{A_{H_2O}} = \text{water vapor pressure,}$$
$$RQ = \text{respiratory quotient} = 0.8. \quad (3.4)$$

For a patient breathing 100% oxygen (FIO$_2$ = 1) at sea level (barometric pressure [PB] = 760 mm Hg), the saturated water vapor pressure (PAH$_2$O = 47 mm Hg at 37°C) must be taken into account (inhaled gases are humidified in the respiratory tract) and subtracted from the barometric pressure. About 20% more oxygen is consumed than carbon dioxide produced, resulting in a respiratory quotient (RQ) of 0.8. For example, the calculated Pao$_2$ in a normally ventilated patient (Paco$_2$ = 40 mm Hg) breathing room air (21% O$_2$) at sea level is 99.7 mm Hg.

$$P_{AO_2} \text{ (room air, normal ventilation)}$$
$$= 0.21 \times (760 \text{ mm of Hg} - 47 \text{ mm Hg})$$
$$- (40 \text{ mm Hg}/0.8) = 99.7 \text{ mm Hg} \quad (3.5)$$

In a normally ventilated patient, Pao$_2$ may be estimated by multiplying the FIO$_2$ by 5. The expected Pao$_2$ on room air is estimated to be 105 mm Hg (21% × 5) (Equation 3.6) using this rule of thumb.

$$P_{ao_2} = F_{IO_2} \times 5 \quad (3.6)$$

The Role of Ventilation in Hypoxemia

Hypoventilation in a patient breathing room air may be life-threatening (Equation 3.7), whereas hypoventilation with 100% O$_2$ will decrease the pH over time but does not reduce Pao$_2$ significantly (Equation 3.8).

$$P_{AO_2} \text{ (room air, hypoventilation)}$$
$$= 0.21 \times (760 \text{ mm Hg} - 47 \text{ mm Hg})$$
$$- (60 \text{ mm Hg}/0.8) = 74.7 \text{ mm Hg} \quad (3.7)$$

$$P_{AO_2} \text{ (100\% O}_2\text{, hypoventilation)}$$
$$= 1 \times (760 \text{ mm Hg} - 47 \text{ mm Hg})$$
$$- (60 \text{ mm Hg}/0.8) = 638 \text{ mm Hg} \quad (3.8)$$

DIFFERENTIALS AND TREATMENT FOR HYPOXEMIA

The importance of examining and understanding the differentials for hypoxemia relates to selection of treatment, if treatment is possible. Hypoventilation is typically treatable and has been discussed. If hypoventilation is not the etiology of hypoxemia, other differentials should be considered: decreased FIO$_2$ (less than 0.21), diffusion barrier to uptake of oxygen, $\dot{V}/\dot{Q}$ mismatch (physiologic shunt), anatomic right-to-left shunt, or some combination of these. Decreased cardiac output is often included in the differential list for hypoxemia. Decreased cardiac output directly impairs arterial oxygenation and exacerbates existing $\dot{V}/\dot{Q}$ abnormalities. Improving cardiac output may increase Pao$_2$, decrease Pao$_2$, or result in no change in Pao$_2$. For clinical purposes, decreased cardiac output is considered a form of $\dot{V}/\dot{Q}$ mismatch and is discussed later.

> Differentials for hypoxemia are hypoventilation, decreased FIO$_2$, diffusion barrier to uptake of oxygen, $\dot{V}/\dot{Q}$ mismatch (including low cardiac output), anatomic right-to-left shunt, or some combination of these.

Decreased FIO$_2$ is easily treated by increasing the concentration of oxygen in the inspired gases. Decreased FIO$_2$ is uncommon in anesthetized veterinary patients that are orotracheally intubated and being maintained with an inhalant drug in 100% oxygen. If the patient is not intubated and is being maintained by mask, the FIO$_2$ is lower because room air may be entrained. Still, Pao$_2$ should be adequate if Equation 3.6 is applied (i.e., 40% $F_{IO_2} \times 5 = 200$ mm Hg). If nitrous oxide is used at a $1:1$ or $2:1$ nitrous oxide/oxygen ratio, the Pa_{O_2} is expected to be 250 mm Hg or 165 mm Hg, respectively. If there is a mistake and the nitrous oxide/oxygen ratio is greater than $3:1$, hypoxemia due to decreased F_{IO_2} is likely. There are safeguards (e.g., color code, label designating the gas, diameter-index safety system [DISS], and pin-index safety system connectors to prevent inadvertent interchange of gases, or "quick connectors" that allow for rapid attachment of hoses) for medical gases that should not allow oxygen and nitrous oxide (or other wrong gas) to be interchanged. However, inappropriate connections may be made forcibly or with some ingenuity. An increase in CO_2 (as described previously) may also contribute to decreased F_{IO_2}. Veterinarians should not blindly trust the anesthesia system.

A diffusion barrier to uptake of oxygen occurs when the transfer of gas across the alveolar wall to the capillary membrane is diminished. Passive diffusion of gas through tissue occurs according to Fick's law. *Fick's law* states that diffusion of gas through tissue is directly proportional to the area, a diffusion constant (proportional to the gas solubility and inversely proportional to the square root of its molecular weight), and the difference in partial pressure; diffusion is inversely proportional to the thickness (West and West 2004). Clinically, a diffusion barrier to uptake may occur with fibrosing lung disease.

The two extremes of $\dot{V}/\dot{Q}$ mismatch are *shunt* and *dead space ventilation* (Fig. 3.3). The depicted shunt unit demonstrates blood traversing pulmonary capillaries without oxygen uptake due to atelectasis. Shunt may also refer to blood that has had no opportunity for gas exchange ($\dot{V}/\dot{Q} = 0$) (e.g., bronchial, thebesian, anterior cardiac veins).

In young patients, anatomic right-to-left shunts (e.g., tetralogy of Fallot, reversed patent ductus arteriosus) may be the cause for decreased Pa_{O_2}. Venous admixture refers to areas of lung with low $\dot{V}/\dot{Q}$. In dead space ventilation, ventilation is normal and perfusion is decreased, as would be the case in thromboembolic disease ($\dot{V}/\dot{Q} = \infty$).

Ventilation/perfusion mismatch is increased with abnormal positioning. In sternal recumbency, $\dot{V}/\dot{Q}$ is closest to 1. In lateral recumbency, the down lung is best perfused and the up lung is best ventilated. Desaturation may occur if the patient is then turned to the alternate side, exacerbating $\dot{V}/\dot{Q}$ mismatch. Dorsal recumbency exacerbates $\dot{V}/\dot{Q}$ mismatch due to atelectasis. A head-down position also exacerbates $\dot{V}/\dot{Q}$ mismatch. With extended surgeries, the effect of gravity on $\dot{V}/\dot{Q}$ mismatch may be enhanced. Other conditions which may contribute to $\dot{V}/\dot{Q}$ mismatch include diaphragmatic hernia, pregnancy, and a full gastrointestinal tract. It is difficult to overcome the closing pressure of the alveoli, so hypoxemia due to atelectasis is difficult to treat in the anesthetized patient. Recruitment maneuvers may be used to temporarily resolve some atelectasis but are not without risk and offer only temporary relief. In a patient with areas of chronically atelectic lung (e.g., chronic diaphragmatic hernia), care should be taken to avoid acutely and completely inflating the lungs to prevent reexpansion pulmonary edema. The ideal practice is slow reexpansion over 24 to 48 hours or longer using low negative pressure applied to the pleural space.

> To avoid reexpansion pulmonary edema, do not reexpand chronically atelectic lung during anesthesia and surgery.

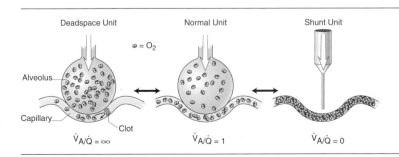

| Deadspace Unit | Normal Unit | Shunt Unit |

○ = O_2

Alveolus

Capillary

Clot

$\dot{V}_A/\dot{Q} = \infty$ $\dot{V}_A/\dot{Q} = 1$ $\dot{V}_A/\dot{Q} = 0$

Figure 3.3. Alveolar units are depicted: shunt ($\dot{V}/\dot{Q} = 0$), dead space ($\dot{V}/\dot{Q} = \infty$), and normal ($\dot{V}/\dot{Q} = 1$). (Illustration by Mark M. Miller, Miller Medical Illustration & Design.)

There may be a combination of factors leading to hypoxemia. It is best to treat the treatable causes and minimize the time the patient is hypoxemic. In patients with preexisting lung pathology, oxygenation prior to anesthetic induction helps maintain Pa_{O_2}. Such patients tend to do well breathing an enriched oxygen environment (sternal recumbency is best for avoiding atelectasis). Because anesthesia results in a decreased response to CO_2, it may be very difficult to wean the patient from oxygen. Recovering a hypoxemic patient with nasal oxygen or in an oxygen cage may improve the outcome (Table 3.2).

Table 3.2. Flow-by values for enriching the oxygen environment ($F_{IO_2} > 0.21$).

Weight (kg)	F_{IO_2}* 0.50	F_{IO_2}* 0.80	F_{IO_2}* 1.00
2.5	0.3 L	0.5 L	0.7 L
5.0	0.6 L	1.25 L	1.5 L
10.0	1.0 L	2.0 L	2.9 L
15.0	1.7 L	3.2 L	4.3 L
20.0	2.2 L	4.3 L	5.7 L
25.0	2.8 L	5.3 L	7.2 L
30.0	3.5 L	6.5 L	8.6 L
35.0	3.9 L	7.5 L	10.0 L†
40.0	4.4 L	8.7 L	10.0 L†
50.0	5.5 L	10.0 L†	10.0 L†
60.0	6.5 L	10.0 L†	10.0 L†
70.0	7.7 L	10.0 L†	10.0 L†
80.0	8.8 L	10.0 L†	10.0 L†

*F_{IO_2} = fraction of inspired oxygen.
†Flow rates greater than 10 L/min may cause trauma to the nasal mucosa.

Hypoxic Pulmonary Vasoconstriction

Historically, hypoxic pulmonary vasoconstriction (HPV), an important protective mechanism, was believed to function improperly during inhalant anesthesia. A normal respiratory unit ($\dot{V}/\dot{Q} = 1$) is illustrated in Figure 3.4. In a normal patient, in the presence of hypoxia, local blood vessels in the lungs vasoconstrict and blood is shunted away from the silent respiratory unit. The decreased blood supply matches the decreased oxygen in the alveoli. This contributes to maintaining a normal $\dot{V}/\dot{Q}$ ratio. A normal circulatory response to decreased alveolar oxygenation is illustrated in Figure 3.4. In the absence of this protective mechanism, $\dot{V}/\dot{Q}$ mismatch occurs with potentially important clinical significance. In isolated perfused lung preparations, sevoflurane and desflurane inhibit HPV. However, HPV was demonstrated to be maintained in sevoflurane- and desflurane-anesthetized intact dogs (Lesitsky et al. 1998).

Diagnosing Hypoxemia

As discussed earlier, hypoxemia may be diagnosed by arterial blood gas analysis. The Pa_{O_2} may be estimated using pulse oximetry, which gives an estimated beat-to-beat arterial saturation (Sp_{O_2}) when placed in an area where a pulse may be detected (see Chapter 2). The human eye is not particularly good at visualizing changes in the color of mucous membranes related to hypoxemia. In an anemic animal in which there is 5 g/dl or less of hemoglobin, cyanosis will not occur. Electrocardiographic changes may be associated with hypoxemia too late to intervene. With acute hypoxemia, there is usually transient tachycardia and accompanying hypertension. The first noticeable ECG changes include

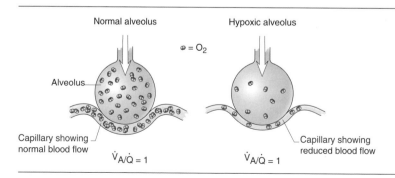

Normal alveolus   Hypoxic alveolus

● = O_2

Alveolus

Capillary showing normal blood flow

$\dot{V}_A/\dot{Q} = 1$

Capillary showing reduced blood flow

$\dot{V}_A/\dot{Q} = 1$

Figure 3.4. Hypoxic pulmonary vasoconstriction (HPV) keeps the $\dot{V}/\dot{Q}$ ratio near 1 in an awake patient with normal lungs. (Illustration by Mark M. Miller, Miller Medical Illustration & Design.)

ST-segment changes and T-wave changes (e.g., inversion, biphasic). Severe bradycardia may develop with continuing desaturation of hemoglobin. If hypoxemia is not corrected, asystole usually ensues. Absolute or relative hypoxemia can be diagnosed by blood gas analysis (Pao$_2$). Arterial blood gas monitoring does not provide real-time, beat-to-beat values for saturation of hemoglobin with oxygen. Pulse oximetry offers a beat-to-beat estimate of oxygen saturation with hemoglobin (Spo$_2$) and serves well as a monitor in critical situations. Pulse oximetry, ECG, and blood gas analyses were discussed earlier (see Chapter 2).

Oxyhemoglobin Dissociation Curve

The oxyhemoglobin dissociation curve describes the relationship between the Pao$_2$ and the affinity of oxygen for hemoglobin. The saturation of hemoglobin for a range of Pao$_2$ values is illustrated in Figure 3.5A.

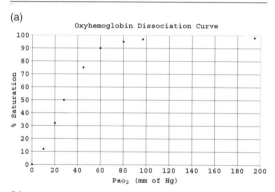

(a)

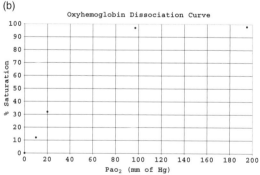

(b)

Figure 3.5. The approximated sigmoid oxyhemoglobin dissociation curve (*A*) illustrates the relationship between the Pao$_2$ and the affinity of oxygen for hemoglobin. (*B*) Fill in and label the points on the chart that are missing (e.g., Pao$_2$ = "y").

There are several clinically important aspects of the oxyhemoglobin dissociation curve. If the Pao$_2$ is 97 mm Hg, the normal arterial oxygen saturation (Sao$_2$) is about 97%. In an anesthetized patient breathing 100% oxygen (an expected Pao$_2$ of 500 mm Hg), the Sao$_2$ = 99 – 100%. A huge change in Pao$_2$ (97 mm Hg to 500 mm Hg) results in little change in Sao$_2$ because the change from 97 mm Hg to 500 mm Hg is on the flat part of the curve. The added oxygen content from 100 mm Hg to 500 mm Hg is a result of dissolved oxygen, which is discussed under oxygen content.

The actual Pao$_2$ may be lower than expected (a relative hypoxemia) without clinical relevance. If the Pao$_2$ is expected to be 500 mm Hg but is actually 200 mm Hg, saturation of hemoglobin is not a clinical problem. If a patient's Pao$_2$ is lower than 80 mm Hg and on the steeper part of the oxyhemoglobin dissociation curve, a small change in Pao$_2$ results in a much larger change in Sao$_2$. In Figure 3.5A, compare the saturation of hemoglobin at a Pao$_2$ value of 80 mm Hg to the Sao$_2$ of a patient with a Pao$_2$ of 60 mm Hg (absolute hypoxemia). The partial pressure of oxygen in venous blood (Pvo$_2$) is 45 mm Hg, which results in a saturation of about 75%. In a hypoxemic patient, there is very little gradient for diffusion of oxygen between arterial blood (Pao$_2$ of 60 mm Hg, 90% saturated) and venous blood (Pvo$_2$ of 45 mm Hg, 75% saturated). The P$_{50}$ is the Pao$_2$ in which hemoglobin saturation is 50% and is associated with a Pao$_2$ of about 28 mm Hg.

> The hemoglobin saturation in a hypoxemic patient (Pao$_2$ equals 60 mm Hg or less) is 90% or less.

Several factors can change the affinity of hemoglobin for oxygen. Shifting the curve to the right results in faster off-loading of oxygen from hemoglobin. During exercise, muscle requires more oxygen. An exercising muscle produces more CO$_2$, increases temperature, and decreases pH. All shift the oxyhemoglobin curve to the right, resulting in less affinity of oxygen to hemoglobin and greater availability of oxygen to tissue. Another situation with beneficial off-loading of hemoglobin at lower saturations (less affinity of oxygen for hemoglobin) occurs with increased 2,3-diphosphoglycerate

(DPG) in red cells. 2,3-DPG is a byproduct of red cell metabolism and increases in chronic hypoxia and in anemia. To increase delivery of oxygen to tissue in chronic hypoxia or anemia, a reasonable physiologic response would be more efficient off-loading of O_2.

Factors resulting in shifting the oxyhemoglobin curve to the right (increased CO_2, increased temperature, decreased pH, and increased 2,3-DPG) are the opposite of those that shift the curve to the left (decreased CO_2, decreased temperature, increased pH, and decreased 2,3-DPG), plus fetal hemoglobin. Obviously, to provide oxygen to fetal tissue, fetal hemoglobin requires greater affinity for oxygen than maternal hemoglobin.

> Factors that shift the oxyhemoglobin curve (change the affinity of hemoglobin for oxygen) are easily remembered if the situations in which the benefit of efficient holding and unloading of oxygen are understood.

OXYGEN CONTENT AND HYPOXIA

The roles of hypoxemia and anemia in oxygen delivery to tissue are best understood by examining the oxygen content of arterial blood. Oxygen content is the sum of bound and dissolved oxygen (Equation 3.9). Anemia impacts the amount of bound oxygen; hypoxemia impacts the amount of dissolved oxygen. Hypoxia results from decreased delivery of oxygen to tissue due to anemia, hypoxemia, both, or other reasons such as poor circulation.

$$O_2 \text{ content} = \text{bound } O_2 + \text{dissolved } O_2 \quad (3.9)$$

The bound (Equation 3.10) and dissolved (Equation 3.11) oxygen may be calculated.

Bound O_2 (ml O_2/dl) =
% saturation × [Hb] g/dl × 1.34 ml O_2/g
(1 g saturation Hb can carry 1.34 ml O_2)   (3.10)

Dissolved O_2 (ml O_2/dl) =
Pa_{O_2} × 0.003 ml O_2/dl (For each 100 ml of blood, 0.003 ml O_2 may be dissolved for each mm Hg O_2 tension)   (3.11)

The oxygen content (ml O_2/dl) in a normal animal (Hb = 15 g/dl; Pa_{O_2} = 100 mm Hg; Sa_{O_2} = 100%) breathing room air (21% O_2; FI_{O_2} = 0.21) is 20.4 ml O_2/dl. Of that, 20.1 ml O_2/dl is bound and 0.3 ml O_2/dl is dissolved (Equation 3.12).

O_2 content in normal animal
(Sa_{O_2} = 100%; 15 g/dl Hb) breathing
room air (FI_{O_2} = 0.21; Pa_{O_2}
= 100 mm Hg):

Bound O_2 (ml O_2/dl)
= 100 (% saturation) × 15 g/dl
    × 1.34 ml O_2/g = 20.1 ml O_2/dl
Dissolved O_2 (ml O_2/dl)
= 100 (mm Hg)
    × 0.003 (ml O_2)/(mm Hg)
= 0.3 ml O_2/dl
Oxygen content = 20.1 ml O_2/dl
    + 0.3 ml O_2/dl = 20.4 ml O_2/dl   (3.12)

The oxygen content of an anemic animal (Hb = 5 g/dl; Pa_{O_2} = 100 mm Hg; Sa_{O_2} = 100%) breathing room air (21% O_2; FI_{O_2} = 0.21) is 7.0 ml O_2/dl (Equation 3.13) and may be increased to 8.2 ml O_2/dl by enriching the oxygen environment to 100% (FI_{O_2} = 1.0) (Equation 3.14).

O_2 content in an anemic animal
(Sa_{O_2} = 100%; 5 g/dl Hb) breathing
room air (FI_{O_2} = 0.21;
Pa_{O_2} = 100 mm Hg):

Bound O_2 (ml O_2/dl) = 100 (%sat)
    × 5 g/dl Hb × 1.34 ml
O_2/g = 6.7 ml O_2/dl
Dissolved O_2 (ml O_2/dl) = 100 mm Hg
    × 0.003 ml O_2/dl = 0.3 ml O_2/dl
Total O_2 content = 7.0 ml O_2/dl   (3.13)

O_2 content of an anemic animal
(Sa_{O_2} = 100%; 5 g/dl Hb) breathing
100% O_2 (FI_{O_2} = 1.0; Pa_{O_2}
= 500 mm Hg):

Bound O_2 (ml O_2/dl) = 100 (%sat)
    × 5 g/dl Hb × 1.34 ml O_2/g = 6.7 ml O_2/dl
Dissolved O_2 (ml O_2/dl)
    = 500 mm Hg × 0.003 ml O_2/dl
    = 1.5 ml O_2/dl
Total O_2 content = 8.2 ml O_2/dl   (3.14)

Anemia impacts the delivery of oxygen to tissues, not the Pa_{O_2}. The Pa_{O_2} impacts the amount of dissolved oxygen and can be increased by enriching the oxygen environment.

OXYGEN TOXICITY

Is it possible to have too much oxygen in the body? Generation of oxygen-derived free radicals increases at high Pa_{O_2} tensions. Factors associated with increased production of oxygen free radicals include ferrous iron and hemoglobin, paraquat, NADPH oxidase and phagocytosis, complement activation, xanthine oxidase, glucose oxidase, and ionizing radiation (Lumb 2005). Oxygen free radicals are a major mechanism for tissue damage resulting from lipid peroxidation.

Extended exposure to high oxygen concentrations may injure the lung. In people, exposure for 30 hours results in impaired gas exchange (West and West 2004). Due to the difference in Pv_{O_2} and trapped Pa_{O_2}, absorption atelectasis may occur in which rapid diffusion of oxygen from the alveolus to the blood collapses the alveoli (West and West 2004). Stimulation of the central nervous system occurs when the Pa_{O_2} exceeds 760 mm Hg. This type of oxygen toxicity usually causes convulsions, which may be preceded by nausea, tinnitus, and facial twitching (West and West 2004). In premature human infants, retrolental fibroplasia may occur as a result of vasoconstriction caused by the high PO_2 (FI_{O_2}) in the incubator; maintaining the Pa_{O_2} below 140 mm Hg prevents this complication (West and West 2004).

An additional complication from oxygen therapy may occur in patients nonresponsive to the carbon dioxide drive to breathe. If a patient is nonresponsive to the carbon dioxide drive to breathe and relies on the hypoxic drive to breathe, the patient suffers severe ventilatory depression in the presence of enriched oxygen environments.

Treatment of severe hypoxemia (Pa_{O_2} equals 60 mm Hg or less) is paramount. However, in a given patient, a compromise between an acceptable Pa_{O_2} value (usually 75 mm Hg or greater) and a dangerously high inspired oxygen (60% oxygen; FI_{O_2} greater than 0.6) that may be required to keep the patient's Pa_{O_2} at an acceptable pressure may be needed. Other aspects of patient care such as bronchodilators, coupage, IPPV, or positive end-expiratory pressure ventilation should be considered to decrease the FI_{O_2} while maintaining an acceptable Pa_{O_2}.

Hyperbaric oxygen may be used to speed healing and decrease infection in gas gangrene, to treat carbon monoxide poisoning, decompression sickness, and occasionally as a therapy in an anemic crisis. Fire hazards are a real concern with use of 100% oxygen, especially at an increased barometric pressure (West and West 2004).

ENDNOTES

1 Much to the chagrin of parents, children readily discover that they can hold their breath longer underwater if hyperventilating before submerging.
2 Mr. Pickwick was a character from Charles Dickens *Mr. Pickwick's Papers/Pickwick Papers* (New York, 1906). The Pickwickian syndrome relates to hypercarbia, hypoxemia, polycythemia, hypersomnolence, pulmonary hypertension, and biventricular failure. Certainly, obese animals must be manually ventilated in order to maintain Pa_{CO_2}.
3 Henry's law states that the concentration of a gas dissolved in liquid is proportional to its partial pressure.
4 Some calculations for replacement bicarbonate therapy use: $0.08 \times BE \times BW$ (kg) (see Chapter 12). The results are similar if one half to one third of the calculated deficit using $0.3 \times BE \times BW$ (kg) is administered.

REFERENCES

Lesitsky, M.A., Davis, S., and Murray, P.A. 1998. Preservation of hypoxic pulmonary vasoconstriction during sevoflurane and desflurane anesthesia compared to the conscious state in chronically instrumented dogs. *Anesthesiology* 89:1501–1508.

Lumb, A. 2005. *Nunn's Applied Respiratory Physiology*. London: Butterworths.

Morandi, F., Mattoon, J.S., Lakrita, J., et al. 2003. Correlation of helical and incremental high-resolution thin-section computed tomographic imaging with histomorphometric quantitative evaluation of lungs in dogs. *Am J Vet Res* 64:935–944.

Pappenheimer, J.R., Comroe, J.H., Cournand, A., et al. 1950. Standardization of definitions and symbols in respiratory physiology. *Fed Proc* 9:602–605.

Shapiro, B.A., Peruzzi, W.T., and Kozlowski-Templin, R. 1994. *Clinical Application of Blood Gases*, 5th ed. Chicago: Year Book Medical Publishers.

Stoelting, R.K., and Hillier, S.C. 2006. *Pharmacology and Physiology in Anesthetic Practice*, 4th ed. Philadelphia: Lippincott Williams & Wilkins.

West, J.B., and West, J.B.B. 2004. *Respiratory Physiology: The Essentials*, 7th ed. Baltimore: Williams & Wilkins.

Chapter 4
Preoperative Preparation

Gwendolyn L. Carroll

Proper preoperative patient evaluation is required in order to develop the components of a complete anesthetic care plan. Patient evaluation includes history, signalment, physical exam, laboratory findings, and diagnostics. Additionally, the American Society of Anesthesiologists (ASA) has developed an ASA classification of patient status that is a predictor of outcome, and it is discussed later in this chapter. The anesthetic plan includes choices for premedication, maintenance anesthesia, intraoperative monitoring, fluid therapy, and postoperative care. The type of procedure, your skill, and the available equipment should be considered. With experience, anesthetic complications may be anticipated and potentially avoided.

PATIENT EVALUATION

In a busy practice, it is possible to make an error regarding anesthetic case management as a result of distraction with surgical management of the case, a packed waiting room, or any of the numerous concerns of daily practice. Fairly regularly, the American Veterinary Medical Association's Professional Liability Trust (PLIT) publishes a brochure outlining the various reasons a veterinarian may be sued and updates their Website.[1] Failure to confirm the patient identification, performing an incorrect procedure, and operating on the wrong limb are avoidable mix-ups. An arithmetic error (e.g., converting pounds [lb] to kilograms [kg]) or a miscalculation in drug dosage (e.g., calculator error resulting in a decimal place error) may contribute to patient morbidity or mortality. Developing a routine approach to each anesthesia case will help protect against mistakes that result from being too tired, too busy, or too stressed.

> Failure to confirm the patient identification, surgery, and correct limb are avoidable grounds for litigation.

History

There are several opportunities to gain valuable patient information that will assist in the development of an anesthetic plan. A detailed patient history is vital, particularly for new patients. Some questions that are pretty clear cut may be addressed using a standardized form during admission (Figure 4.1). For example, sex, reproductive history, heartworm status, vaccination history, activity level, exercise tolerance, exercise-induced hyperthermia, malignant hyperthermia (rare), seizure history, insurance coverage, appetite, weight loss or gain, time of previous meal, a history of vomiting or diarrhea, frequency of urination, increase in water consumption, current medications, and previous surgical procedures may be addressed with an admission form.

If clarification is needed, the owner or agent may be asked about their responses during the appointment and physical exam. A detailed medical history may be obtained from the owner during the office visit. It may be difficult to get consistent answers to routine questions (e.g., owners who report their dog is 4 years old and they have owned him for 6 years). However, if the owner is allowed to explain what is wrong, rather than responding to leading questions, the interview will provide a great deal of information.

Determine how long the chief problem has persisted. If there has been a chronic or recurrent condition, what event triggered the office visit? Asking

Patient Information Worksheet
Texas A&M University
Veterinary Medical Teaching Hospital
Small Animal Hospital

Stamp Firmly With Case Card

o   **Directions: To aid the doctor in reaching an accurate diagnosis, a complete background on your pet is essential. Please fill out the following questionnaire to the best of your ability using a ballpoint pen. When you are finished, return the form to the receptionist.**

How long have you owned your pet? _____
Where was your pet obtained? _____
Is your animal kept primarily out of doors or in the house? _____

Is your animal allowed to roam free?	YES	NO	
Has your animal been boarded or hospitalized recently?	YES	NO	Unknown
Are there any other animals in your household?	YES	NO	

         If Yes, What? _____

Has your pet's appetite either increased or decreased? (circle one)	YES	NO	Unknown
Has your pet lost or gained any weight recently? (circle one)	YES	NO	Unknown

What is your pet's diet? _____
How much and how often does your pet eat? _____

Is your animal ever fed table food?	YES	NO	Unknown
Has your pet been treated for any major medical problems?	YES	NO	Unknown

         If Yes, What? _____
If you animal is neutered, what was his/her age of alteration? _____

Has your pet ever undergone surgery?	YES	NO	Unknown

         If Yes, What and when? _____
If female and not neutered, when was her last heat? _____

If female, has she had any litters?	YES	NO	Unknown

         If Yes, when_____

Is your pet now taking medication to prevent heartworm disease?	YES	NO	Unknown
Has your animal traveled out-of-state?	YES	NO	Unknown
Has your pet lost any stamina lately?	YES	NO	Unknown
Is your pet drinking more water than usual?	YES	NO	Unknown
Is your pet urinating more frequently than usual?	YES	NO	Unknown
Has your pet vomited frequently?	YES	NO	Unknown
Have there been any recent changes in your pet's bowel movements?	YES	NO	Unknown
Has your pet been scratching?	YES	NO	Unknown
Has your pet had any seizures or convulsions?	YES	NO	Unknown
Has your pet had any change in attitude or behaviors?	YES	NO	Unknown
Has there been change in your pet's walking?	YES	NO	Unknown
Have you noticed any abnormal swellings?	YES	NO	Unknown

         If Yes, where? _____

If female, has your pet had any abnormal vaginal discharge?	YES	NO	Unknown
Has your pet had unusual/unexpected reactions to medications?	YES	NO	Unknown
Has your pet had any discharge from the eyes or nose?	YES	NO	Unknown
Has your pet had any coughing or breathing difficulty?	YES	NO	Unknown

Vaccination History: (please write down date of last vaccination, if know)
Dog: Rabies_____ DHLPP_____
Cat: Rabies_____ FVRCP_____ FeLV_____ FIV_____ FIP_____

Figure 4.1. A standard admissions form may be filled out by the owner or agent prior to the physical exam.

"What brings you in today?" will focus the owner on the primary complaint.

A detailed history will include previous medical conditions, drugs taken in the last month, previous anesthesia/surgery, and a resuscitation code (see Chapter 12). For established clients, much of the information needed will be in the patient's medical record and only a brief update will be needed. For new clients, sufficient time should be allowed to cover medical history. If available, previous anesthetic records should be reviewed for drugs, dosages, and endotracheal (ET) tube size. Specifically, any problems during induction or recovery and any misadventures during anesthetic maintenance should be evaluated. The anesthetic history will advise you of potential difficulties that might recur during a subsequent anesthetic episode. For example, asthma, regurgitation, seizure, hypotension, arrhythmia, or arrest may be averted by changing the anesthetic protocol, administering protective drugs, improving monitoring, or employing different techniques.

Any current or recent drug[2] or herbal[3] therapy, including over-the-counter drugs[4] (e.g., aspirin), should be recorded. Some drugs interact with enzymes and electrolytes, or affect acid-base status, seizure or arrhythmogenic threshold, neuromuscular transmission, respiration, or the cardiovascular system (e.g., chloramphenicol prolongs barbiturate anesthesia, streptomycin prolongs neuromuscular blockade, ketamine lowers the seizure threshold, digoxin lowers the arrhythmogenic threshold, β-blockers decrease contractility of the heart). Some drugs act directly with anesthetics (e.g., cimetidine increases the toxicity of lidocaine, patients receiving aminophylline and ketamine have a greater decrease in seizure threshold than either drug alone). More dogs and cats are receiving behavior-modifying drugs such as tricyclic antidepressants (e.g., amitriptyline, doxepin) and selective serotonin uptake inhibitors (SSRIs; e.g., fluoxetine). Fewer monoamine oxidase inhibitors (MAOIs) are prescribed in veterinary medicine, presumably due to the dietary restrictions and drug interactions that occur with the MAOIs. There are concerns regarding the use of anticholinergics and some opioids such as meperidine (inhibits serotonin uptake) with tricyclic, SSRI, and MAOI antidepressants. Serotonin syndrome[5] may occur if tramadol, a nonopiate μ-agonist that has some serotonin-uptake inhibition, is administered with an SSRI.

The medical history also provides an opportunity to find out health information that may have gone undetected (e.g., heartworm status). It is a Herculean task to keep all possible drug reactions and interactions with anesthetics and analgesics as "walk-around knowledge." If unsure about a drug, check a reference to make sure there will be no surprises. A few drugs (e.g., amitriptyline, aspirin) should be discontinued for some time before elective anesthesia and surgery.

> Prior to anesthesia and surgery, consult a pharmacology reference if patient is receiving an unfamiliar medication. Explore effects and interactions of unfamiliar herbs.

Any relevant organ system history and any specific problems of the patient should be evaluated prior to anesthesia. For trauma victims (especially hit-by-car [HBC]), several considerations should be routine. The patient should be evaluated for pulmonary trauma (e.g., pneumothorax, bulla, hemorrhage, fractured ribs), cardiovascular stability, urinary tract integrity, abdominal hemorrhage, and body wall or diaphragmatic hernias. Texts on anesthesia and concurrent disease exist (Barasch et al. 2001; Roizen 2000) and should be consulted if a patient suffers from an unfamiliar disease. The following brief organ system review (Table 4.1) is not meant to be exhaustive but to help describe the thought process required to anesthetize patients with concurrent disease, such as asthma.

Similarly, specific problems such as coughing (Table 4.2) that may exist on presentation prior to anesthesia should be determined and their effect on anesthesia and anesthetic choices considered. If preoperative treatments are possible, patients should be stabilized before anesthesia. Again, the list of specific problems is not complete but should help illustrate the thought process used in developing an individualized anesthetic care plan.

Informed owner consent for anesthesia, surgery, and any alternative or complementary practices such as physical therapy should be obtained. The extent to which an owner wants resuscitation procedures (e.g., resuscitation code; see Chapter 12) to be performed should be documented in the record. The risks of anesthesia and the particular surgery or diagnostic procedure should be carefully outlined.

Table 4.1. Limited review of organ systems determined by history or physical exam and potential anesthetic concerns.

Organ System	History or Physical Exam	Potential Impact
Cardiovascular	Arrhythmia	Anesthetic drug choices, cardiac or extra cardiac origin (e.g., pain, GDV), treatment (e.g., analgesia antiarrhythmic, oxygen); check blood pressure
	Hypotension	Anesthetic drug choices, CVP, volume status, fluid choices, inotropy
	Hypertension	Anesthetic drug choices, rule out cardiac, renal, brain, or endocrine disease, hypoxemia, hypercarbia, pain
	Murmur	Decrease fluid administration if mitral insufficiency or PDA; ECG
	Heartworm disease	Concerns vary from increased risk for arrhythmias to caval syndrome
Respiratory	Asthma	Anesthetic choices, preoperative preparation, support (e.g., bronchodilators, steroids, oxygen)
	Pulmonary compromise	Rapid sequence IV induction, oxygen support
	Nasal obstruction	Support (e.g., bite block to keep mouth open on extubation, oxygen)
	Elongated soft palate	Prepare for reintubation and tracheotomy in recovery (e.g., induction agent and laryngoscope) or surgical correction
	Laryngeal mass	Guide tube, assorted sized endotracheal tubes
	Pneumothorax/bulla	Decreased inspiratory pressure; prepare thorax for emergency thoracotomy
	Diaphragmatic hernia	Chronic—poor prognosis due to reexpansion pulmonary edema. Steroids ± antihistamines, decreased inspiratory pressure
Central nervous system	Seizures	Drug choices, elevation of head after myelogram
	Increased intracranial pressure; fontanel	Mild hyperventilation, drug choices
	Pre-existing nerve dysfunction	Document on record (e.g., facial nerve paralysis); adequate padding intraoperatively
Hepatic	Liver compromise, jaundice, clotting issues, low albumin, anemia	Drug choices, buccal mucosal bleeding time, clotting profile, glucose, fluid choices (e.g., plasma, colloid, blood products)
Gastrointestinal	Full stomach, megaesophagus, parasites, anemia, NSAIDs,	Rapid sequence induction, early inflation of the pilot balloon, fluid choices (e.g., plasma, colloid, blood products)

Table 4.1. *Continued.*

Organ System	History or Physical Exam	Potential Impact
Endocrine	Adrenals, thyroid, pancreas	Check blood pressure, ECG, thromboembolic disease, electrolytes, glucose, support (e.g., nitroprusside)
Renal	Polyurea, polydipsia, proteinuria, isosthenuria	Check blood pressure, PCV, phosphorus and electrolytes. Support (e.g., dopamine, mannitol, inotropy)
Integument	Atopy, petechiation, edema, dehydration	Past steroid use, clotting profile, liver function, cardiac evaluation, immune function

This table is not inclusive but is intended to demonstrate the process involved in preoperative preparation.

Table 4.2. Specific problems that may impact preoperative preparation and anesthetic choices.

Problem	Considerations
Volume depletion → hypotension	Fluid and drug choices (e.g., colloids, local anesthetic epidurals compound hypotension). Correct prior to anesthesia
Hemorrhage	Cross match (consider reproductive history and previous transfusions if female). Check compatibility in all cats! See volume depletion
Anemia	Fluid choices, enrich oxygen environment pre- and postoperatively, see hemorrhage
Hypoproteinemia, hypoalbuminemia	Fluid choices, drug choices
Vomiting → aspiration, volume depletion, electrolyte disturbances	Keep patient sternal, inflate cuff of endotracheal tube quickly, remove endotracheal tube with pilot balloon slightly inflated. Check electrolytes. No mask or chamber inductions. See volume depletion
Coughing	Etiology (e.g., collapsing trachea, parenchymal disease, cardiogenic or neurogenic edema, laryngeal paralysis, asthma)
Atrial fibrillation	Avoid drugs that speed AV nodal conduction (e.g., dobutamine) or that increase heart rate (e.g., atropine). Use opioids such as sufentanil
Anorexia/cachexia	Check glucose, albumin, and electrolytes; provide extra padding; support body temperature
Obesity	Difficult ventilation will probably need IPPV, other cardiovascular changes that accompany "Pickwickian" syndrome

Continued

57

Table 4.2. *Continued.*

Problem	Considerations
Infection, sepsis	Limit local techniques (e.g., local anesthetics do not work in an acid pH (infection), epidurals should be carefully considered if there is local infection or in sepsis; disseminated intravascular coagulation, hyper-, hypoglycemia, fluid choices
Cancer	Radiography-metastasis check; ultrasonography; analgesia
Fever	Malignant hyperthermia (e.g., dantrolene), monitor ETCO$_2$, avoid triggers; exercise-induced hyperthermia, heat exhaustion
Disseminated intravascular coagulation, thrombocytopenia	Fluid choices (e.g., fresh frozen plasma, fragmin, heparinized plasma); anesthetic techniques (e.g., no epidurals); support (e.g., preoxygenate and recover on nasal oxygen is possible)

This table is not inclusive but is intended to demonstrate the process involved in preoperative preparation for specific problems.

Different surgical procedures will require different questions. For example, when performing a cesarean section, in the rare event that the life of the patient and the offspring cannot both be saved, the owner's wishes should be determined before surgery. Similarly, the owner should be asked if the reproductive capability the pregnant patient should be preserved if possible. A contact number should always be available in order to contact the client in the case of an unforeseen complication.

Patient Signalment

A great deal of information may be obtained from the patient signalment. Patient identification has been discussed. A failsafe method of identification should be employed and each staff member trained in its routine use to identify patients. An accurate body weight provides information for accurate drug dosing. Additionally, body condition is an indicator of support that may be needed. For emaciated patients, impaired hepatic function may lead to hypoglycemia, extra padding should be provided to protect pressure points, especially nerves, and steps to maintain normothermia should be taken. For overweight patients, intermittent positive-pressure ventilation (IPPV) will be required in order to maintain normocapnia and smooth the anesthetic plane. "Pickwickian"[6] patients may also suffer from hyper-

carbia, hypoxemia, polycythemia, hypersomnolence, pulmonary hypertension, and biventricular failure. In heavily muscled animals or pregnant patients, mean arterial blood pressure should be maintained a little higher (80 mm Hg) than that typically required for renal perfusion (60 mm Hg). Other patient signalment such as species, breed, sex, temperament, and age offer additional information that should be considered in development of the anesthetic care plan.

SPECIES CONCERNS

Veterinarians are exposed to a variety of species (Fig. 4.2), but this chapter concentrates on anesthetic choices in cats and dogs. In general, cats seem to be more sensitive to side effects of some drugs (e.g., lidocaine). Cats are obligate carnivores. As such, they respond to drugs differently than omnivores or herbivores respond. Cats' inability to glucuronide conjugate makes several drugs very toxic (e.g., acetaminophen). Some drugs seem to be acceptable for short-term use in cats but not extended daily use (e.g., propofol).

In cats, ketamine is excreted unchanged by the kidney and is contraindicated in renal failure. In dogs, ketamine is ultimately metabolized and should be used cautiously in dogs with liver failure. Propylene glycol, a carrier in many drug formulations

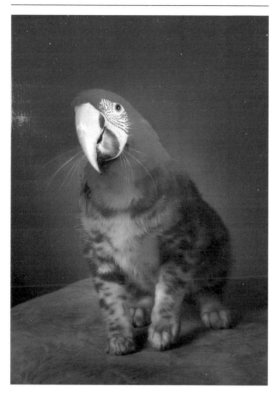

Figure 4.2. Although many species exist, this text concentrates on anesthetic choices for cats and dogs. ("Bird cat" photograph generously provided by Larry Wadsworth, Medical Photographer II, at the College of Veterinary Medicine and Biomedical Sciences, Texas A&M University.)

(e.g., diazepam, etomidate), may cause hemolysis in many species. The effect in cats seems to be more prevalent.

There are also differences in anatomy and physiology in cats and dogs that should be appreciated (e.g., the dural sac in cats extends caudally one more vertebra than in dogs, so an epidural performed at the L-S junction in cats is more likely to be a spinal than in dogs).

Distribution of opioid receptors in cats and dogs is believed to contribute to the different responses that are seen after opioid administration (e.g., occasional excitement in cats).

Unlike dogs, thyroid tumors in cats tend to be hormone producing. A hyperthyroid cat needs to have a cardiac evaluation. Similarly, cats that have murmurs are more likely to have significant cardiac disease than dogs with murmurs. Practically that

means that a small older dog with mitral regurgitation that is not in failure should do well with a regular anesthetic protocol, as long as the fluid administration is judicious and sympathomimetic drugs are avoided (e.g., ketamine). In cats with murmurs, there is likely to be significant cardiac disease and they should be evaluated with an electrocardiogram (ECG), radiographs, and possibly an echocardiogram.

Behavioral differences in cats and dogs make many assessments difficult. Cats are very stoic and their behavior is not easy to understand, making pain assessment more difficult than in dogs.

BREED CONCERNS

Breed concerns may be more of an issue in dogs than cats because purebred dogs are more likely to be registered and are more common. Brachycephalic dogs and cats should be observed closely after premedication for respiratory difficulty. A rapid intravenous induction protocol should be used. The soft palate and laryngeal function should always be evaluated before recovery. A laryngoscope, guide tube (e.g., polypropylene urinary catheter) or stylet, ET tube, and a short-acting induction drug should be available for reintubation if needed (see Chapter 15). Once reintubated, a decision can be made regarding whether a tracheotomy or other intervention would be needed before another attempt at extubation. Brachycephalic cats and dogs often have difficult recoveries. Cats do not do well with tracheotomies. Oxygen should be available for recovery.

Other breed concerns include extended recoveries in sight hounds after barbiturate anesthesia (also after propofol, but not clinically significant), malignant hyperthermia in Greyhounds, and von Willebrand's disease in Doberman Pinschers. Some anesthesiologists avoid drugs like acepromazine that may decrease platelet aggregation in Doberman Pinschers. There is a line of Boxers that allegedly respond poorly to acepromazine.

The impact of any disease that may influence anesthesia and that is prevalent in a breed should be pursued. Members of dog breeds (e.g., Doberman Pinchers, Rottweilers, Great Danes, Newfoundlands, Cocker Spaniels, King Charles Cavalier Spaniels, Boxers) or cat breeds (e.g., Maine Coon, Persian) that are commonly at risk for heart disease should have careful auscultation and an ECG prior to anesthesia. A radiograph and perhaps echocardiogram should be performed if the results of the auscultation, ECG, or history are suspicious. Even at a young age, breeds that may suffer from cardiomyopathy should have a careful auscultation and ECG prior to anesthesia. Other breeds such as Cocker Spaniels or Schnauzers that may have conduction disturbances (e.g., sick sinus syndrome) should have an ECG preoperatively. Other criteria for conducting an ECG prior to anesthesia include presence of a murmur, radiographic evidence of heart enlargement or pulmonary edema, and advanced age (6 years or older, unless a breed at risk). Often mitral regurgitation will be an incidental finding in dogs and judicious fluid administration may be all that is needed. Several breed concerns regarding anesthesia that have not been validated appear in lay literature or on the Internet.

PATIENT SEX

The sex of the patient is important, particularly if the anesthesia planned is for surgical neutering. Although hermaphrodites do occur in dogs, surgical neutering mistakes are rarely made in dogs. In cats, mistakes occur more frequently. Even though the sex of the patient may be reported by the client, the sex should be confirmed on physical exam.

For female patients undergoing nonreproductive surgery (e.g., fracture repair), it is important to determine if they are pregnant. Anesthesia increases the risks to the fetuses, particularly if the patient becomes hypoxemic or hypotensive. Generally, higher arterial blood pressures and enriched oxygen environments are maintained in pregnant patients to ensure good circulation and oxygen delivery. Other risks to the fetus include side effects from the drugs administered to the pregnant female. Almost all drugs administered to the adult will cross through the placenta and into the milk.

As for risk to the pregnant adult, increased uterine size and weight may decrease the functional residual capacity during ventilation. The large uterus may contribute to silent regurgitation and decrease venous return (even though less so than in humans). High concentrations of circulating progesterone decrease the minimum alveolar concentration (MAC) of the inhalant so the anesthetic plane must be critically evaluated for each patient.

PATIENT AGE

Age is not an illness, nor a contraindication for anesthesia, but it may be a significant risk factor for development of perianesthetic complications in some species. In any case, coexisting disease, whether degenerative or not, increases the risk of anesthesia. Despite a potentially prolonged anesthetic course, maintaining adequate circulating blood volume, addressing any underlying health issues, precautions to keep the patients warm, decreasing unnecessary anesthetic time, and adequate padding will contribute to successful outcomes.

Several considerations exist for neonates (see Chapter 13). Neonates do not appear to autoregulate blood pressure in the same range that adults autoregulate. The response curve to $PaCO_2$ is shifted to the right when compared to adults and the PaO_2 tends to be lower than an adult. Youngsters respond differently to drugs based on different size drug distribution compartments. The plasma protein tends to be lower which will impact protein bound drugs. Inadequate liver glycogen stores make youngsters prone to hypoglycemia. Young patients thermoregulate poorly. Youngsters are dependent on heart rate rather than contractility for their cardiac output. Their stiff ventricles do not respond well to inotropy. Heart rate can be maintained with anticholinergics if normothermic.

TEMPERAMENT

The last relevant patient signalment is temperament. It is important to determine if the patient can be safely handled. For veterinarians just starting out, an experienced technician is invaluable. Historically, a combination of fentanyl (an opioid) and droperidol (a butyrophenone) (i.e., Innovar-Vet) was used in savage dogs. Because this drug combination is no longer available, Telazol, a combination of tiletamine (a phencyclidine) and zolazepam (a benzodiazepine), has been used alone or with butorphanol for savage dogs. If the dog is muzzled, remove the muzzle after drug administration in case the dog vomits. Once chemically restrained, the dog can be more safely handled; always exercise caution.

Although I am not an advocate of chamber inductions, cats that are difficult or impossible to restrain for injection without injury to the cat or personnel may be captured in an induction chamber. Once they can be safely removed from the chamber, drug(s) to lower the amount of inhalant required or to protect against bradycardia may be administered and intravenous access gained.

Rambunctious dogs will benefit from a sedative or tranquilizer to make the experience less stressful on patient and staff. The shy or stoic dog that is very anxious but cooperative should not be denied pre-medicants to calm anxiety. The catecholamine and cortisol stress response to anxiety can actually be greater than that to pain. Techniques for addressing treatment of anxiety are covered in Chapter 5.

Physical Examination

The physical examination prior to anesthesia should concentrate particularly on organ systems impacted by anesthesia. Vital signs include body temperature, heart rate, respiratory rate, arterial blood pressure (if applicable), and pain score (see Chapter 9). Body weight and condition, sex, and reproductive status should be confirmed. The thorax and abdomen should be evaluated for loss of integrity, fractured ribs or vertebra, subcutaneous air, masses, free fluid, organomegaly, and presence of a bladder.

CARDIOVASCULAR SYSTEM

The cardiovascular system may be evaluated by several methods. The pulse should be palpated for rhythm (e.g., bradycardia, tachycardia, sinus arrhythmia) and quality (e.g., strong, thready, defi-cient). The palpable pulse pressure represents the difference between the systolic and diastolic arterial blood pressure and may provide a false sense of comfort or needless concern. The mean arterial blood pressure (MAP) is determined by use of an equation:

$$MAP = DAP + \frac{1}{3}(SAP - DAP) \qquad (4.1)$$

where MAP represents the mean arterial blood pressure, SAP represents the systolic arterial blood pressure, and the DAP represents the diastolic arterial blood pressure.

The pulse pressure may feel good, but if the diastolic pressure (DAP) is low and the systolic pressure (SAP) modest, the resulting mean arterial pressure (MAP) will be low. Similarly, the pulse pressure may feel bad, but if the patient is vasoconstricted and the systolic (SAP) and diastolic (DAP) pressures are both elevated, the difference between the two may be small. In this instance, the pulse will feel poor, but the MAP will actually be high.

The heart should be ausculted and evaluated for murmurs, absence of heart sounds in areas of the thorax where heart sounds should be ausculted (e.g., diaphragmatic hernia, pleural effusion) or a quiet heart (e.g., pericardial effusion). The pulse should be palpated and the heart should be ausculted simultaneously to determine if pulse deficits are present.

Some indications for performing an ECG were evaluated earlier (e.g., breed, age). Other indica-tions for performing a preoperative ECG include trauma such as HBC, in which traumatic myocardi-tis may occur as late as 72 hours after the incident. Diseases such as gastrointestinal dilation and vol-vulus, splenic tumor, and pancreatitis should also trigger a preoperative ECG. Patients with great pain, hypoventilation, or hypoxemia may also have arrhythmias due to high sympathetic tone. The administration of an analgesic and oxygen may improve the arrhythmias; often, the arrhythmias disappear under anesthesia. Patients with electro-lyte disturbances such as hyperkalemia from hypoadrenocorticism or urinary obstruction, or hypercalcemia from hypoadrenocorticism or adeno-carcinoma may have arrhythmias that will require treatment prior to anesthesia.

If the heart rate is high (e.g., tachycardia) or low (e.g., bradycardia), differentials should be exam-ined and potential causes ruled out. Differentials for tachycardia include the following:

- Sympathetic stimulation (e.g., pain, hypercap-nia)
- Hypotension (e.g., volume depletion)
- Too deep anesthetic plane
- Hyperthermia
- Drugs (e.g., anticholinergics, β-agonists, ket-amine)
- Acute hypoxemia

Differentials for bradycardia include the following:

- Hypothermia
- Hypertension
- Drugs (e.g., opioids, α_2-agonists, β-blockers, acute administration of calcium)
- Hyperkalemia

- Vagally mediated reflexes (e.g., oculocardiac reflex, carotid massage, micturition syncope)
- Increased intracranial pressure (Cushing reflex)
- Terminal hypoxemia

Recognition of aberrant ECG tracings is important preoperatively for stabilization of a patient prior to anesthesia (e.g., hyperkalemia) and for choice of premedicants. As stated earlier, pulse pressure is not always reflective of arterial blood pressure (see Chapter 2). In clinics that have the capability, arterial blood pressure should be evaluated prior to anesthesia, particularly if there is a history of cardiac disease, hyperadrenocorticism, or renal disease or if a pheochromocytoma or increased intracranial pressure is suspected (see Chapter 13).

The etiology of the hypertension should be determined and treatment instigated preoperatively if warranted. If hypertension is documented, there are some precautions that should be taken. A retinal exam is indicated if one has not been performed. Depending on the etiology of the hypertension, there are some drugs that might be needed (e.g., nitroprusside, esmolol), which may not typically kept in the practice and should be ordered.

Other indicators of cardiovascular function include examination of the mucous membranes for color and capillary refill time (CRT). Normal mucous membrane color should be pink. A penlight should be used to evaluate mucous membrane color. When a mucous membrane is compressed with the finger, it should blanch and return to pink in less than 2 seconds. One caution regarding using CRT without considering other measures: although not common, CRT may remain normal for some minutes after death. Pale mucous membranes may indicate anemia or vasoconstriction (e.g., painful patients may be very pale due to vasoconstriction). Cyanotic mucous membranes reflect desaturated hemoglobin; at least 5 g/dl of reduced hemoglobin is required for the human eye to perceive cyanosis. An anemic patient may never become cyanotic (e.g., anemic patients may only have 5 g/dl of hemoglobin). If mucous membranes are bright red and injected, the patient may be hypercarbic or vasodilated (e.g., septic); if extreme, the cherry red mucous membranes may result from carbon monoxide poisoning; chocolate cyanosis results from methemoglobinemia. Jaundiced mucous membranes indicate hepatic compromise.

RESPIRATORY SYSTEM

The respiratory system should be carefully examined. The respiratory rate should be counted and a subjective evaluation of adequacy of chest excursions compared to expected tidal volume (V_T). Dyspnea may result from laryngeal paralysis, obstruction, alveolar or parenchymal disease, pleural masses or fluid, and pneumothorax. Stress should be avoided in dyspneic patients, often making diagnosis and treatment problematic. Enriching the oxygen environment and allowing the patient to calm down or sedating the patient may be required. Careful auscultation should reveal lung sounds in all expected areas (e.g., quiet lung sounds may indicate a pneumothorax). Abnormal auscultation such as rales, rhonchi, or wheezing may indicate lung disease. Further diagnostics such as radiography may be warranted. For trauma patients, a thoracic radiograph to determine the presence of a pneumothorax or bullae will help guide ventilatory support of the anesthetized patient. Often, anesthesia and surgery may be postponed until the thoracic trauma is resolved.

If surgery cannot be postponed, the thorax should be clipped and prepared for a chest tap if needed after induction or during maintenance and recovery. The patient should be allowed to spontaneously ventilate or, if IPPV is needed, hand ventilation rather than mechanical ventilation is indicated and the inspiratory pressure should be carefully monitored. If chest compliance changes during the procedure or the patient desaturates, the thorax is already prepared tapping.

CENTRAL NERVOUS SYSTEM AND SPECIAL SENSES

The central nervous system (CNS) and special senses should be carefully evaluated. There are specific recommendations for anesthetic management of patients with increased intracranial pressure. Although controversial, modest hyperventilation appears to protect the brain from the vasodilation that occurs with increased $Paco_2$ and the vasodilatory effects of the inhalant anesthetics. Because there is typically a 5–mm Hg difference between $Paco_2$ and ETCO₂ (dead space ventilation), an ETCO₂ maintained between 27 and 32 mm Hg should correlate with a $Paco_2$ between 32 and 37 mm Hg. The $Paco_2$ will always be higher than the ETCO₂ (concentration gradient will go from high to low). An arterial blood gas may be drawn simultaneously with the ETCO$_2$ and the difference compared to confirm the amount of dead space ventilation. If the patient is not moved, dead space ventilation (PaCO$_2$ − ETCO$_2$) should remain pretty constant at the value derived.

There are also drugs (e.g., ketamine) that are contraindicated in the presence of increased ICP or increased intraocular pressure (IOP; e.g., glaucoma, descemetocele). Drugs that promote hypoventilation (e.g., μ-agonists, α$_2$-agonists) should be avoided as premedicants. Anesthetic techniques also vary with increased ICP or IOP. Patients should not be heavily restrained by occluding jugular flow. Patients should be intubated at a deep anesthetic plane to prevent coughing. Mask and chamber inductions are contraindicated.

For patients that have vertebral instability (e.g., atlantoaxial subluxation, fractured back or neck) positioning for intubation and physical support are very important. Once anesthetized, muscles are relaxed and can no longer protect the spine from destabilization, and it is the responsibility of the anesthetist to maintain normal alignment. Similarly, for patients with cervical instability, extreme care should be used when intubating the patient, to avoid worsening the patient's condition. It is extremely important to determine if the cervical patient is able to ventilate after surgery. These patients may need ventilatory support for 24 hours after surgery to provide an opportunity for postsurgical spinal swelling to decrease.

Perhaps one of the most difficult treatment decisions required is the level of anesthesia that is needed for comatose patients. Often for diagnostic procedures, anesthesia is not required. For invasive procedures, the patient must be appropriately analgesed. A combination of an opioid and benzodiazepine may be sufficient if ventilation is supported and ETCO$_2$ monitored.

RENAL DISEASE

Patients suffering from renal disease face many obstacles. Hypotension is the worst possible complication for patients with compromised renal function. Preoperative arterial blood pressure, urine specific gravity, protein, and a BUN/creatinine ratio will assist the clinician in determining the severity of the renal compromise. Direct arterial pressure should be measured if possible. Concerns for dogs and cats vary slightly based on metabolism and

elimination of anesthetic drugs (e.g., ketamine) as well as their response to drugs used for diuresis (e.g., dopamine). Urine output should be measured (normal 1 ml/kg/hr or greater). Anesthetic management of patients with renal disease is discussed later (see Chapters 11 and 13).

LIVER DISEASE

Liver or biliary disease may result in jaundice, coagulopathy, seizures, and hypoalbuminemia. Examining bile acids may be indicated in addition to routine serum chemistries. A buccal mucosal bleeding time (or toenail clip) in addition to a clotting profile may be indicated. Drug metabolism may be altered (e.g., ketamine in dogs) or patient response to drugs may vary with the condition (e.g., benzodiazepine should be avoided in patients with portosystemic shunt). Fluid selection will be determined by the clotting profile, the albumin, and the glucose concentration. Some people recommend avoiding lactate (e.g., using Normasol-R or Ringer's solution rather than lactated Ringer's solution) for patients with compromised liver function. Arterial blood pressure should be measured directly if possible. Anesthetic management for patients with liver disease is discussed later (see Chapter 13).

GASTROINTESTINAL DISEASE

Gastrointestinal disease may result from infection, parasites, obstruction (e.g., intussusception, gastric dilatation and volvulus, hernia, foreign body), trauma, or degenerative disease (e.g., tumor, protein losing enteropathy). The medical concerns are as varied as the etiologies and range from anemia to shock. The anesthetic concerns impact drug selection based on patient safety (e.g., no mask inductions with vomiting) or clinician convenience (e.g., widely held view by endoscopists that μ-agonists make it difficult to traverse the gastroduodenal sphincter). Anesthetic management for patients with specific gastrointestinal disease is addressed later (see Chapter 13).

ENDOCRINE SYSTEM

Derangements in the endocrine system are more difficult to diagnose on physical exam and usually require laboratory testing. There are established protocols used for patients with endocrine disease that offer a starting point for anesthetic management (see Chapter 14).

INTEGUMENTARY AND MUSCULOSKELETAL SYSTEMS

A close evaluation of the integument may reveal clotting issues (e.g., petechiation or ecchymosis), lacerations, edema, burns, atopy, tumors (e.g., mast cell tumor), infection, or dehydration. Analgesics that are good for visceral pain are often ineffective for somatic pain. For example, ketamine, a poor visceral analgesic, is very good for somatic pain. Ketamine is used in burn patients, with skin grafts, and for bandage changes.

Evaluating the musculoskeletal system and joints may reveal muscle weakness or atrophy, spasms, fractures, lameness, tumors, and hematomas. Underlying systemic illnesses such as systemic lupus erythematosus may be suspected in cases of myositis. Myasthenia gravis (MG) may present as muscle weakness. Medication such as aminoglycosides that may exacerbate MG should be avoided; iodinated contrast agents, quinine, quinidine or procainamide, β-blockers (propranolol, timolol maleate eyedrops), and calcium channel blockers should be avoided. Neuromuscular blocking agents such as succinylcholine and vecuronium should only be used by an anesthesiologist familiar with MG. Anesthetic precautions such as orotracheal intubation in sternal recumbency and inflation of the pilot balloon prior to securing the ETT should be used in patients suspected of MG to avoid aspiration from regurgitation.

Laboratory Evaluation

When deciding what diagnostic tests to perform, the results of the history and physical exam, patient age, and the procedure being performed should be considered. There are few rules that dictate what tests should be performed. Typically, tests that are economically justified and that will impact the anesthetic management of a case should be considered. If an abnormal value will not change what you do, an owner may elect to avoid a test. If the tests and their impact are explained, most owners are grateful for the opportunity to decide whether or not to authorize a test. Document the discussion in the patient record. Age may impact the tests that are recommended. Glucose, total protein, and packed cell volume (PCV) should be checked in young patients, particularly neonates. Parasites and heartworm disease are more of a concern in juveniles and young adults. Tests that might uncover degenerative diseases would be more appropriate for middle-aged or geriatric dogs. Cardiopulmonary, liver, renal, and thyroid function should be assessed in older patients.

There are rarely indications for beginning an anesthetic procedure without a PCV and total protein (TP). The "big four," a PCV, TP, an Azostick (Bayer, Elkart, IN), and a blood glucose (commercially available blood glucometer) are collected on most elective procedures. In this clinic, for a small price difference, a Nova analysis (Nova Biomedical Corporation, Waltham, MA) may be run, which provides pH and blood gas results, Hct, Hb, Na^+, K^+, Cl^-, Ca^{2+}, Mg^{2+}, glucose, lactate, and BUN. A complete blood count (CBC) and a serum chemistry profile will provide adequate baseline information for most compromised or older patients. Depending on the patient and the procedure, a clotting profile, bile acids, Chagas titer, and thyroid test may also be needed.

In addition to laboratory evaluation, other helpful diagnostics may include an ECG, echocardiogram, radiography, ultrasound, and thoracocentesis or abdominocentesis. Thoracocentesis may be needed for diagnosis but is usually conducted to correct free fluid or free air in thorax that is compromising ventilation prior to anesthesia. If thoracic pathology exists that may require intraoperative tapping, the thorax should be clipped and prepared prior to draping. Abdominocentesis is usually done for diagnostic purposes and is not recommended for anesthesia, unless the fluid volume is large and compromising ventilation (see Chapter 3).

Risk and Physical Status

Risk and physical status are impacted by both non-patient and patient factors. Factors unrelated to the patient include the surgeon's competence and the anesthetist's competence. The type of surgery and length of surgery also impact risk. Patients undergoing longer surgeries are more likely to become infected than patients having shorter procedures. Some surgeries are more difficult and have inherently more risk. The patient's physical status, which is an assessment of the patient as a candidate for anesthesia is easily assigned, using the ASA patient status classification. The ASA status (Table 4.3) is

Table 4.3. ASA Physical Status Classification System.

Category	Description
1	Normal healthy patient
2	Patient with mild systemic disease
3	Patient with severe systemic disease
4	Patient with severe systemic disease that is a constant threat to life
5	Moribund patient not expected to survive without the operation
6	Declared brain-dead patient whose organs are being removed for donor purposes
E	An "E" may be added to categories 2–6 to indicate an emergency

based on history, physical exam, and laboratory data. The ASA status will facilitate drug and technique selection and is a predictor of perioperative complications. Age is a significant risk factor for development of perianesthetic complications in dogs even when ASA status is considered (Hosgood and Scholl, 1998). However, conditions in the dog that increased the ASA status by 1 (e.g., going from ASA Class 2 to ASA Class 3) had more impact on the odds of serious complications than the odds of serious complications of an old dog compared to a young or middle-aged dog. In cats, the ASA risk assessment is a better predictor of risk for minor or serious complications than is age (Hosgood and Scholl, 2002).

Although the ASA indicates that there is no need for further description of ASA status than that provided in Table 4.3, it may be helpful to look at examples. Patients in Class 1 are normal, healthy patients with no organic disease. Class 1 typically applies to elective surgeries such as surgical neutering. Patients in Class 2 may have a mild abnormality that does not compromise systemic health, such as an uncomplicated bone fracture or benign skin tumor. Patients in Class 3 have systemic disease that may limit activity or may become incapacitating but is presently compensated by intrinsic physiologic mechanisms (e.g., mild to moderate dehydration, subclinical heartworm disease, hyperthyroidism, fever, dehydration, anemia). Patients in Class 4 have life-threatening uncompensated systemic

disease that is presently altering their activity (e.g., congestive cardiomyopathy, hepatic encephalopathy, severe dehydration). Moribund patients that are not expected to live 24 hours with or without surgery are classified as Class 5 (e.g., extreme shock after HBC, septic with multiorgan failure and disseminated intravascular coagulation, gastric dilation and volvulus). A newer category in human medicine that may apply to veterinary medicine in the near future is Class 6, which applies to patients that are clinically dead but are being maintained for organ harvest. The addition of an "E" to Classes 2 through 6 indicates that the procedure is an emergency. Emergency anesthesia has a much greater risk than elective anesthesia (Gannon 1991).

Preanesthetic Preparation and Recovery
The environment can play an important role in the anesthetic experience for the patient. Patients should be induced and recovered in a warm, quiet area. Housing for dogs and cats should be separate if possible. Patients that may need time to adjust to the hospital or patients that need companions should be allowed time to adjust to the environment.

> Develop a plan for each patient that includes preoperative preparation, monitoring and equipment, premedicants, analgesia, anesthetic induction, maintenance, and recovery. Have a plan and carry it out!

Fasting requirements will vary based on the patient. The benefits of fasting include decreased stomach contents, which will reduce vomiting and regurgitation, and decreased bloating. An empty stomach does not contribute to impaired venous return (clinically, during endoscopy, increasing stomach air appears to compromise venous return). For adult dogs and cats, an 8- to 12-hour fast with ad libitum water is sufficient. For young patients (and some adult toy breeds), a briefer fast is indicated due to smaller glycogen stores. Patients with high metabolic rates do not tolerate long fasts. Requirements for patients with diabetes or insulinomas are discussed in greater detail later (see Chapter 13). Unless contraindicated by the surgical procedure (e.g., enterotomy or gastrotomy), food and water should be provided as soon as the patient is awake and able to protect their airway (generally 3 to 5 hours after extubation).

Assign an ASA score based on history, physical exam, laboratory results, and additional diagnostics. The anesthetic plan should reflect the patient ASA status. Drug choices include premedicants (see Chapter 5), induction drugs (see Chapter 6), maintenance (see Chapter 7), and analgesics (see Chapter 9). Local anesthetic techniques (see Chapter 8) may be used to provide analgesia and to decrease the amount of other drugs needed. Balanced anesthesia is similar to multimodal analgesia. A combination of drugs and techniques are used to minimize the amount of any one drug and the attendant side effects from a particular drug or technique. The customary equipment needed should be gathered (e.g., intravenous catheters, drugs, fluids, endotracheal tube, stylet or guide tube, anesthetic machine, monitoring equipment, external heat source [Bair Hugger {Arizant Healthcare Inc., Eden Prairie, MN}], special supplies as needed for local techniques or constant rate infusion [CRI]). Consider how body position will impact ventilation or circulation (e.g., patient in head-down position needs IPPV).

All abnormal body systems should be normalized if possible. For example, hyperkalemia from urinary obstruction is a medical emergency rather than a surgical emergency. If the bladder can be emptied by catheter or in rare circumstances by cystocentesis, the patient's electrolytes should be normalized and hydration should be corrected in order to prepare for the best surgical outcome. Patients should be premedicated with appropriate drugs to relieve anxiety or to treat pain. A patent intravenous catheter should be in place and fluid administration initiated.

A plan for recovery should also be made prior to surgery. Anticipate the special needs of patients. Patients recovering from myelograms should have their heads elevated for about 30 to 45 minutes after the myelogram to decrease the possibility of seizures. Patients for whom tourniquets have been placed should be monitored closely for cardiac arrhythmias and hypotension during tourniquet release. In patients in which respiratory obstruction or arrest are likely, a mouth gag (Fig. 4.3), an ET tube, laryngoscope, and induction drug should be

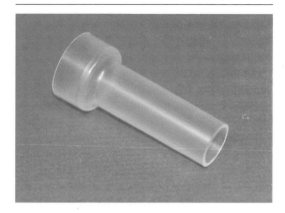

Figure 4.3. Cats are especially prone to obstruction if they have nasal disease. Until they are awake enough to breathe through their mouth, a mouth gag should be available. This is a 3-ml syringe case that has been shortened and filed so the cut edge is not sharp. The smaller opening (cut edge) fits easily in the mouth opening formed by the upper and lower canines and incisors. Cats tolerate it better than most commercially available cat mouth gags.

available. If a bandaged patient is dyspneic, the bandage (e.g., head, belly, chest) should be blamed until proved otherwise.

Governing vessel 26 (GV 26; see Chapters 12 and 14) should be located in case of arrest or respiratory failure.

An individualized "Emergency Drug Sheet" may be prepared for each patient. The drugs and doses of emergency drugs should be calculated and available (see Chapter 12). Drugs and fluids needed for cardiovascular collapse, shock, and hemorrhage should be available. A stocked "crash cart" should be portable or present in areas of the hospital in which arrest may be anticipated (Fig. 4.4). In most practices, a tackle box is sufficient to keep drugs available. There should be a mechanism to keep track of drugs that are removed from the box or are out of date.

A plan for recovery should include oxygen for anemic or hypotensive patients. A quiet, warm, dimly lit area should be available for recovery. Adequate padding should be provided. Good nursing care, including emptying the bladder and providing nonabsorbent liners, lubricating the eyes, turning a patient unable to turn them-

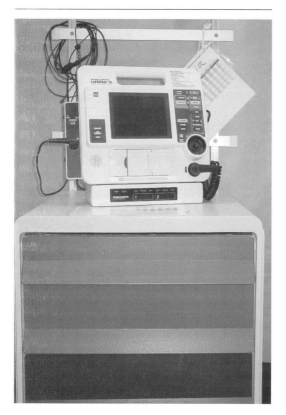

Figure 4.4. Anything from a stocked tackle box up to a crash cart with a defibrillator, emergency drugs, fluids, a laryngoscope, endotracheal tubes, and oxygen tubing should be portable or present in areas of the hospital where arrests might occur.

selves, and comfortable dry bandages, should be employed.

Of great importance is the provision of postoperative analgesics (see Chapter 9). Every time the patient is examined, assign a "pain score" and document your treatment and the patient response in the record! Be prepared to sedate the patient if needed to control activity or dysphoria.

At the end of the day, the patient should be resting but arousable. All vital signs should be normal and the pain score addressed if needed. Normal grooming and interest in the environment and in eating and drinking are important indicators of well-being.

ENDNOTES

1 See http://www.avmaplit.com/.
2 Physicians' Desk Reference 2006 (60th Edition), Thomson/PDR staff.
3 Physicians' Desk Reference for Herbal Medicines 2004 (3rd Edition), Medical Economics.
4 PDR Guide to Over-the-Counter Drugs (PDR Family Guide to Over-the-Counter Drugs) 1997, *Physicians' Desk Reference.*
5 Serotonin syndrome is generally caused by a combination of two or more drugs, one of which is often a selective serotonergic medication. The combination of MAOIs, tricyclic antidepressants, and SSRIs most frequently contributes to this condition; lithium, tryptophan, serotonin agonists, and perhaps tramadol are also implicated. Any drug that enhances serotonin neurotransmission can contribute to this syndrome. This toxic hyperserotonergic condition is very dangerous and potentially fatal.
6 Mr. Pickwick was a character from Charles Dickens' *Pickwick Papers.* The Pickwickian syndrome relates to hypercarbia, hypoxemia, polycythemia, hypersomnolence, pulmonary hypertension, and biventricular failure.

REFERENCES

Barash, P.G., Cullen, B.F., and Stoelting, R.K. 2001. *Clinical Anesthesia*, 4th ed. Philadelphia: Lippincott Williams & Wilkins.

Gannon, K. 1991. Mortality associated with anaesthesia. A case review study. *Anaesthesia* 46:962–966.

Hosgood, G., and Scholl, D.T. 1998. Evaluation of age as a risk factor for perianesthetic morbidity and mortality in the dog. *J Vet Emerg Crit Care* 8:222–236.

Hosgood, G., and Scholl, D.T. 2002. Evaluation of age and American Society of Anesthesiologists (ASA) physical status as risk factors for perianesthetic morbidity and mortality in the cat. *J Vet Emerg Crit Care* 12:9–16.

Roizen, M.F. 2000. Anesthetic implications of concurrent diseases. In *Anesthesia* edited by R.D. Miller, 5th ed. Philadelphia: Churchill Livingstone, pp. 903–1016.

Stoelting, R.K., and Hillier, S.C. 2006. *Pharmacology and Physiology in Anesthetic Practice.* Philadelphia: Lippincott Williams & Wilkins.

West, J.B., and West, J.B.B. 2004. *Respiratory Physiology—The Essentials*, 7th ed. Baltimore: Williams & Wilkins.

required to reveal ketamine's sympathomimetic effects. The literature is split concerning the arrhythmogenicity of ketamine. There are better choices for patients with cardiac arrhythmias. Ketamine is also a bronchodilator. When used in conjunction with aminophylline, the seizure threshold may be significantly lowered.

The dose of ketamine is variable depending on the desired outcome. In a fractious cat, ketamine may be squirted in the open mouth. Ketamine (2 to 10 mg/kg transmucosally [TM]) is well absorbed through the buccal mucosa and may be administered by this route in traumatized patients where administration of other agents or restraint for injection is not realistic. Ketamine at low dosages (0.5 to 1.0 mg/kg IM) may be used to provide somatic analgesia without cataleptoid effects; 2 to 4 mg/kg intravenously or intramuscularly may provide 30 minutes of somatic analgesia. Ketamine boluses or CRI is particularly helpful in patients with burns or skin wounds and in patients with chronic pain due to the effect of NMDA antagonists on "windup." A priming dose of ketamine (0.2 to 0.5 mg/kg IV) followed by a ketamine infusion (2 to 10 μg/kg/min IV) may be used intraoperatively or postoperatively, particularly in patients with chronic pain. Larger doses (10 to 20 mg/kg IM) are used for immobilization, particularly in cats. These higher doses are associated with recoveries that are often objectionable. The cats appear to startle to noise and display some stereotypy. Occasionally, the patients will have seizure-like activity or increased body temperature postoperatively. Anecdotally, permanent behavior changes have been reported.

> Avoid ketamine in cats with renal failure and dogs in liver failure and in animals with increased intraocular or intracranial pressure, seizure history, or mitral regurgitation. Ketamine may or may not be associated with arrhythmias.

Tiletamine, a component of Telazol, is rarely used alone. The indications and contraindications of Telazol are similar to those of ketamine and diazepam, but the duration of Telazol is longer and the routes of administration are more flexible than those of ketamine and diazepam. The volume of injectate of Telazol is smaller unless ketamine has been desiccated and reconstituted to a smaller volume. When administering a drug combination, the half-life of each drug should be similar. As discussed earlier, in the case of Telazol, if it is necessary to redose, ketamine rather than Telazol may be administered. Telazol with or without butorphanol is relatively predictable when administered to savage dogs.

SEDATIVE/ANALGESICS

In small animal veterinary medicine, there are two main classes of drugs with sedative and analgesic properties (i.e., α_2-agonists and opioids). Sedative/analgesics may be used preoperatively for their calming effect or for preemptive analgesia. Used in combination, an α_2-agonist and an opioid provide neuroleptic analgesia that may be used for restraint (e.g., radiographs). When used in combination for restraint in the absence of a painful procedure, both the α_2-agonist and opioid may be antagonized when no longer needed (discussed under each drug). An α_2-agonist and an opioid may also be combined to perform minor procedures (e.g., epidural administration of an analgesic), or if combined with a local anesthetic technique (e.g., lidocaine block) may be used to accomplish minor surgical procedures (e.g., pin removal, wound suture).

α_2-Agonists

α_2-Agonists are used extensively in large animal anesthesia, but their use in dog and cat anesthesia has been limited due to their profound cardiopulmonary effects. When administered epidurally, α_2-agonists have some local anesthetic effects. When used for analgesia, α_2-agonists act spinally, but there is evidence for supraspinal effects. Typically, α_2-agonists cause a vagally mediated bradycardia and depression of ventilation. The bradycardia results from a baroreceptor-mediated response to increase peripheral resistance (e.g., vasoconstriction). The transient vasoconstriction is followed by vasodilation and hypotension. The resistance of some anesthesiologists to the perioperative use of α_2-agonists results from the occasional difficulty encountered when managing intraoperative hypotension in normal healthy patients. Xylazine was associated with cardiac arrhythmias which might occur several hours after xylazine administration. Arrhythmias do not seem to be an issue with medetomidine.

intravenously to avoid histamine release. Most synthetic opioids do not result in histamine release. The duration of action of morphine is about 3 to 4 hours. Morphine may be administered subcutaneously, intramuscularly, intravenously (caution), orally, epidurally, intra-articularly (IA), or topically (cornea). Oral administration results in a great deal of first-pass metabolism. Epidural administration is effective for caudal abdominal and hind limb procedures, as well as forelimb and thoracic procedures. Because morphine is not lipid soluble, it migrates craniad when administered epidurally, rather than glomming onto the epidural fat and affecting only the hind limbs and abdomen. The onset of action of epidural morphine is about 1 hour; duration of action of epidural morphine is also about 24 hours. There are two incidences of respiratory depression. The first respiratory depression occurs in a timeframe consistent with the systemic absorption of morphine; the second respiratory depression occurs at about 10 hours, when the morphine is believed to have reached the brain. In veterinary patients, respiratory depression is not as critical a complication as in humans. It may be necessary to supplement a patient with oxygen (e.g., flow-by with 40% oxygen) to improve Pao_2, but it is rarely needed for longer than 24 hours. Oxygen toxicity has not proven to be as large an issue in adult veterinary patients as in humans. Although all opioids may result in urinary retention, epidural administration accounts for increased occurrence. The bladder should not be manually expressed, but should be catheterized.

Peripheral μ-receptors have been identified in the synovium and on the cornea of dogs. As a result, topical morphine is effective in intra-articular injection and topical ocular application. Morphine receptors have not been found in the thoracic pleura.

Other μ-agonist opioids that do not precipitate significant histamine release and are similar to morphine in duration of action and efficacy include oxymorphone, hydromorphone, and methadone. Similarly, fentanyl is not associated with histamine release but has a brief duration of action, making it suitable for intravenous CRI or transdermal application. Generic transdermal patches are now available. Because the efficacy of these commonly used μ-agonists is similar, preference is based on lipid solubility, ease and route of administration, personal bias, and cost. Codeine is a μ-agonist rarely used preoperatively. The schedule for codeine depends on the formulation. Because codeine is indicated for mild to moderate pain, it is best reserved for chronic pain.

PARTIAL μ-AGONISTS, κ-AGONISTS AND μ-ANTAGONISTS, AND NONOPIOID μ-AGONISTS

Partial μ-agonists (e.g., buprenorphine) are opioids that have a great affinity for the μ-receptor, but once on the receptor have little intrinsic activity. As a result, a partial μ-agonist may be quite difficult to remove from the receptor, but while on the receptor, does not do very much (provides modest analgesia). κ-Agonists and μ-antagonists (e.g., butorphanol, nalbuphine) provide modest analgesia through the κ-receptor and antagonize activity of μ-receptor agonists. The partial μ-agonists behave similarly to the κ-agonist and μ-antagonists in two respects: both groups may antagonize pure μ-agonists by removing them from the receptor and both are only indicated for mild to moderate pain.

Clinically, these groups of drugs seem to have a "ceiling effect" on some of the untoward side effects associated with administration of pure μ-agonists. For example, butorphanol has a "ceiling effect" on ventilatory depression. Increasing the dose that is administered does not increase the ventilatory depression. Although the potential bradycardia that occurs may be clinically relevant, it is not as frequently significant as that for μ-agonists. Similarly, marked sedation is not as common. However, all these partial μ and κ effects are accompanied by an attendant modest MAC decrease.

Buprenorphine, a partial μ-agonist is a Schedule III opioid. Buprenorphine may be administered intravenously, intramuscularly, subcutaneously (clinically seems less efficacious), transmucosally, or epidurally. The onset of action is about 20 to 30 minutes and the duration of action is about 6 to 8 hours; if administered epidurally, about 18 hours of analgesia may be provided. Interestingly, when administered transmucosally, it is important to squirt the drug into the cheek pouch or under the tongue for absorption (to avoid first pass) rather than in the back of the throat where it may be swallowed. It is also important to distinguish dogs from cats for transmucosal administration. In cats, the pH of the saliva is alkaline and the bioavailability of transmucosal buprenorphine is close to 100%. The bioavailability of transmucosal buprenorphine in dogs has not been determined but may be different from the cat if there is a difference in saliva pH. A special note for cats administered transmucosal buprenorphine is that the taste is not objectionable. The salivation and frothing that occurs after an objectionable taste is given to a cat does not occur after buprenorphine.

When administered after a μ-agonist, buprenorphine may antagonize the μ effects. Similarly, although not common, if there is significant respiratory depression after buprenorphine administration, it may be difficult to antagonize its effects, even with naloxone, a μ-antagonist.

Butorphanol, a κ-agonist and μ-antagonist, is a Schedule IV opioid and is approved for use as an analgesic in cats and an antitussive in dogs and cats. Butorphanol does not provide much sedation but also does not produce much excitement. Butorphanol may be administered intravenously, subcutaneously, intramuscularly, and orally. The onset of action is about 10 to 15 minutes, but the duration is relatively short. There is a difference in dosing and duration for visceral and somatic pain and a difference in species efficacy and duration. In dogs, the duration of butorphanol is quite short (1 to 2 hours) and the analgesic efficacy is limited. It is not always disadvantageous to have a shorter-acting analgesic available. For example, if attempting to stabilize a trauma patient, a shorter acting opiate without significant μ-mediated side effects may be beneficial. Another role for butorphanol in dogs relates to its use in breeds that are often dysphoric after μ-agonist administration. For example, Labrador Retrievers appear to become dysphoric after μ-agonist administration even if a painful surgical procedure has been performed. Often, these dogs do not respond to tranquilization. A dose of butorphanol may be administered to assess whether the dogs appear more comfortable; if an error in judgment has occurred, the short duration of action will not complicate management for very long. If the dog appears more comfortable after the butorphanol, buprenorphine may be administered to provide longer analgesia. If the dog is not more comfortable, a fentanyl CRI or other μ-agonist may be repeated without much delay.

In cats, butorphanol appears to be a better analgesic and appears to have a longer duration of action than in dogs. In a small pharmacokinetic pilot study in cats, transmucosal butorphanol administration was not different from oral administration but in some instances, the taste was objectionable. In dogs, transmucosal butorphanol administration using a buccal patch resulted in decreased bioavailability (unpublished); a buccal patch is not currently commercially available.

Nalbuphine is a mixed agonist/antagonist that is not scheduled. Nalbuphine is not as efficacious an analgesic as is butorphanol; the duration of action is also shorter. Clinically, the most important use of nalbuphine is to antagonize the effects of μ-agonists. One milliliter (20 mg) of nalbuphine is mixed with 9 ml of saline and administered IV to effect.

Tramadol is a nonopioid μ-agonist that is used mostly for chronic pain. Tramadol may be dispensed after surgery or for chronic pain but is rarely indicated preoperatively for acute pain. Tramadol shares some characteristics of antidepressants because it also inhibits serotonin and norepinephrine reuptake. Tramadol is about 75% bioavailable when administered orally; pharmacokinetic data indicate veterinarians have been underdosing tramadol. Tramadol may be associated with some side effects common to μ-agonists, but clinically these side effects do not seem to be as significant. The change in heart rate and respiratory depression is less than seen with morphine. Similarly, the gastrointestinal side effects are milder. Tolerance is not as likely as that for μ-agonists. In humans, tramadol lowers the seizure threshold. In chronic pain management it is often combined with an antiepileptic such as gabapentin, which will help protect against lowering the seizure threshold.

μ-ANTAGONISTS

Antagonism of μ-agonists in painful animals is discouraged because antagonism includes the analgesia as well as the sedation and cardiopulmonary effects. Pure μ-antagonists (e.g., naloxone 5 to 15 μg/kg IV) cannot really be titrated to antagonize the side effects without impacting the analgesia. One milliliter (0.4 mg) may be diluted in order to attempt to titrate the naloxone just to arousal. The acute awareness of pain may be associated with increased concentration of circulating catecholamines and the side effects associated with sympathetic stimulation.

Naltrexone is a μ-antagonist with a longer duration of action than naloxone. The duration of action for naltrexone may be 1 to 2 hours as compared to

Table 5.1. Commonly used premedicants in cats and dogs.*

Anticholinergics
Atropine: Dog (D) and cat (C) 0.02–0.04 mg/kg IV, SQ, IM
Glycopyrrolate: (D and C) 0.005–0.011 mg/kg IV, SQ, IM

Tranquilizers
Acepromazine: (D and C) 0.025–0.05 mg/kg SQ, IV, IM (not to exceed 1 mg)
Midazolam: (D and C) 0.2 mg/kg SQ, IV, IM
Diazepam: (D and C) 0.2 mg/kg IV, IM

Opioids

μ-Agonists
Morphine: (D) 0.4–1 mg/kg IM, SQ (higher doses appear in the literature); (C) 0.05–0.2 mg/kg IM, SQ
Constant rate infusion (CRI): (D) 0.1 mg/kg IV every 3–5 minutes until the appropriate dose is found,
    then that dose is administered IV by a syringe pump or added to 4 hours of fluids and administered IV.
Oxymorphone: (D) 0.05–0.1 mg/kg IM, SQ, IV; (C) 0.05 mg/kg IM, IV, SQ
Hydromorphone: (D) 0.1–0.2 mg/kg IM, IV, SQ; (C) 0.05–0.1 mg/kg IM, IV, SQ
Methadone: (D) 1–1.5 mg/kg SQ, IM, IV
Fentanyl: (D) 2–5 μg/kg IM, IV, SQ; (C) 1–2 μg/kg IM, IV, SQ
CRI: (D) a loading dose (0.002 mg/kg IV) is administered followed by an infusion of 0.001–0.006 mg/kg/
    hr IV; (C) a loading dose (0.001–0.002 mg/kg IV) is followed by an infusion (0.001–0.004 mg/kg/hr IV.
For transdermal (TD) use: (D and C) 4 μg/kg/hr

Partial μ agonist and κ-agonist/μ-antagonist
Buprenorphine: (D and C) 5–15 μg/kg IM, IV, SQ, transmucosal (TM)
Butorphanol: (D and C) 0.2–0.4 mg/kg, IM, IV, SQ; up to 1 mg/kg should be used for oral dosing.

NMDA receptor antagonists
Ketamine: (C) 5 mg/kg, IM
CRI: (D and C) 1–2 mg/kg IV, IM or 0.5 mg/kg IV followed by 2–10 μg/kg/min IV

α_2-Agonists
Xylazine: (D and C) 0.1–0.5 mg/kg IM, IV, SQ. The dose should be lowered if administered in
    conjunction with an opioid and lower doses (about half) may be administered postoperatively for
    anxiety.
Medetomidine: (D and C) 0.001–0.010 mg/kg IM, IV, SQ. The dose should be lowered if administered in
    conjunction with an opioid and lower doses (about half) may be administered postoperatively for
    anxiety.

NSAIDs
Carprofen: (D) 1–2 mg/kg PO BID, or 4 mg/kg SQ or PO q day
Deracoxib: (D perioperative) 3–4 mg/kg/day q day for up to 7 days
Meloxicam:(C) ≤0.2 mg/kg SC for acute surgical pain. Label dose = 0.3 mg/kg SQ, for acute surgical pain
but is too high, lower dose 0.2 mg/kg SQ works well.

*Doses for purposes other than premedication may be found elsewhere: Chapter 6 for induction doses,
Chapter 9 for analgesic doses, Chapter 10 for additional NSAID doses.

10 to 20 minutes for naloxone. The extended duration of action of naltrexone makes renarcotization less likely in patients that have been antagonized.

Nonsteroidal Anti-inflammatory Drugs

Nonsteroidal anti-inflammatory drugs (NSAIDs) have been used since the discovery that bark of the willow tree controlled colic (Lees et al. 2004a, 2004b); aspirin was soon synthetically prepared. Aspirin as well as other NSAIDs (e.g., flunixin, piroxicam, phenylbutazone, dipyrone) have been historically used in dogs and cats, but safety concerns have limited their perioperative use. References describing the earlier drugs are available (Lees et al. 1991; Mathews 2000; McKellar et al. 1991; Nolan 2000). Even though there are NSAIDs approved for use as preoperative analgesics in dogs and cats, the use of NSAIDs is probably best restricted to postoperative use. Because the anesthetic course cannot be predicted, it is impossible to predict which patients will suffer from blood loss or hypotension and which patients should not be administered preoperative analgesics. If reserved for postoperative use, NSAIDs may be administered to patients who have not had significant blood loss, hypotension, or other contraindication to NSAID administration. Please see Chapter 10 for an in-depth analysis of NSAIDs approved for use in dogs and cats in the United States.

> NSAIDs should not be used in conjunction with steroids or other NSAIDs.

Miscellaneous Premedicants

Antibiotics may be indicated in contaminated surgeries or in dentals in which the patient has preexisting mitral regurgitation or some type of cardiac disease that lends itself to pooling and infection.

Antihistamines may be indicated in mast cell tumor manipulation and in chronic diaphragmatic hernia repair. In situations where there is the potential for histamine release or reperfusion of tissue that may have been without circulation for some time, the administration of antihistamines may protect against histamine release and reperfusion injury.

Glucocorticoids inhibit the arachadonic acid cascade and have anti-inflammatory, antipyretic, and analgesic effects. Corticosteroids inhibit phospholipase A_2, thereby limiting production of arachidonic acid. Arachidonic acid is the precursor of both prostaglandins, which lower nociceptive thresholds potentiating the effects of agents like bradykinin, serotonin, and histamine that do cause pain and of leukotrienes that also cause hyperalgesia. Corticosteroids may reduce bone pain, increase appetite and weight gain, and produce polyuria and polydipsia. Corticosteroids have been historically used for the treatment of osteoarthritis. Long-term use of parenteral corticosteroids may cause iatrogenic hyperadrenocorticism. Intra-articular administration of corticosteroids may accelerate cartilage damage and may precipitate adverse systemic affects. Corticosteroids should not be used in conjunction with NSAIDs due to the increased risk of gastrointestinal ulceration and perforation.

REFERENCES

Lees, P., Giraudel, J., Landoni, M.F., et al. 2004b. PK-PD integration and PK-PD modeling of nonsteroidal anti-inflammatory drugs: Principles and applications in veterinary medicine. *J Vet Pharmacol Ther* 27:490–502.

Lees, P., May, S.A., and McKellar, Q.A. 1991. Pharmacology and therapeutics of non-steroidal anti-inflammatory drugs in the dog and cat: 1. General pharmacology. *J Small Anim Prac* 32:183–193.

Lees, P.L., Taylor, P.M., Landoni, F.M., et al. 2003. Ketoprofen in the cat: Pharmacodynamics and chiral pharmacokinetics. *Vet J* 165:21–35.

Mathews, K.A. 2000. Non-steroidal anti-inflammatory analgesics: Indications and contraindications for pain management in dogs and cats. *Vet Clin North Am Small Anim Prac* 30:783–804.

McKellar, Q.A., May, S.A., and Lees, P. 1991. Pharmacolgy and therapeutics of non-steroidal anti-inflammatory drugs in the dog and cat: 2 Individual agents. *J Small Anim Prac* 32:225–235.

Nolan, A.M. 2000. Pharmacology of analgesic drugs. In *Pain Management in Animals,* edited by P. Flecknell and A. Waterman-Pearson, pp. 21–52. London: W.B. Saunders,

ADDITIONAL READING

Balmer, T.C. 1997. Analgesia in cats. *Vet Rec* 140: 435.

Balmer, T.V., Jones, R.S., Roberts, M.J., et al. 1998. Comparison of carprofen and pethidine as postoperative analgesics in the cat. *J Small Anim Prac* 30:11158–11164.

Bennett, J.S., Daugherty, A., Herrington, D., et al. 2005. The use of nonsteroidal anti-inflammatory drugs (NSAIDs). *Circulation* 111:1713–1716.

Brideau, C., Van Staden, C., and Chan, C.C. 2001. In vitro effects of cyclooxygenase inhibitors in whole blood of horses, dogs, and cats. *Am J Vet Res* 1755–1760.

Brune, K. 2003. COX-2 inhibitors and the kidney: A word of caution. *Pain Clinical Updates* 11.

Carroll, G.L., Howe, L.B., and Peterson, K.D. 2005. Analgesic efficacy of preoperative meloxicam or butorphanol in onychectomized cats. *J Vet Med Assoc* 226:913–919.

Castro, E., Soraci, A., Fogel, F., et al. 2000. Chiral inversion of R(−)fenoprofen and ketoprofen enantiomers in cats. *J Vet Pharmacol* 23:265–271.

Chandrasekharan, N.V., Dai, H., Roos, K.L., et al. 2002. COX-3, a cyclooxygenase-1 variant inhibited by acetaminophen and other analgesic/antipyretic drugs: Cloning, structure, and expression. *Proc Natl Acad Sci* USA 99:13926–13931.

David, A., and Simon, T. Use of Rimadyl in cats. 2000. *Vet Rec* 147:283–284.

Dobromylskyj, P., Flecknell, P.A., Lascelles, B.D., et al. 2000. Management of postoperative and other acute pain. In *Pain Management in Animals,* edited by P. Flecknell and A. Waterman-Pearson, pp. 81–145. London: W.B. Saunders.

DuBois, R.N., Abramson, S.B., Crofford, L., et al. 1998. Cyclooxygenase in biology and disease. *FASEB J* 12:1063–1073.

Engelhardt, G., Bogel, R., Schnitzer, C., et al. 1995. Meloxicam: Influence on arachidonic acid metabolism. Part 1. In vitro findings. *Biochem Pharm* 51:21–28.

Finco, D.R., Duncan, J.R., Schall, W.D., et al. 1975. Acetaminophen toxicosis in the cat. *J Vet Med Assoc* 166:469–472.

Giraudel, J.K., Toutain, P.I., and Lees, P. 2003. Development and application of in vitro assays for the evaluation of inhibitors of constitutive and inducible cyclooxygenase. *J Vet Pharmacol Ther* 26(Suppl 1):173–174.

Giraudel, J.K., Toutain, P.I., and Lees, P. 2005. Development of in vitro assays for the evaluation of cyclooxygenase inhibitors and application for predicting the selectivity of NSAIDs in the cat. *Am J Vet Res* 66:700–709.

Glew, A., Aviad, A.D., Keiser, D.M., et al. 1996. Use of ketoprofen as an antipyretic in cats. *Can Vet J* 37:222–225.

Hampshire, V.A., Doddy, F.M., Post, L.O., et al. 2004. Adverse drug event reports at the United States Food and Drug Administration Center for Veterinary Medicine. *J Am Vet Med Assoc* 225:533–536.

Hardie, E.M. Management of osteoarthritis in cats. 1997. *Vet Clin North Am Small Anim Prac* 27:945–953.

Horspool, L.J.I., Hoejimakers, M., Van Laar P., et al. 2001. The efficacy and safety of vedaprofen gel in postoperative pain management in cats. *Proceedings of the Voorjaarsdagen International Veterinary Congress*, p. 161. Amsterdam.

Hugonnard, M., Leblond, A., Keroack, S., et al. 2004. Attitudes and concerns of French veterinarians towards pain and analgesia in dogs and cats. *Vet Anaes Anal* 31:154–153.

Isaacs, J. 1996. Adverse effects of non-steroidal anti-inflammatory drugs in the dog and cat. *Aust Vet Practit* 26:180–186.

Johnston, S.A., and Fox, S.M. 1997. Mechanisms of action of anti-inflammatory medications used for the treatment of osteoarthritis. *J Am Vet Med Assoc* 210:1486–1492.

Jones, C.J., and Budsberg, S.C. 2000. Physiologic characteristics and clinical importance of the cyclooxygenase isoforms in dogs and cats. *J Am Vet Med Assoc* 217:721–729.

Jones, R.D., Baynes, R.E., and Nimitz, C.T. 1992. Nonsteroidal anti-inflammatory drug toxicosis in dogs and cats: 240 Cases (1989–1990). *J Am Vet Med Assoc* 201:475–477.

Justus, C., and Philipp, H. 1994. Multi-centre study on clinical efficacy and tolerance of meloxicam (Metacam®) in cats with acute locomotor disorders [abstract]. *Br Small Anim Vet Assoc* 175.

Justus, C., and Quirke, J.F. 1995. Dose-response relationship for the antipyretic effect of meloxicam in an endotoxin model in cats. *Vet Res Commun* 19:321–330.

Kore, A.M. 1990. Toxicology of nonsteriodal antiinflammatrory drugs. *Vet Clin North Am Small Anim Prac* 419–430.

Kyles, A.E. 1995. Clinical pain management. *Perspectives* March/April 6–12.

Lamont, L.A. 2002. Feline perioperative pain management. *Vet Clin North Am Small Anim Prac* 747–763.

Lascelles, B.D.X., Cripps, P., Mirchandani, S., et al. 1995. Carprofen as an analgesic for postoperative pain in cats. *J Small Anim Pract* 36:535–541.

Lascelles, B.D.X., Henderson, A.J., and Hackett, I.J. 2001. Evaluation of the clinical efficacy of meloxicam in cats with painful locomotor disorders. *J Small Anim Prac* 42:587–593.

Lascelles, D., and Waterman, A. 1997. Analgesia in cats. *Practice* 19:203–213.

Lee, V.C., and Rowlingson, J.C. 1995. Pre-emptive analgesia: Update on nonsteroidal anti-inflammatory drugs in anesthesia. In *Advances in Anesthesia,* pp. 69–110. St. Louis: Mosby.

Lees, P., Landoni, M.F., Giraudel, J., et al. 2004a. Pharmacodynamics and pharmacokinetics of nonsteroidal anti-inflammatory drugs in species of veterinary interest. *J Vet Pharmacol Ther* 27:479–490.

Livingston, A. 2000. Mechanism of action of nonsteroidal anti-inflammatory drugs. *Vet Clin North Am Small Anim Prac* 30:773–781.

Maddison, J.E. 1992. Adverse drug reactions: Report of the Australian Veterinary Association Adverse Drug Reaction Subcommittee. *Aust Vet J* 69:288–291.

Mathews, K.A. 1997. Erratum. *Compend Contin Educ Pract Vet* 19:69.

Mathews, K.A. 1996a. Nonsteroidal anti-inflammatory analgesics in pain management in dogs and cats. *Can Vet J* 37:539–545.

Mathews, K.A. 1996b. Nonsteroidal anti-inflammatory analgesics to manage acute pain in dogs and cats. *Compend Contin Educ Pract Vet* 18:1117–1123.

McMichael, M. 2005. Toxicology. In *Veterinary Emergency Protocols 2004–2005*, pp. 103–117. College Station: Texas A&M University.

Möllenhoff, A., Nolte, I., and Kramer, S. 2005. Antinociceptive efficacy of carprofen, levomethadone and buprenorphine for pain relief in cats following major orthopaedic surgery. *J Vet Med* 52:186–198.

Muir, W.M., Wiese, A.J., and Wittum, T.E. 2004. Prevalence and characteristics of pain in dogs and cats examined as outpatients at a veterinary teaching hospital. *J Am Vet Med Assoc* 224:1450–1463.

Papich, M.G. 2000. Pharmacologic considerations for opiate analgesic and nonsteroidal anti-inflammatory drugs. *Vet Clin North Am Small Anim Prac* 30:815–837.

Parton, K., Balmer, T.V., and Boyle, J. 2000. The pharmacokinetics and effects of intravenously administered carprofen and salicylate on gastrointestinal mucosa and selected biochemical measurements in healthy cats. *J Vet Pharmacol Ther* 23:73–79.

Poulson, N.B., and Justus, C. 1999. Effects of some veterinary NSAIDs on ex vivo thromboxane production and in vivo urine output in the dog. In *Proceedings of the Symposium on Recent Advances in Non-steroidal Anti-inflammatory Therapy in Small Animals*, pp. 25–28. Paris.

Rainsford, K.D., Skerry, T.M., et al. 1999. Effects of the NSAIDs meloxicam and indomethacin on cartilage proteoglycan synthesis and joint responses to calcium pyrophosphate crystals in dogs. *Vet Res Commun* 23:101–113.

Robinson, S.A. Managing pain in feline patients. 1997. *Vet Clin North Am Small Anim Prac* 27:945–953.

Runk, A., Kyles, A.E., and Downs, M.O. 1999. Duodenal perforation in a cat following the administration of nonsteroidal anti-inflammatory medication. *J Am Anim Hosp Assoc* 35:52–55.

Slingsby, L.S., and Waterman-Pearson, A.E. 1997. Post operative analgesia in the cat: A comparison of pethidine, buprenorphine, ketoprofen and carprofen. *J Vet Anaesth* 24:43.

Slingsby L.S., and Waterman-Pearson, A.E. 1998. Comparison of pethidine, buprenorphine, and ketoprofen postoperative analgesia ovariohysterectomy in the cat. *Vet Rec* 143.

Slingsby, L.S., and Waterman-Pearson, A.E. 2000. Postoperative analgesia in the cat after ovariohysterectomy by use of carprofen, ketoprofen, meloxicam or tolfenamic acid. *J Small Anim Prac* 41:447–450.

Slingsby, L.S., and Waterman-Pearson, A.E. 2002a. Comparison between meloxicam and carprofen for postoperative analgesia after feline ovariohysterectomy. *J Small Anim Prac* 43:286–289.

Slingsby, L.S., and Waterman-Pearson, A.E. 2002b. Comparison of pethidine, buprenorphine, and ketoprofen postoperative analgesia ovariohysterectomy in the cat. *Vet Rec* 43:185–189.

Stoelting, R.K., and Hillier, S.C. 2006. *Pharmacology and Physiology in Anesthetic Practice*. Philadelphia: Lippincott Williams & Wilkins.

Taylor, P.M. Newer analgesics: Nonsteroidal anti-inflammatory drugs, opioids, and combinations. 1999. *Vet Clin North Am Small Anim Prac* 29:719–735.

Taylor, P.M. 1996. Pharmacodynamics and enantioselective pharmacokinetics in the cat. *Res Vet Sci* 60:133–151.

Tjälve, H. 1997. Adverse reactions to veterinary drugs reported in Sweden during 1991–1995. *J Vet Pharmacol* 20:105–110.

USP Veterinary Pharaceutical Information Monographs. Anti-inflammatories. 2004. *J Vet Pharmac Ther* 27:1–109.

Wallace, J.L., and Fiorucci, S. 2003. A magic bullet for mucosal protection . . . and aspirin is the trigger! *Trends Pharmacol Sci* 24:323–326.

Wallace, J.L. 2003. Meloxicam. *Compen Cont Educ Prac Vet* 25:64–65.

Watson, A.D.J., Nichlson, A., Church, D.B., et al. 1996. Use of anti-inflammatory and analgesic drugs in dogs and cats. *Aust Vet J* 74:203–210.

Wiese, A.J., Muir, M.W., and Wittum, T.E. 2005. Characteristics of pain and response to treatment in dogs and cats examined at a veterinary teaching hospital emergency service. *J Vet Med Assoc* 226: 2004–2009.

Wilke, J.R. 1984. Idiosyncracies of drug metabolism in cats. *Vet Clin North Am Small Anim Prac* 14:1345–1354.

Wright, B.D. 2002. Clinical pain management techniques for cats. *Clin Techn Small Anim Prac* 17: 151–157.

Chapter 6
Induction Agents and Total Intravenous Anesthesia

Kris T. Kruse-Elliott

Drugs described herein are those used for intra-venous (IV) induction of general anesthesia, occasional short-term maintenance of anesthesia by either intermittent or continuous IV infusion, and total intravenous anesthesia (TIVA) in dogs and cats. For the most part, these drugs induce an unconscious state suitable for intubation and minor nonpainful procedures. More commonly, they are used to induce anesthesia and transition to inhalant anesthesia for maintenance.

Intravenous administration of drugs results in a smooth, predictable, and safe induction of general anesthesia when properly applied. The rapid induction achieved with IV agents allows for fairly immediate control of the airway and intubation usually with a smooth transition to inhalant anesthesia for maintenance. Because there is no absorption required for intravenously administered drugs the onset of action is rapid and generally predictable.

> The availability of noncumulative intravenous hypnotics has reduced the attractiveness of inhalant ("mask") inductions.

Considerations regarding drug selection include knowledge of basic pharmacology of the various drugs commonly used in veterinary medicine in conjunction with information on patient physical status—specifically deviations from normal physiology that may negatively impact responses to the drugs selected or available. All injectable anesthetics have significant depressive effects on major organ function. The goal is to optimize drug utilization to minimize the potential for negative outcome in each individual patient. This includes proper selection and dosing of

the injectable anesthetic as well as selection of appropriate analgesic and muscle relaxant drugs that balance the anesthetic episode and supplement the desirable central nervous system (CNS) effects of the primary induction drug being used.

> Titration of intravenous induction agents coupled with appropriate adjunct drugs, individualized for each patient, can be used to optimize the desired effect and minimize potential for negative outcomes.

Drugs discussed here are primarily used as induction agents to enable intubation and transition to inhalant anesthesia for maintenance. In certain situations they may be used as the sole general anesthetic agent for very short nonpainful procedures or as part of a TIVA protocol for longer procedures. The tendency for some of these drugs to be cumulative and their negative effects on major organ function preclude prolonged use for anesthetic maintenance in all but the most healthy patients.

If simultaneous IV drug administration or dilution of an injectable agent is necessary, compatibility of the solutions should be known. Trissell (2005) provides an extensive reference for investigating drug data (e.g., compatibility, storage, light sensitivity) for all injectable drugs. Most compatibility studies are conducted with the original formulation. Generic drugs may not be the same formulation and may have a different compatibility profile.

HYPNOTICS

For practical purposes, this class will be limited to those hypnotic agents that are still readily available and in common use in veterinary medicine. This includes the ultrashort-acting barbiturates (thiopental and methohexital), propofol, and etomidate. These drugs are used for both induction of general anesthesia and short-term maintenance. While the exact mechanisms of all of their individual actions are not known, a common theme of these hypnotic drugs is their modulation of γ-aminobutyric acid (GABA)-mediated neurotransmission in the central nervous system via drug-specific mechanisms. GABA acts postsynaptically to increase chloride conductance and thus hyperpolarize the neuron and inhibit transmission. Other less well defined mechanisms appear to play a role in some or all of their depressive effect on major organ systems.

All the drugs in this class cause depression of the CNS in a dose-dependent manner. They reduce cerebral blood flow and metabolism (oxygen consumption), consequently decreasing intracranial pressure and cerebral spinal fluid pressure. These effects may be brain protective in patients with CNS disease. Of the drugs described later, thiopental is considered to be the "gold standard" for cerebral protective effects and the best choice for patients with CNS disease in many settings. Etomidate also has excellent CNS protective effects and is a very good choice in these patients.

Thiopental—The Gold Standard

Thiopental (Schedule III) is an ultrashort-acting thiobarbiturate with very rapid onset of action (15 to 30 seconds) and short duration of action (15 to 20 minutes). Initial recovery and awakening from an induction dose of thiopental occurs by redistribution of the drug from the CNS to primarily lean body tissues (muscle), viscera, and fat. Thiopental is ultimately metabolized by the liver and excreted via the kidneys. While thiopental may be used as the sole anesthetic for short procedures, its effects are cumulative. Repeated administration of thiopental (exceeding 20 mg/kg IV) will saturate the major redistribution sites and prolong CNS effects. Significantly prolonged and difficult recoveries and cardiopulmonary depression may be a hazard of multiple top-up[1] doses of thiopental. Consequently, thiopental should only be used for induction, not maintenance, of anesthesia. Thiopental does not provide any analgesia.

While thiopental does not directly impact hepatic or renal function, the negative hemodynamic effects

of thiopental can reduce function in these organs due to reduced perfusion. Patients with profound liver dysfunction, such as portosystemic shunt, may have a prolonged recovery from thiopental induction. Aging may be associated with reduced hepatic blood flow, and this may contribute to somewhat longer recovery periods in geriatric patients. In coursing (sight) hounds, there is reduced activity of the hepatic P450 enzyme, which results in slower metabolism of thiopental and can significantly prolong recovery unless very low doses are used.

Depression of cardiopulmonary function is the major side effect with thiopental usage. Respiratory center depression occurs in a dose-dependent manner leading to reduced responsiveness to hypoxemia or hypercarbia and a reduction in overall minute volume. Apnea may be observed after the initial induction dose of thiopental, although it can be minimized with judicious titration of thiopental to yield the desired anesthetic effect. Laryngeal reflexes appear to be depressed to a lesser extent with thiopental compared to some other induction agents, making it a good choice for examination of arytenoid function (Gross et al. 2002; Jackson et al. 2004). Laryngospasm and coughing may be more likely to occur with thiopental induction, although this is usually a minor issue and thiopental is generally considered a good drug choice for patients anticipated as difficult to intubate. Because thiopental is cumulative, if an extended airway exam is anticipated, a noncumulative hypnotic such as propofol may be used.

Cardiovascular responses to thiopental are somewhat variable depending on the patient's physical status and ancillary drugs. There is typically a reduction in stroke volume due to decreased myocardial contractility. Decreases in peripheral vascular resistance result in an initial hypotension with a baroreceptor-mediated reflex increase in heart rate. Consequently, overall cardiac output and blood pressure may actually be maintained near normal following thiopental administration to healthy animals. However, in hemodynamically unstable patients, induction with thiopental is often associated with systemic hypotension. In patients with preexisting volume depletion, cardiovascular disease, or other hemodynamically unstable patients, higher doses of thiopental are associated with cardiac arrhythmias, including sinus tachycardia, ventricular premature complexes, ventricular bigeminy, ventricular tachycardia, or, rarely, ventricular fibrillation (see Chapter 2). These arrhythmias are more likely to occur in the presence of α_2-agonists such as xylazine (which sensitize the myocardium to epinephrine-induced arrhythmias, or when there is concomitant administration of epinephrine. The arrhythmias are usually short-lived and frequently resolve within 15 to 20 minutes as blood and myocardial tissue levels of thiopental are reduced by redistribution. Consequently, pretreatment or post-treatment with a single dose of lidocaine is often sufficient to prevent or resolve thiopental-induced ventricular arrhythmias. Adequate premedication to reduce the dose of thiopental is often an effective preventative measure. Alternating lidocaine (7 mg/kg IV) and thiopental (7 mg/kg IV) is a satisfactory induction protocol for premedicated arrhythmic patients (described later).

Thiopental is unstable in solution and so is supplied in powder form with a diluent that requires refrigeration once mixed. It can be mixed in concentrations from 1% to 5%; however, the lower concentration is more desirable due to its potential for perivascular tissue damage at higher concentrations. In solution, thiopental is highly alkaline and will cause tissue necrosis and perivascular sloughing if administered outside the vein. The site of inadvertent perivascular administration of thiopental should be infiltrated with an equal or greater volume of saline[2] to dilute the tissue concentration to below 1%.

Thiamylal (Schedule III) is another ultrashort-acting thiobarbiturate that is more potent than thiopental. It has not been available in the United States for several years.

Methohexital

Methohexital (Schedule IV) is an ultrashort-acting oxybarbiturate. Its duration of action (5 to 10 minutes) is approximately half that of thiopental. Very rapid redistribution accounts for the majority of its very short duration of action, although it is also rapidly metabolized by the liver. Unlike thiopental, methohexital may be used for short-term maintenance of anesthesia as it has less of a cumulative effect. Methohexital is preferred over thiopental for induction of anesthesia in sight hounds due to its rapid redistribution and metabolism.

While recovery from methohexital anesthesia is very rapid, it is not necessarily smooth and can be associated with excitation, muscle tremors, and occasionally seizures. These side effects may also be observed during induction. While appropriate premedication diminishes the frequency of adverse effects, the use of methohexital is generally limited to induction prior to gas anesthesia and it is not recommended as the sole anesthetic for even short procedures. It is not recommended in animals with a predisposition toward seizure activity. The poor quality of induction and recovery observed with methohexital have tended to limit its usefulness and application in veterinary medicine.

Dose-related respiratory depression and cardiovascular depression are observed with methohexital administration but are more short-lived than with thiopental, due to methoxexital's shorter duration. The effects of methohexital on cardiovascular and respiratory system function are generally similar to those observed in response to thiopental administration. Because of the rapid recovery, including respiratory system function, methohexital may be a good choice for short anesthesia of brachycephalic breeds. In these dogs, rapid recovery to preanesthetic levels of respiratory system function is desirable.

Methohexital is supplied as a powder and reconstituted to 2.5% for IV administration. Inadvertent perivascular administration is not associated with the same tissue necrosis as is observed with thiopental. Moreover, it appears to be more stable following reconstitution with an approximately 4- to 6-month shelf-life.

Pentobarbital

Pentobarbital (Schedule II) is a short-acting oxybarbiturate (compared to phenobarbital, which is a long acting). The dose in unpremedicated small animals (15 to 26 mg/kg IV) provides about 1 hour of surgical anesthesia with no analgesia. In some instances, pentobarbital may be used to maintain ventilator patients, but it is otherwise rarely indicated in clinical veterinary small animal medicine. Recoveries are violent and prolonged.

Propofol

Propofol[3,4] (not scheduled) is a lipid-soluble drug formulated in a solution of soybean oil, egg lecithin, and glycerol at a 10 mg/ml concentration. It is an ultrashort-acting nonbarbiturate hypnotic agent with rapid onset of action and recovery. There is substantially less residual CNS depression at recovery compared with the other hypnotic agents. Recovery is related to an initial redistribution to lean tissues and rapid, primarily hepatic, metabolism. There is evidence of extrahepatic metabolism as clearance of propofol exceeds hepatic blood flow. Propofol is often used in sight hounds as an alternative induction agent. Even so, recovery from propofol is slower in sight hounds than in other breeds, related to a slower rate of hepatic metabolism in these dogs. Always dose propofol to effect. Other conditions (e.g., sepsis) or premedicants (e.g., medetomidine) will alter the required induction dose of propofol.

> As with any hypnotic, the dose of propofol should be decreased in septic, multiorgan failure, or geriatric patients. Appropriate premedicants will further decrease the dose of propofol required.

In cats, the consecutive use of propofol over several days is not recommended due to the development of Heinz body anemia. Phenolic compounds such as propofol cause oxidative injury to feline red blood cells due to the cat's diminished capacity to conjugate phenol. Cats given propofol over 6 to 7 consecutive days exhibited Heinz body formation, anorexia, diarrhea, and lethargy. The study was discontinued prematurely due to the clinical deterioration of the cats; all cats recovered 1 or 2 days after the daily injections were discontinued. A second study using a different formulation of propofol (i.e., metabisulfate as a bacterial retardant), lower dose, and only 3 consecutive days of anesthesia did not reproduce the results found in the first cats. Evidence suggests that propofol should not be given to cats for more than 3 consecutive days (see Andress et al. 1995, and Matthews et al. 2004).

Due to its rapid clearance, propofol may be used to aide in maintaining anesthesia by either intermittent bolus or continuous rate infusion (IV), with duration and quality of recovery similar to those observed for a single induction dose of propofol. There is no analgesia with hypnotics, so combination with an analgesic agent such as an opioid is required for any painful procedures where propofol will be the sole anesthetic agent.

When used for anesthetic induction in dogs and cats, adverse events may occur. Most events may be eliminated or diminished by premedication. If acepromazine alone or in combination with butorphanol is administered as a premedicant prior to propofol induction (IV) and maintenance with isoflurane in oxygen, significant hypotension occurs; volume replacement is generally effective treatment. Irrespective of premedicant, apnea, pain on injection, ventricular premature depolarizations, and metabolic changes (i.e., Pv_{CO_2} increases and pH decreases) may occur. Other side effects seen include: muscle fasciculations, paddling, muscle rigidity, opisthotonus, seizures, emesis, retching, and salivation. Clinically, seizure-like activity that is responsive to diazepam has been observed after propofol induction; propofol may also be used to anesthetize patients in status epilepticus. Anesthetic recovery from propofol varies with premedication.

> Because hypnotics do not provide analgesia, an analgesic (e.g., opioid, nonsteroidal anti-inflammatory drug) is required for any painful procedures when propofol will be the sole anesthetic agent.

Propofol generally causes greater cardiovascular and respiratory depression than thiopental at equipotent anesthetic doses. There is a reduction in cardiac output and blood pressure following propofol administration that is not accompanied by an increase in heart rate as is observed with thiopental. In hypovolemic or other cardiovascular-compromised patients, these alterations in cardiovascular function may be severe. Because these effects are dose dependent, they are of lesser magnitude during a continuous infusion or with smaller boluses of propofol to maintain anesthesia.

Respiratory depression in propofol results in an initial and profound apnea immediately following induction of anesthesia, with transient cyanosis at higher doses of the drug. The occurrence of apnea and cyanosis can be reduced by careful and slow titration of the drug to achieve the desired depth of anesthesia, as opposed to rapid bolus administration of large doses. If injected too slowly (greater than 90 seconds), additional propofol (about 1 mg/kg IV) may have to be administered for orotracheal intubation or transition to inhalant. Preoxygenation is recommended in some patients to further reduce the likelihood of cyanosis. At lower doses, such as continuous infusion, there is a reduction in tidal volume and rate of respiration leading to reduced overall minute volume of ventilation that is dose related.

> Careful, slow titration of propofol decreases the occurrence of apnea and cyanosis. Do not administer propofol as a rapid bolus.

The original emulsion formulation of propofol is without preservatives. Consequently bacterial growth may occur in opened vials, leading to significant quantities of endotoxin in the solution. The formulation, which contains a bacterial retardant, is still at risk for contamination. Injection of contaminated solutions can lead to development of sepsis syndrome and associated cardiovascular collapse. Filter needles (5 μm; Braun, Products Unlimited, Justin, TX 76247; Fig. 6.1) should be used to draw the contents of a vial into a sterile syringe. Even if a rubber stopper is in place rather than a vial, the bottle is not intended for multiple uses. The potential for contamination limits the shelf-life of propofol. Unused portions of propofol should be discarded after 6 hours. Similarly, a propofol CRI should be completed and replaced within the 6-hour window. When careful aseptic technique (alcohol swab of vial; *one-time only* use vial) is used to draw propofol into a syringe it has been stored for several days without evidence of contamination; some efficacy is lost when stored in plastic. Some have also advocated refrigerated storage overnight. However, in either case the risk for bacterial growth remains, particularly if aseptic technique has not been used while handling the drug. Propofol may be diluted with 5% dextrose but should not be diluted further than 2 mg/ml.

When propofol is used for prolonged anesthetic maintenance (e.g., ventilator patient), the patient's plasma may become hyperlipemic. The type of IV catheter and duration of lipid infusion or diazepam for *long-term* administration CRIs may impact the occurrence of sepsis. However, induction with propofol or diazepam and propofol through a catheter should not be an issue. Extravasation of propofol is not associated with skin sloughing, but infiltrating the area with saline seems reasonable.

Etomidate

Etomidate is also a nonscheduled, nonbarbiturate IV hypnotic agent that comes as a 2 mg/ml concentration in 35% propylene glycol. This solution does not contain preservatives; daily discard of open [used] etomidate is recommended. Unlike propofol emulsions, solutions of etomidate have not been known to support bacterial growth.

As with the other drugs in the hypnotic group, the initial recovery and awakening from etomidate occur through rapid redistribution, followed by metabolism via hydrolysis in the liver and by plasma esterases. Recovery is somewhat quicker than is observed with thiopental, with a clearance rate of etomidate that is three to five times faster. Recovery may be rougher than expected with propofol. Initial recovery may be accompanied by periods of myoclonus and excitement, particularly in patients that were not premedicated with an anxiolytic/analgesic. During induction, it is important to dose etomidate adequately in order to avoid retching and potential vomiting that may occur in lightly anesthetized patients during intubation. Premedication significantly reduces the side effects described earlier, and the use of a benzodiazepine, such as diazepam or midazolam, is highly recommended prior to the administration of etomidate.

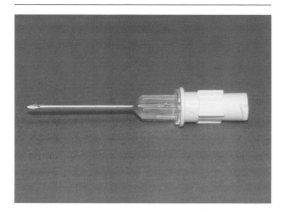

Figure 6.1. Filter needles (5 μm) should be used to draw the contents of a glass vial into a sterile syringe. The outside of the vial should be swabbed with alcohol.

Etomidate is the drug of choice in patients with extracardiac arrhythmias (e.g., gastrodilitation volvulus, pyometra) and in patients with cardiovascular disease (e.g., systolic dysfunction). Cardiovascular depression is virtually nonexistent with etomidate use. There is only minimal alteration in stroke volume, heart rate, and cardiac output when etomidate is used for induction of anesthesia. There is minimal to no change in systemic vascular resistance and blood pressure; both renal and hepatic blood flow are well maintained. In patients with renal or hepatic compromise, etomidate is an excellent choice to ensure maintenance of major organ perfusion.

> Patients that are likely to develop oxygen deficits (e.g., shock) during or after surgery should be anesthetically induced with etomidate (intravenous).

Respiratory depression occurs with an induction dose of etomidate but is much less than that observed with thiopental and is of very short duration. The degree of depression is dose dependent and correlated with the rate of administration. As with the other hypnotic agents, the slower rate of administration yields less respiratory depression.

A notable side effect with etomidate is suppression of adrenocortical function. Surgical stimulation is generally associated with increases in plasma cortisol. Administration of etomidate suppresses cortisol production by dose-dependently inhibiting the enzymes involved in adrenocortical production of cortisol. This includes inhibition of the response to ACTH stimulation. Adrenocortical inhibition by etomidate is reversible and of short duration (up to 6 hours following a single induction dose). Patients with adrenocortical insufficiency or those being treated with glucocorticoids are not necessarily at any greater risk, as it is anticipated they will be supplemented with glucocorticoids regardless of the induction agent or anesthetic protocol being used. However, long-term continuous infusion of etomidate or consecutive daily administration will necessitate glucocorticoid supplementation in patients that might not otherwise require it. Dexamethasone (0.1 to 0.25 mg/kg IV) may be administered at induction to "cover" the suppression of corticosteroid production resulting from etomidate administration.

Acute hemolysis has been observed in plasma from patients given etomidate. This is likely a result of an osmotic effect of propylene glycol causing rupture of red blood cells. At typical doses, induction with etomidate is not associated with significant or measurable free hemoglobin in plasma. Hemolysis may become an issue if a continuous infusion of the drug is employed. At very high doses or infusion rates, hemoglobinuria may occur and this should be avoided, particularly in patients with renal disease.

Clinical Use of Hypnotic Agents

In unpremedicated dogs and cats, the doses of thiopental, methohexital, propofol, and etomidate are all 1.5 to 2 times the dose used when patients are premedicated (see Table 6.1). As described earlier, the majority of negative side effects, particularly

Table 6.1. Dosing (mg/kg, IV) of hypnotic and dissociative induction agents in unpremedicated or premedicated dogs or cats.

Drug	Unpremedicated dose (mg/kg IV)	Premedicated dose (mg/kg IV)
Thiopental	18–20	6–12
Methohexital	8–10	4–5
Propofol	6–10	4–6
Etomidate	3	1–2
Diazepam/ketamine*	Diazepam 0.28, plus ketamine 5.5	To effect
Zolazepam/tiletamine	2–4	To effect

*Diazepam/ketamine: immediately before use, mix equal volume of ketamine (1 ml) and diazepam (1 ml) = 2 ml **total** volume, which is a new concentration of ketamine 50 mg/ml and diazepam 2.5 mg/ml). Then administer 1 ml/10 kg IV to effect (OR, 1 ml/20 lb IV to effect).

cardiovascular dysfunction, arrhythmias, and respiratory depression, are dose dependent and can be significantly lessened by judicious use of premedication prior to induction of general anesthesia. Moreover, the recovery period can often be smoothed by administration of a premedicant.

Premedication can be either intramuscular (IM) or subcutaneous given 15 to 20 or 20 to 30 minutes, respectively, before induction. Alternatively, IV premedication immediately preceding administration of the hypnotic agent may be quite effective in tractable dogs and cats. For nonpainful procedures IM or subcutaneous acepromazine or an IV benzodiazepine may be administered. However, most patients will benefit from the additional sedation and pain relief that result when an opioid is added to the premedication protocol. Common IM or subcutaneous premedication protocols include acepromazine, acepromazine with an opioid; midazolam or diazepam with an opioid; or butorphanol, buprenorphine, oxymorphone, hydromorphone, methadone, or morphine alone (see Chapter 5). These drugs may also be used in varying combinations for IV premedication. Oxygen, a mask, an endotracheal tube, laryngoscope, and potentially an Ambu bag (see Fig. 1.2) should always be available to deliver either flow-by oxygen or intermittent positive-pressure ventilation.

After premedication, one modified induction technique with thiopental is IV administration of midazolam or diazepam (0.2 mg/kg to a maximum dose of 5 mg), followed by lidocaine and thiopental. Lidocaine and thiopental are drawn up at 7 mg/kg each and administered sequentially (lidocaine then thiopental) at one-third to one-half the initial calculated dose followed by additional sequential doses of each as needed to achieve adequate effect. It is important to flush between administration of these drugs as they are incompatible in solution. The advantage of this technique is a further lowering of the thiopental dose as well as antiarrhythmic effect of lidocaine. This makes it a reasonable induction protocol for patients that have compromised cardiovascular or other major organ function by reducing the negative side effects of thiopental.

Combination of propofol (10 mg/ml) with thiopental (25 mg/ml) as a 1 : 1 volume mixture has been reported to be an effective induction technique with induction and recovery qualities similar to those observed with propofol alone. The major advantage of this combination appears to be improved stability of the solution as opposed to propofol alone; thus, there is less likelihood of bacterial growth and endotoxin contamination. Other advantages and disadvantages of this combination remain to be determined.

Both propofol (0.2 to 0.5 mg/kg/min IV following induction) and etomidate (0.05 to 0.2 mg/kg/min IV) have been advocated for use as continuous rate infusion (CRI) for maintenance of anesthesia and as part of a total IV approach to general anesthesia. As described earlier, precautions must be taken when using etomidate for any duration beyond induction due to its adrenocortical suppression. Moreover, the total dose of propylene glycol and associated hemolysis may be problematic with an etomidate CRI. Consequently, it is only recommended as a CRI for very short procedures (usually less than 30 to 60 minutes) as part of a balanced technique for high-risk patients where inhalant anesthesia may not be a viable option to preserve major organ function and homeostasis. With propofol CRI, attention must be paid to possible cardiorespiratory depressant effects; the lowest dose required for maintenance should be used. Due to their lack of analgesic activity, any CRI with these drugs must include analgesic agents when it is anticipated that pain will be associated with the procedure.

DISSOCIATIVES

Induction drugs in this class differ from the hypnotics in their mechanism of action and effect on the CNS and consciousness. Some of the CNS effect of dissociatives is attributed to antagonism of *N*-methyl-D-aspartate (NMDA) receptors in the brain and spinal cord. Induction with these drugs yields a dissociated state with varying states of depression or activation in the brain rather than global CNS depression. Analysis of electroencephalograms indicates induction of dissociation between the thalamus and limbic systems of the brain by drugs in this group. In this state, the patient appears cateleptoid with open eyes, nystagmus, hypertonus, and muscle movement that is unrelated to any surgical stimulation. Unlike the hypnotic agents, dissociative induction drugs are potent cerebral vasodilators and cause an increase in cerebral blood flow, intracranial pressure, cerebral spinal fluid pressure, and cerebral oxygen consumption, making them undesirable for patients with head trauma, brain tumors, or other CNS diseases with the potential for elevated intracranial pressure as well as certain ocular disorders (due in part to the increase in intraocular pressure associated with increases in ocular muscle tone). Controlled ventilation to keep arterial carbon dioxide concentrations at normal or slightly below normal levels will diminish the effects of dissociative agents on intracranial pressure.

Dissociative agents provide intense short-duration somatic analgesia but poor visceral analgesia. This analgesic activity occurs at subanesthetic doses. Analgesic effects of dissociative drugs have been attributed to NMDA receptor antagonism, interaction with opiate receptors, local anesthetic effect, or blockade of α-adrenoceptor pathways. Ketamine in particular has found use as an adjunct analgesic in addition to its role as an induction drug. It can be administered as a low-dose CRI or epidurally for prevention or treatment of pain in dogs and cats.

Ketamine

Ketamine (Schedule III) is a short-acting dissociate agent that has a rapid onset of action and is rapidly redistributed from the CNS and metabolized in the liver. Its duration of action is similar to thiopental, lasting approximately 15 to 20 minutes when given as a single IV induction dose. Ketamine undergoes extensive hepatic metabolism in dogs prior to renal excretion; however, in cats, there is minimal hepatic metabolism and it is excreted mostly unchanged by the kidneys. Recovery quality is extremely poor in dogs when ketamine is used alone, with excitement, violent and excessive movement, extreme muscle tone, and occasionally seizures. Use of a tranquilizer or sedative is required to minimize or eliminate the adverse recovery side effects of ketamine. Recoveries are less violent in cats given ketamine alone; however, adjunct sedation or tranquilization is still recommended to improve muscle relaxation and recovery quality. Sight hounds induced with ketamine have recovery times and qualities similar to other breeds, making this a good induction drug choice in these dogs.

Ketamine causes an increase in sympathetic outflow by direct CNS stimulation. Cardiovascular effects of ketamine that result include increases in

blood pressure, heart rate, cardiac output, and myocardial oxygen consumption. Increases in myocardial contractility occur via this CNS stimulatory effect; however, the direct effect of ketamine on the heart muscle is as a negative inotrope. Consequently, patients that lack the ability to further increase sympathetic outflow (i.e., critically ill or trauma patients with already depleted catecholamines and maximized sympathetic tone) will exhibit reductions in cardiac output and blood pressure in response to ketamine. Arrhythmogenic effects of ketamine are variable and controversial, with some describing increases in epinephrine-induced arrhythmias and others demonstrating decreases. Because the increase in systemic vascular resistance with ketamine increases myocardial work, it is contraindicated in patients with valvular disease.

While ketamine may induce dose-dependent and transient apnea, the degree of ventilatory depression is significantly less than is observed with hypnotic agents. Minute volume is initially slightly reduced following administration of ketamine but returns to normal levels within 15 minutes. Apneustic breathing or a shallow and irregular breathing pattern is common with ketamine. Unlike the hypnotic agents, ketamine does not depress the ventilatory response to hypoxia. There is a substantial increase in salivation and airway secretions following ketamine administration. Anticholinergics may reduce secretions, but they also thicken them, making it more difficult to clear mucus from the airway, and so they are not always beneficial or necessary. Airway reflexes are better maintained with ketamine, although swallowing is diminished. Generally, intubation is easily accomplished following induction with ketamine, particularly in cats (a small amount of topical lidocaine may be swabbed on the arytenoids if necessary) (see Chapter 15).

Ketamine comes as a 10% aqueous solution with preservative and a relatively long shelf-life. For IV use in cats, it can be diluted (often 1:10) with normal saline to provide more accurate dosing. It is not recommended for IM use in dogs but can be used in this manner in cats, although it does cause noticeable pain on injection due to its acidic pH. For anesthesia induction in dogs, it is most often mixed with either midazolam or diazepam (Schedule IV). In cats, it is either given alone intramuscularly or intravenously or, more commonly, in combination with a benzodiazepine and/or an opioid. It can also be safely used with acepromazine sedation in both dogs and cats, although it is still recommended that a benzodiazepine be included in the induction protocol for dogs regardless of premedication protocol.

Telazol

Telazol (Schedule III) is a 1 : 1 (wt/wt) combination of the dissociative drug tiletamine and the benzodiazepine zolazepam. The drug has limited stability in solution and so is provided as a powder that is reconstituted with an aqueous diluent to yield 5 ml of a 100 mg/ml solution (50 mg/ml of tiletamine and 50 mg/ml of zolazepam). Once reconstituted, it is stable for 4 days at room temperature and 2 weeks if refrigerated. The half-life of each component of Telazol varies with species. In dogs, the half-life of tiletamine is 1.3 hours, and for zolazepam, it is 1 hour. In cats, a longer half-life exists for tiletamine (2.5 hours) and zolazepam (4.5 hours). Tiletamine has a longer duration of action than ketamine and is also more analgesic. Duration of anesthesia is 20 to 30 minutes in dogs and 40 to 50 minutes in cats, depending on the dose used. Analgesia with Telazol is adequate for mildly painful procedures. The benzodiazepine zolazepam is added to provide improved muscle relaxation and smoother induction and recovery.

The cardiorespiratory effects of Telazol are similar to those observed with ketamine and are dose dependent. For the most part, the physiologic response to Telazol resembles that observed with ketamine-diazepam or ketamine-midazolam combinations. There is generally good hemodynamic stability at the lower doses of the drug. Respiratory depression can be profound at higher doses in both dogs and cats (15 to 20 mg/kg IM), and it is recommended that dosing be kept below 15 mg/kg in both species to minimize adverse effects. Muscle relaxation is improved over that observed with ketamine as a result of the zolazepam. Maintenance of airway reflexes and excessive salivation are similar to what is observed with ketamine.

Telazol can be given either intramuscularly or intravenously to both cats and dogs. Intramuscular administration is more commonly used in practice. Onset of action is rapid following IM administration, occurring within 6 to 8 minutes on average.

When administering Telazol IV, the onset of action occurs within 60 to 90 seconds. Recovery occurs via redistribution and hepatic metabolism in dogs; both components are excreted in the urine in cats (not suggested in renal insufficiency in cats). Repeated dosing with Telazol is not recommended in dogs or cats due to prolonged recovery and poor recovery quality. Zolazepam appears to be eliminated and metabolized more rapidly, which contributes to the rough recovery due to residual effects of tiletamine in dogs. Premedication with acepromazine[5] or an opioid reduces the dose of Telazol required for induction, improves induction quality, and smoothes recovery from anesthesia.

Clinical Use of Dissociative Agents

For dogs, ketamine is rarely administered by any route other than IV due to the otherwise poor quality of induction and recovery. As described earlier, a benzodiazepine should be added to ketamine when used in dogs to smooth out the otherwise rough recovery. Either diazepam or midazolam is added to ketamine in a 1 : 1 (vol/vol) mixture. This yields a solution that is 2.5 mg/ml of diazepam or midazolam and 50 mg/ml of ketamine and is administered at 1 ml of the mixture per 10 kg of body weight. In normal healthy dogs, a more rapid and smooth induction will be achieved by administering the total calculated dose as an IV bolus. Duration of action is somewhat longer with the diazepam-ketamine combination versus the midazolam-ketamine combination. There is only very mild respiratory depression at this dose and good maintenance of cardiovascular function as described earlier. In compromised patients, the dose should be reduced and titrated to effect. Premedication with acepromazine[5] or an opioid will further smooth induction and recovery and slightly reduce the total required dose. Combinations with α_2-agonists such as xylazine or medetomidine have been used to provide a better quality IM induction in dogs as well as IV induction. The effect of these combinations causes depression of cardiovascular function and overall recovery will be much longer, so they may not be an optimal choice for dogs or cats.

In cats, ketamine can be given either intramuscularly or intravenously for induction of general anesthesia, usually in combination with a benzodiazepine, acepromazine, and/or an opioid and frequently a combination of more than one class of sedative and analgesic drug. For IM use, it is dosed at 5 to 20 mg/kg depending on ancillary drugs being used. Combinations commonly used are xylazine-ketamine, acepromazine-ketamine, midazolam- or diazepam-ketamine, and any of these combinations with butorphanol, oxymorphone, hydromorphone, or buprenorphine added. Such IM cocktails are commonly used for short mild to moderately painful procedures (e.g., feline castration, wound lavage) as they provide adequate anesthesia and analgesia with relatively rapid recoveries.

Telazol is perhaps best used IM in both dogs and cats as either a premedication or induction agent. In fractious or savage dogs, Telazol has been used at 4 to 6 mg/kg IM (with or without butorphanol [0.2 to 0.4 mg/kg IM]) to achieve adequate restraint and venous access. Additional IV Telazol (1 to 4 mg/kg IV to effect) or any of the other induction drugs at low doses may then be administered to allow intubation and transition to inhalant anesthesia as needed. In cats given 2 to 4 mg/kg IM, similar results are obtained. If Telazol is combined with opioids, minor surgical procedures may be accomplished in cats similar to those described for ketamine earlier. When using IV Telazol for induction of dogs or cats, the dose is reduced to 1 to 3 mg/kg with appropriate premedication. Because the duration of action is longer and the cost is greater with Telazol versus ketamine, Telazol has not been as commonly used as an IV induction drug in dogs or cats. The short shelf-life of Telazol also limits its use in small animal patients.

OPIOID BENZODIAZEPINE COMBINATIONS AND TIVA

In critically ill patients, trauma cases, emergency cesarean sections, patients with cardiovascular disease, etc. there is often a need to minimize the negative effects of induction drugs and inhaled anesthetics in order to maximally preserve homeostasis. With TIVA, intravenously administered drugs are used to achieve general anesthesia. Protection of the airway must be a consideration regardless of the use of inhaled anesthetic. The patient may be intubated and placed on supplemental oxygen or ventilated. TIVA may also be used in a modified approach or "balanced anesthesia" technique whereby the use of inhaled anesthetics is kept to a bare minimum (often less than 0.25 to 0.5 times MAC[6]). Again, the goal is to minimize the negative

effects on major organ function by reducing or eliminating the more noxious agent, inhaled anesthetics.

> Balanced anesthesia contributes to patient safety by decreasing the negative effects of each drug that must be administered.

For TIVA, combinations of drugs are used to achieve unconsciousness, muscle relaxation, attenuation of autonomic reflexes, and analgesia sufficient for the procedure or surgery to be performed. Local anesthetic techniques (see Chapter 8) may be employed as needed. Benzodiazepines (diazepam or midazolam) provide minimal sedation in dogs and cats but do provide some degree of muscle relaxation and act synergistically with opioids to enhance sedation from these drugs. Moreover, they have minimal effect on cardiovascular or respiratory system function or other major organs, and they aid in reducing the dose of drugs required for induction and maintenance of anesthesia. Pure μ-agonists (oxymorphone, hydromorphone, fentanyl, or sufentanyl) are the opioids of choice for TIVA given their synergistic activity with benzodiazepines to induce sedation and a near-anesthetic state, profound analgesia, and minimal effect on blood pressure. While opioids do cause vagally mediated bradycardia and some respiratory depression, these side effects are generally dose dependent and easily controlled by flow-by oxygen, orotracheal intubation and IPPV with oxygen, or administration of anticholinergics, having minimal impact on overall homeostasis. Pretreatment with an anticholinergic (e.g., glycopyrrolate [0.011 mg/kg IV]) prior to administration of sufentanyl is recommended due to the more profound effect of sufentanyl on heart rate compared to the other opioids. Because the benzodiazepines and opioids are dosed and administered individually, there is good control over the total amount of each drug administered and better ability to anticipate any side effects. In very ill patients, the use of a benzodiazepine-opioid combination may be sufficient for minor procedures. These drugs may be given individually as an IV bolus or as a CRI (Table 6.2).

Additional anesthetic effect is achieved by a small induction dose of a hypnotic or dissociative

Table 6.2. Selected balanced or total intravenous anesthesia protocols for dogs and cats for procedures lasting less than 2 hours.

	Initial dose, IV	CRI dose, IV
Benzodiazepine		
Diazepam	0.1–0.2 mg/kg	0.2–0.5 µg/kg/hr
Midazolam	0.05–0.2 mg/kg	0.2–0.5 µg/kg/hr
Opioid		
Fentanyl	5–10 µg/kg	1–20 µg/kg/hr
Sufentanil	2–5 µg/kg	0.1–0.2 µg/kg/min
Induction/maintenance		
Propofol	1–4 mg/kg	0.2–0.5 mg/kg/min
Etomidate	1–2 mg/kg	0.02–0.3 mg/kg/min†
Midazolam (M)/Fentanyl (F)‡	M: 0.2 mg/kg plus	M: 8 µg/kg/min Plus
	F: 5–10 µg/kg*	F: 0.8 µg/kg/min

*Depending on the health of the animal, an induction agent such as etomidate (0.5 to 2 mg/kg IV) may be needed. In critically ill patients, the hypnotic agent will not be required.
†Rarely indicated due to adrenal suppression.
‡Duration of infusion for longer than 2 hours begins to impact length of recovery and the infusion should be discontinued sooner than 30 minutes prior to recovery.

agent that is carefully selected based on patient status and followed by a CRI when indicated. This is usually limited to propofol, etomidate (for short durations), or ketamine. Alternatively, intubated patients may be maintained on a small amount of inhalant anesthetic, often 0.25 to 0.5 times MAC[6] or less, in 100% oxygen. If needed, in some patients, a neuromuscular blocking agent (e.g., atracurium 0.2 to 0.4 mg/kg IV every 30 to 45 minutes to effect; see Chapter 11) may be administered to improve muscle relaxation. However, it is imperative that adequate analgesia, amnesia, and unconsciousness be ensured when using neuromuscular blocking agents. By carefully selecting each drug for its desired effect, appropriate timing and dosing, and titration to effect as required, a safe and balanced period of general anesthesia may be achieved while maintaining relative homeostasis of major organ systems. Given the number of drugs available, the possible combinations to achieve balanced anesthesia or TIVA are numerous; knowledgeable application of pharmacology will aid appropriate choices in individual settings.

ENDNOTES

1 *Top-up dose* is a dose needed to restore anesthesia to its original plane.

2 Lidocaine may be substituted for saline after thiopental extravasation because it neutralizes pH and decreases vasospasm. To prevent sloughing and necrosis, it is important to dilute the concentration of thiopental to less than 1%.
3 PropoFlo: Abbott Laboratories, North Chicago IL 60064. Does not contain benzyl alcohol.
4 Rapinovet: Schering-Plough, Kenilworth NJ 07033. Does not contain benzyl alcohol.
5 Some caution is suggested with the use of phenothiazines and Telazol due to respiratory and myocardial depression.
6 In the absence of additional drugs, 0.4 MAC ≈ MAC awake.

REFERENCES

Andress, J.L., Day, T.K., and Day, D. 1995. The effects of consecutive day propofol anesthesia on feline red blood cells. *Vet Surg* 24:277–282.

Benson, G.J. 2002. Intravenous anesthetics. In *Veterinary Anesthesia and Pain Management Secrets*, edited by S.A. Greene, pp. 91–95. Philadelphia: Hanley and Belfus.

Dodam, J.R., Kruse-Elliott, K.T., Aucoin, D.P., et al. 1990. Duration of etomidate-induced adrenocortical suppression during surgery in dogs. *Am J Vet Res* 51:786–788.

Gross, M.E., Dodam, J.R., Pope, E.R., et al. 2002. A comparison of thiopental, propofol, and diazepam-ketamine anesthesia for evaluation of laryngeal function in dogs premedicated with butorphanol-glycopyrrolate. *J Am Hosp Assoc* 38:503–506.

Jackson, A.M., Tobias, K, Long, C., et al. 2004. Effects of various anesthetic agents on laryngeal motion during laryngoscopy in normal dogs. *Vet Surg* 33:102–106.

Kruse-Elliott, K.T., Swanson, C.R., and Aucoin, D.P. 1987. Effects of etomidate on adrenocortical function in canine surgical patients. *Am J Vet Res* 48:1098–1100.

Lin, H.C. 1996. Dissociative anesthetics. In *Lumb and Jones Veterinary Anesthesia*, 3rd ed., edited by J.C. Thurmon, W.J. Tranquilli, and G.J. Benson, pp. 241–296. Baltimore: Williams & Wilkins.

Matthews, N.S., Brown, R.M., Barling, K.S., et al. 2004. Repetitive propofol administration in dogs and cats. *J Am Anim Hosp Assoc* 40:255–260.

Pablo, L.S., and Bailey, J.E. 1999. Etomidate and telazol. In *Veterinary Clinics of North America: Small Animal Practice*, Vol. 29, No. 3, edited by N.S. Matthews, pp. 779–792. Philadelphia: W.B. Saunders.

Robertson, S.A., Johnston, S., and Beemsterboer, J. 1992. Cardiopulmonary, anesthetic, and postanes-thetic effects of intravenous infusions of propofol in greyhounds and non-greyhounds. *Am J Vet Res* 53:1027–1032.

Short, C.E., and Bufalari, A. 1999. Propofol anesthe-sia. In *Veterinary Clinics of North America: Small Animal Practice*, Vol. 29, No. 3, edited by N.S. Matthews, pp. 747–778. Philadelphia: W.B. Saunders.

Smith, J.A., Gaynor, J.S., Bednarski, R.M., et al. 1993. Adverse effects of administration of propofol with various preanesthetic regimens in dogs. *J Am Vet Med Assoc.* 202(7):1111–1115.

Thurmon, J.C., Tranquilli, W.J., and Benson, G.J. 1996. Injectable anesthetics. In *Lumb and Jones Veterinary Anesthesia*, edited by J.C. Thurmon, W. J. Tranquilli, and G.J Benson, 3rd ed., pp. 210–240. Baltimore: Williams & Wilkins.

Thurmon, J.C., Tranquilli, W.J., and Benson, G.J. 1999. *Essentials of Small Animal Anesthesia and Analgesia*. Baltimore: Lippincott Williams & Wilkin.

Trissell, L.A. 2005. *Handbook on Injectable Drugs*, 13th ed., Bethesda: Special Publishing and American Society of Health System Professionals.

Chapter 7
Inhalant Anesthetics

Gwendolyn L. Carroll

The ideal inhalant has not yet been discovered. Before the development of injectable anesthetics for which there is greater control, the idea of administration of an inhalant anesthetic was very attractive. Administration of inhalants appeared to be "safer" because most currently used inhalants are minimally metabolized. Recovery from the inhalant requires discontinuation and ventilation (e.g., spontaneous or controlled) with oxygen, a mixture of gases containing at least 21% oxygen, or air. All inhalants have some disadvantages, particularly cardiopulmonary effects. Inhalant anesthetics with unique or particularly bothersome side effects have been used minimally or are no longer available in this country; such undesirable effects include the following:

- Sensitization of the myocardium to epinephrine-induced arrhythmias (e.g., halothane)
- Necrotizing hepatitis (e.g., halothane)
- Malignant hyperthermia (e.g., all inhalants, but particularly halothane)
- Seizures (e.g., enflurane)
- Flammability (e.g., ether, cyclopropane)
- Renal compromise (e.g., methoxyflurane with concurrent flunixin administration)

This chapter addresses the common potent inhalant anesthetics that practicing veterinarians are likely to use (e.g., isoflurane, sevoflurane) in the United States. Another potent inhalant commonly used in human medicine (e.g., desflurane) will be introduced, but the expense of the vaporizer precludes its use in many practices. Methoxyflurane and halothane, two older inhalant anesthetics, are no longer commercially available in the United States. Even though the use of nitrous oxide in veterinary medicine has declined in recent years, there

are some indications for its use. Xenon is used in human medicine.

This chapter offers practical information that is needed to appropriately deliver a reasonable and relatively constant concentration of inhalant anesthetic to the brain. Excellent and thorough reviews of inhalant anesthesia (Stoelting and Hillier 2006; Keegan 2005; Eger 1974) are available for the engaged reader.

UPTAKE AND DISTRIBUTION

In the same manner that *pharmacokinetics* describes the action of injectable drugs in individuals, *uptake* and *distribution* assist in the understanding of the onset and actions of inhalant anesthetics in the body. Several terms are important when considering uptake and distribution of inhalants. The partition coefficient, partial pressure, equilibrium, and their relationship are described. The solubility of an inhalant in blood and tissue is represented by a partition coefficient. A partition coefficient describes the distribution of an inhalant anesthetic between two phases at equilibrium (Fig. 7.1). It depicts the ability of two phases to accept anesthetic and is temperature dependent.

> A partition coefficient (λ) reflects the relative capacity of each phase to accept inhalant anesthetic at equilibrium.

The partial pressure of a gas represents the tendency for the gas to leave a phase. Equilibrium is reached when the partial pressures in two adjacent phases equalize (see Fig. 7.1). The same concentration of anesthetic may not be present in the two phases even though the partial pressures are the same. The distribution of two inhalant anesthetics

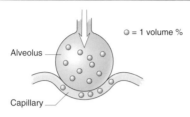

Figure 7.1. A blood-gas partition coefficient of 0.5 is attained when the same partial pressure is attained in two phases. Note that the concentrations in the two media or phases are different even though the partial pressures are identical in the two phases. In this example, at equilibrium (equal partial pressures), the blood volume percent is 5% and the alveolar gas volume is 10%. (Illustrations by Mark M. Miller, Miller Medical Illustration & Design.)

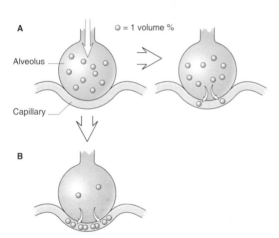

Figure 7.2. Beginning with introduction of an inhalant of 10% into the alveolus: the alveolus then equilibrates with blood; that is, the blood and alveoli have equal partial pressures of the inhalant. (*A*) Blood-gas partition coefficient = 0.25. (*B*) Blood-gas partition coefficient = 4. (Illustrations by Mark M. Miller, Miller Medical Illustration & Design.)

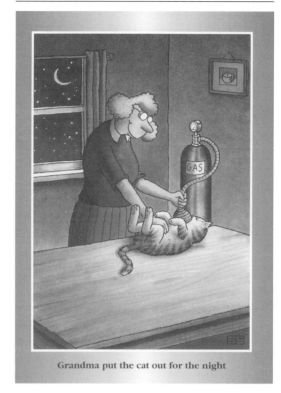

Grandma put the cat out for the night

Figure 7.3. Terminology is very important in anesthesia. Patients are anesthetized, or in slang are "slept." (From Stan Eales, "Grandma put the cat out for the night," at stan@staneales.freeserve.co.uk.)

with different blood-gas partition coefficients is illustrated in Figure 7.2.

> Partial pressure of a gas represents the tendency for the gas to leave a phase.

> Equilibrium is reached when the partial pressures in two adjacent phases equalize.

The blood-gas partition coefficient describes the "solubility" of an inhalant anesthetic in a patient's blood. The inhalant's solubility will greatly affect the rate at which the alveolar concentration (P_A) will rise toward the inspired concentration (P_I). The more soluble anesthetics (e.g., methoxyflurane) have a very slow rate of rise of P_A. Nitrous oxide, sevoflurane, and desflurane are not very soluble and have a rapid alveolar rate of rise; that is, P_A of the inhalant increases rapidly to equalize with the inspired partial pressure of the anesthetic. Isoflurane has intermediate solubility. See Table 7.1 for comparative solubilities.

The goal of inhalant anesthesia is to establish an anesthetic state by delivering an appropriate and constant partial pressure of inhalant anesthetic to the brain; the state of anesthesia produced is reversible when the partial pressure of anesthetic in the brain is reduced (see Equation 7.1).

Table 7.1. Physical properties of inhalant anesthetics.

Inhalant	Boiling point (°C)	Vapor pressure (mm Hg) 20°C	Partition coefficients 37°C				
			Blood-gas	Brain-blood	Muscle-blood	Fat-blood	Oil-gas
Halothane	50.2	244	2.4–2.5	2.6	3.5	60	224
Isoflurane	48.5	240	1.4	3.7	4.0	45	98
Sevoflurane	58.5	170	0.65	1.7	3.1	48	53
Desflurane	22.8	669	0.42–0.45	1.3	2.0	2.0	19
Nitrous oxide		Gas	0.47–0.63	1.1	1.2	2.3	1.4
Xenon		Gas	0.115				

(See references.)

Factors influencing the transfer of inhalant anesthetic from the vaporizer of an anesthesia machine to the patient's brain

$$\text{Anesthetic} \Longleftrightarrow P_A \Longleftrightarrow P_a \Longleftrightarrow P_{br}$$
Machine

P_I Blood-gas λ Brain-blood
V_A λ
Machine (e.g.   (e.g., solubility)   Cerebral
   volume,   CO   blood
   fresh gas flow, D_{A-v} D_{a-v}
   solubility in
   system
(e.g., rubber)

Inspired partial pressure (P_I) of the inhalant anesthetic, alveolar ventilation (V_A), alveolar partial pressure (P_A) of the inhalant anesthetic, partition coefficient (λ) of the inhalant anesthetic, cardiac output (CO), alveolar-to-venous partial pressure difference (D_{A-v}), arterial-to-venous partial pressure difference (D_{a-v}).

$$(7.1)$$

In order to reach appropriate and constant partial pressure in the brain, the anesthetic must move from the vaporizer through the breathing system, respiratory system, and cardiovascular system to the brain; when the vaporizer is turned off, anesthetic is removed from the body by moving in the reverse direction. Diffusion of the inhalant is dependent on partial pressure gradients rather than concentration gradients; it moves from an area of higher partial pressure to an area of lower partial pressure.

The partial pressure of a gas is the product of the fractional concentration of the gas and the total pressure (barometric pressure). As illustrated earlier, the partial pressure represents the tendency of the gas to escape that phase. A partial pressure may produce different concentrations in different phases. The relationship between partial pressure (tension) and concentration is illustrated in Equation 7.2.

Calculation of the percentage of a gas if the tension (mm of Hg) of the gas and the barometric pressures are known [the assumption is that the gases are dry]

$$\text{Concentration (\%)} = (\text{Tension/Barometric pressure}) \times 100 \quad (7.2)$$

The P_I of the inhalant anesthetic determines the amount of inhalant that will be delivered to the alveolus. Greater partial pressure of anesthetic in inhaled gases produces a larger gradient for diffusion of the inhalant to the alveolus and causes a more rapid rise in the alveolar partial pressure (e.g., the Fick principle). The oxygen moving from the lungs into the arterial blood minus the oxygen returning to the lungs from venous blood equals the oxygen removed from the lungs. The oxygen taken up by the lungs is the difference in the oxygen presented to the lungs by ventilation minus the amount of oxygen leaving the lungs by ventilation.

The rate of diffusion is inversely proportional to molecular weight (Graham's law), or the heavier molecule is less diffusible. A high initial P_I of an anesthetic will offset the effect of uptake of the inhalant. In order to maintain a constant P_A over time as the rate of uptake slows, the P_I (practically, the vaporizer concentration) should be decreased.

The concentration effect and second gas effect impact the effect P_I has on the alveolar rate of rise.

The concentration effect means that a higher P_I produces a faster rise in P_A. Once there is uptake of anesthetic gas and oxygen, the remaining anesthetic gas is in a smaller volume of total gas, resulting in a higher concentration of anesthetic gas in the alveoli.

> The concentration effect is applied in practical anesthesia when higher P_I values are used to produce faster inductions due to the faster rate of rise in P_A.

The second gas effect indicates that the high volume uptake of one gas (e.g., nitrous oxide) accelerates the rate of rise of a second concurrently administered gas (e.g., potent inhalant). A recent investigation indicates that the large volume uptake of nitrous oxide alone does not explain the second gas effect of nitrous oxide on sevoflurane during constant inspired ventilation (Hendrickx et al. 2006). Concentrations of nitrous oxide previously thought to be too small to result in a second gas effect may actually produce an effect.

> The high volume of uptake of one gas accelerates the alveolar rate of rise of a second gas administered concurrently (second gas effect).

Similar to the effect of increasing P_I, increasing alveolar ventilation (V_A) enhances the movement of anesthetic into the lung and offsets increased uptake of anesthetic into the blood. Changes in V_A affect the alveolar rate of rise of a very soluble anesthetic more than a less soluble gas. With spontaneous ventilation, the inhalant influences its own uptake by decreasing ventilation as anesthetic depth increases.

Inhalants enter the body through the lungs by ventilation. Changes in ventilation influence the rate of rise of P_A more with a soluble anesthetic than with a poorly soluble anesthetic. With a poorly soluble inhalant, the effect of ventilation is trivial. A large functional residual capacity (FRC) slows the alveolar rate of rise compared to a small FRC. Smaller more frequent alveolar breaths speed attainment of P_A more than do fewer large breaths (minute ventilation being equal). Positive-pressure ventilation that increases minute ventilation will produce more rapid changes in P_A than will spontaneous ventilation.

The anesthetic breathing system influences the rate of rise of P_A. Use of a nonrebreathing system results in essentially no difference between the concentration of anesthetic exiting the vaporizer and the anesthetic P_I. In a circle breathing system, the volume of the system, the rubber-gas partition coefficient, and the fresh gas flow rate (oxygen and anesthetic) impact the rate of rise of P_A. With a vaporizer outside the breathing system, increasing the flow rate (increases delivery of oxygen and inhalant anesthetic) will overcome the effect of the volume of the breathing system based on the time constant (e.g., volume of the machine divided by the flow rate equals one time constant, which changes the concentration in the breathing circuit by 63% if there is no uptake of inhalant) (Table 7.2).

> After one time constant, the concentration of inhalant that is presented to a patient breathing on a circle system is 63% of the vaporizer setting (e.g., wash-in/wash-out function).

Conversely, with a vaporizer inside the circle, increasing the fresh gas flow rate (increases delivery of oxygen only) decreases the inhalant concentration inspired. Higher solubility of the inhalant in rubber slows the rate of rise of P_A compared to an agent with lower solubility in rubber. Alternatively,

Table 7.2. The relationship between the capacity of the anesthetic machine and the oxygen flow rate to the percentage change of inhalant delivered to the patient (P_I) is described by the time constant.

Capacity of Anesthetic Machine/Fresh Gas Flow (Time Constant [t])	Percentage Change of Inhalant Anesthetic Delivered to the Patient (P_I)
One t	63%
Two t	86%
Three t	95%
Four t	98%

when the vaporizer is turned off, elution of anesthetic from rubber slows the decrease in P_A.

The transfer of the inhaled anesthetic from the alveoli to arterial blood is determined by the blood-gas partition coefficient (λ), the cardiac output (CO), and the difference between the alveolar and venous partial pressures ($D_{[A-v]}$) of anesthetic. Absorption is determined by blood-gas solubility, blood flow (CO) through the lungs, perfusion of other tissue by blood, tissue-blood solubility, and tissue mass. When anesthesia has been induced, the alveolar partial pressure (P_A) approaches equilibrium with the arterial partial pressure (P_a) and the brain partial pressure (P_{br}) of the inhalant anesthetic. The partial pressure gradients of the anesthetic gas are as follows: delivered > inspired > alveolar > arterial > tissue. Until equilibrium is reached, the gradients continue to exist. At equilibrium, the P_A of the anesthetic may be used to estimate anesthetic depth based on the potency of the inhalant anesthetic (minimum alveolar concentration [MAC]).

Cardiac output affects the alveolar rate of rise of an inhalant anesthetic more for very soluble anesthetics than for poorly soluble inhalants. An increase in CO enhances anesthetic uptake and distribution, slowing the rate of rise of P_A, because of greater uptake by tissues such as muscle. Conversely, if CO decreases, the P_I increases but the distribution of anesthetic to tissues such as muscle is delayed. With a poorly soluble anesthetic agent, the rate of rise is inherently fast and a change in CO has little impact. If using a soluble agent for a patient with low cardiac output (e.g., shock), a faster rate of rise for P_A should be anticipated and the P_I should be decreased.

Alveolar concentrations of soluble inhalant anesthetics rise quickly in patients with low cardiac output.

Another determinant of alveolar rate of rise is the difference between the P_A and P_v values which reflect tissue uptake of the drug. The vessel-rich group (VRG; well-perfused tissues [e.g., brain, heart, kidneys]) accounts for less than 10% of the body mass but receives 75% of total blood flow. The VRG equilibrates rapidly with the inhaled anesthetic. It takes about three time constants for

about 75% of the returning venous blood to approach the P_A. Skeletal muscle and fat represent about 70% of the body mass but receive only 10 to 20% of the cardiac output. As a result, time is required for tissues to approach saturation with anesthetic and uptake from the lung continues. The uptake of inhalant is represented by the alveolar-to-venous partial pressure difference (D_{A-v}). The amount of inhalant that diffuses into the blood (P_a) is affected by the same factors that are responsible for the uptake of inhalant by the lung (P_A) from the inspired gases (P_I). The P_A and P_I become closer to each other with time, indicating that the uptake of inhalant by the blood decreases over time. The VRG tissues (less than 10% of body weight and receiving about 75% of the CO) require about three time constants to equilibrate with P_a.

The rate of decline of the partial pressure (P_A) of the inhalant anesthetic determines the rate of recovery. Continued uptake of inhalant by tissues that have not equilibrated when the inhalant is turned off will speed the decrease of P_A. As long as a gradient exists between P_a and P_{tissue}, anesthetic continues to be absorbed, speeding the decline of P_A. For poorly soluble inhalants, the effect of anesthetic time is minimized and the rate of decline of P_a is fast. Recovery may be hastened by turning off the inhalant and turning up the oxygen flow rate.

The rate of change of P_A during recovery depends on the length of anesthesia and the solubility of the inhalant. With very soluble anesthetics, there may be adequate tissue concentrations to maintain P_A when the vaporizer is turned off ($P_I = 0$). For insoluble drugs, the rate of change in P_A is fast regardless of the length of anesthesia. Metabolism of inhalants will theoretically speed the decrease in P_A.

INHALANT ANESTHETICS

Nitrous oxide is a lowly potent inhalant anesthetic that is generally combined with a potent inhalant to supplement analgesia and decrease the amount of the more potent primary anesthetic. Nitrous oxide does not provide skeletal muscle relaxation, amnesia, or loss of consciousness sufficient to produce general anesthesia. Increased awareness of the potential complications associated with the use of nitrous oxide has decreased its popularity. The potent inhalants used in veterinary medicine in the United States include isoflurane, sevoflurane, and, to a lesser extent, desflurane. These anesthetics may have profound cardiopulmonary effects. They produce analgesia, amnesia, and muscle relaxation but do not prevent the volley of afferent and efferent nervous impulses produced by noxious stimuli (e.g., "windup").

Many potential side effects of potent inhalant anesthetics may be avoided by not allowing the vaporizer and oxygen flow to be on for extended time periods when not connected to a patient ("Monday morning phenomenon").[1]

Minimum Alveolar Concentration

The minimum alveolar concentration (MAC) is defined as the inhalant concentration at which 50% of individuals move in response to a noxious stimulus[2] at one atmosphere (Table 7.3). MAC is an indication of anesthetic potency. The reciprocal of the partial pressure of an inhalant to produce an effect (e.g., immobility) equals the potency. At 1.3 MAC, 95% of patients do not move in response to a defined stimulus. In veterinary patients, a tail clamp or electrical impulse is used as the stimulus and bracketing is used to determine the MAC value. With bracketing, after a steady anesthetic state is reached at a given inhalant concentration, a noxious stimulus (e.g., tail clamp or electrical impulse) is applied. If there is no movement, the inhalant is decreased to 80% of the concentration that did not produce movement. If movement occurs at 80% of the previous anesthetic concentration, the MAC is said to be midway between the anesthetic concentration at which movement is prevented and at which movement occurred; tighter brackets produce a more accurate determination of MAC. Using smaller brackets increases accuracy but simultaneously increases the time required to determine the MAC value.

In humans, a skin incision is typically used as a noxious stimulus in MAC determination and cannot be repeated. With surgical incision as a stimulus, MAC is determined by population. Several people are administered several predetermined inhalant concentrations above and below the expected MAC concentration. MAC is then established by visualizing the best fit line for the percentage of patients moving at each concentration; the concentration preventing movement in 50% of patients can then be estimated.

MAC is relatively constant within a species and across species. Individual cats have a consistent degree of sensitivity to various inhalants, indicating a possible genetic influence. Sex and type of stimulus do not affect MAC variability. Anesthetic duration, circadian rhythm, and thyroid status have little effect on MAC. Severe acid base changes, hypoventilation or hyperventilation, hypoxemia, hypertension, and anemia only affect MAC if life-threatening variations occur. Aging, hypothermia and hyperthermia, pregnancy, and several drugs alter MAC. Opioid administration in cats decreases the MAC of isoflurane, improves cardiovascular function, and blunts respiratory, hormonal, and cardiovascular responses to noxious stimuli.

MAC may be used to compare inhalant anesthetic potencies for clinical use. For example, if a patient maintained on 2% isoflurane is changed to sevoflurane, an equivalent MAC concentration of sevoflurane may be estimated based on known MAC values (Equation 7.3).

Comparison of the ratios of MAC equivalent concentrations to the MAC values for isoflurane and sevoflurane

$$\frac{\text{Isoflurane\% (vaporizer setting)}}{\text{MAC}_{isoflurane}} =$$
$$\frac{\text{Sevoflurane\% (vaporizer setting)}}{\text{MAC}_{sevoflurane}}$$

$$\frac{2\% \text{ Isoflurane}}{1.3 \text{ (MAC}_{isoflurane})} = \frac{X\% \text{ Sevoflurane}}{2.9 \text{ (MAC}_{sevoflurane})}$$

$$X = \frac{(2.9)(2)}{1.3}, \quad X = 4.5\% \text{ Sevoflurane} \quad (7.3)$$

In order to maintain a stable MAC in a patient on 2% isoflurane in oxygen, a vaporizer setting of 4.5% sevoflurane would be MAC equivalent.

Table 7.3. Minimum alveolar concentrations (MAC) of inhalant anesthetics in dogs and cats.

Inhalant	Dog %	Cat %
Halothane	0.87–0.94	1.14
Isoflurane	1.28–1.3	1.63–1.9
Sevoflurane	2.09–2.9	2.58–3.4
Desflurane	7.2–10.3	9.97–10.27
Nitrous oxide	188–200	250
Xenon	63–71 (human)	

(See references.)

In spontaneously ventilating cats, a desflurane concentration of 1.7 MAC lowers arterial blood pressures but not cardiac index. During controlled ventilation in cats, arterial blood pressure and cardiac index are decreased.

The percentage of inspired desflurane that can be metabolized is 0.02%. Potential toxicities that may occur after desflurane administration may be found in Table 7.4.

MASK OR CHAMBER INDUCTIONS

Mask or chamber inductions were popular before modern injectable anesthetics were made available. The beauty of inhalant induction related to delivery and elimination of anesthetic via the respiratory system, which allowed easy control of anesthetic depth. In the absence of reversible and non-cumulative injectable anesthetics, there appeared to be a greater safety margin since the inhalants could be administered to effect and eliminated quickly if necessary. The anesthetic could be "dialed" to a patient's current health status. When inhalant inductions are used, injectable drugs that lower the MAC of the inhalant should be used. There are advantages to chamber inductions for savage cats. Once the animals are removed from the chamber, MAC-lowering drugs may be administered. There are several disadvantages to inhalant mask or chamber inductions, and the following should be considered:

- A deeper anesthetic plane is needed for orotracheal intubation than for maintenance of anesthesia, which could cause excessive cardiopulmonary depression.
- Rapid control of the airway is important to prevent the opportunity for aspiration of foreign material in patients that are not fasted, are vomiting, or have a megaesophagus.
- The airway should be secured with a cuffed endotracheal tube as quickly as possible in patients with respiratory disease.
- Patients with ocular injuries or facial lesions may be prone to further damaging the site of injury as they move or resist during mask or chamber inductions.
- With current potent, lowly soluble inhalants, very little time is available for orotracheal intubation before anesthetic depth becomes too light and the mask must be replaced.

- Environmental contamination occurs due to the higher fresh gas flow rates and the higher concentrations required to effect induction; this may affect the ozone layer and unnecessarily expose veterinary personnel to waste gases.
- Mask and chamber inductions should be done in a well-ventilated room and ideally in a fume hood to minimize exposure of personnel to waste gases.

> There are few indications for mask or chamber inductions; when used attention should be paid to control of waste gases and minimizing exposure of personnel.

OCCUPATIONAL EXPOSURE

Exposure to waste anesthetic gases is a potential health hazard. For specific recommendations or advice regarding human exposure to waste gases, people at risk should consult their physicians. The following are general recommendations. All waste gases should be scavenged. Vaporizers should be filled under a hood or with a keyed bottle-filler port. In recovery, the patient should remain intubated and breathing oxygen until extubation. Women of child-bearing age should not be allowed in areas of high risk for exposure to waste anesthetic gases (e.g., induction area where mask or chamber inductions may take place or recovery area where several patients may be exhaling inhalant anesthetics). If necessary for persons at risk to be in rooms with volatile halogenated anesthetics, they should wear a charcoal mask. Charcoal will adsorb potent volatile halogenated anesthetics but not nitrous oxide.

The National Institute for Occupational Safety and Health recommends that environmental exposure to halogenated inhalants be 2 ppm or less if used alone. The concentration of nitrous oxide should be 25 ppm or less. If halogenated inhalants are used with nitrous oxide, the concentration should be 0.5 ppm or less.

ENDNOTES

1 "Monday morning phenomenon" refers to the hazards associated with failure to discontinue the oxygen and inhalant after discontinuing administration to a patient. Taking care to discontinue the oxygen and inhalant after disconnecting from a patient decreases the likelihood of carbon monoxide

production, avoiding desiccated carbon dioxide absorbents, especially those with strong bases (e.g., Baralyme), and avoids the production of flammable organic compounds such as methanol and formaldehyde which may spontaneously combust, particularly with the use of sevoflurane.

2 In human MAC determinations, the noxious stimulus is typically surgical.

REFERENCES

Barter, L.S., Ilkiw, J.E., Steffey, E.P., et al. 2004. Animal dependence of inhaled anaesthetic requirements in cats. *Br J Anaesth* 92:275–277.

Barter, L.S., Ilkiw, J.E., Pypendop, B.H., et al. 2004. Evaluation of the induction and recovery characteristics of anesthesia with desflurane in cats. *Am J Vet Res* 65:748–751.

Clarke, K.W. 1999. Desflurane and sevoflurane. *Vet Clin North Am Small Anim Prac* 29:793–810.

Clarke, K.W., Alibhai, H.I.K., Lee, Y.W., et al. 1996. Cardiopulmonary effects of desflurane in the dog during spontaneous and artificial ventilation. *Res Vet Sci* 61:82–86.

Eger, E.I. 1974. *Anesthetic Uptake and Action*. Baltimore: Williams & Wilkins.

Eger, E.I. 1994. New inhaled anesthetics. *Anesthesiology* 80:906–922.

Hendrickx, J.F.A., Carette, R., Lemmens, H.J.M., et al. 2006. Large volume N_2O uptake alone does not explain the second gas effect of N_2O on sevoflurane during constant inspired ventilation. *Br J Anaesth* 96:301–395.

Hikasa, Y., Ohe, N., Takase, K., et al. 1997. Cardiopulmonary effects of sevoflurane in cats: Comparison with isoflurane, halothane, and enflurane. *Res Vet Sci* 63:205–210.

Hikasa, Y., Yamashita, M., Takase, K., et al. 1998. Prolonged sevoflurane, isoflurane and halothane anaesthesia in oxygen using rebreathing or nonrebreathing system in cats. *J Vet Med A* 45:559–575.

Hikasa, Y., Yamashita, M., Takase, K., et al. 1997. Comparison of prolonged sevoflurane, isoflurane, and halothane anaesthesia combined with nitrous oxide in spontaneously breathing cats. *J Vet Med A* 44:427–442.

Keegan, R.D. 2005. Inhalants used in veterinary medicine. In *Recent Advances in Veterinary Anesthesia and Analgesia: Companion Animals*, edited by R.D. Gleed and J.W. Ludders. Ithaca: International Veterinary Information Service (www.ivis.org).

McMurphy, R.M., and Hodgson, D.S. 1996. Cardiopulmonary effects of desflurane in cats. *Am J Vet Res* 57:367–370.

McMurphy, R.M., and Hodgson, D.S. 1995. The minimum alveolar concentration of desflurane in cats. *Vet Surg* 24:453–455.

Merin, R.G., Bernard, J.M., Doursout, M.F., et al. Comparison of the effects of isoflurane and desflurane on cardiovascular dynamics and regional blood flow in the chronically instrumented dog. *Anesthesiology* 74:568–574.

Mutoh, T., Nishimura, R., Kim, H.Y., et al. 1997. Cardiopulmonary effects of sevoflurane, compared with halothane, enflurane, and isoflurane, in dogs. *Am J Vet Res* 58:885–890.

Pagel, P.S., Kampine, J.P., Schmeling, W.T., et al. 1991. Comparison of the systemic and coronary hemodynamic actions of desflurane, isoflurane, halothane, and enflurane in the chronically instrumented dog. *Anesthesiology* 74:539–551.

Pagel, P.S., Kampine, J.P., Schmeling, W.T., et al. 1993. Evaluation of myocardial contractility in the chronically instrumented dog with intact autonomic nervous system function: Effects of desflurane and isoflurane. *Acta Anaesthesiol Scand* 37:203–210.

Pascoe, P.J., Ilkiw, J.E., and Fisher, L.D. 1997. Cardiovascular effects of equipotent isoflurane and alfentanil/isoflurane minimum alveolar concentration multiple in cats. *Am J Vet Res* 58:1267–1273.

Polis, I., Gasthuys, F., Van Ham, I., et al. 2001. Recovery times and evaluation of clinical hemodynamic parameters of sevoflurane, isoflurane and halothane anaesthesia in mongrel dogs. *J Vet Med A* 48: 401–411.

Preckel, B., Müllenheim, J., Hoff, J., et al. 2004. Haemodynamic changes during halothane, sevoflurane and desflurane anaesthesia in dogs before and after the induction of severe heart failure. *Eur J Anaesthesiol* 21:797–806.

Pypendop, B.H., and Ilkiw, J.E. 2004. Hemodynamic effects of sevoflurane in cats. *Am J Vet Res* 65: 20–25.

Souza, A.P., Guerrero, P.N.H., Nishimori, C.T., et al. 2004. Cardiopulmonary and acid-base effects of desflurane and sevoflurane in spontaneously breathing cats. *J Feline Med Surg* 7:95–100.

Stoelting, R.K., and Hillier, S.C. 2006. *Pharmacology and Physiology in Anesthetic Practice*, 4th ed. Philadelphia: Lippincott Williams & Wilkins.

Chapter 8
Local Anesthetic and Analgesic Techniques

Gwendolyn L. Carroll

Local anesthetic and analgesic techniques using local anesthetics, opioids, α_2-agonists, and phency-clidines are being increasingly utilized in small animal medicine and surgery. The early anesthesia texts thoroughly examined local anesthetic techniques. As "safer" injectable and inhalant techniques became available, the use of local anesthetic techniques declined in all except food animal surgery and equine lameness. When it became evident that local anesthetic techniques were important for balanced anesthesia and multimodal pain management they regained importance in small animal medicine and surgery. Analgesia may be provided locally with a peripheral block, epidurally or spinally, and systemically (Berde and Strichartz 2000).

Local anesthetics prevent conduction of electrical impulses along membranes of nerves and muscles at the site of administration (e.g., prevent "windup," the hyperexcitable state of the spinal cord resulting from the volley of afferent impulses originating from a noxious stimulus) (see Chapter 9). When administered systemically, local anesthetics may alter conduction along nerves in skeletal, smooth, and cardiac muscle; electrical impulses in the central nervous system (CNS) and peripheral nervous system and the specialized cardiac conduction system may be changed.

HISTORY

The first use of local anesthetic techniques in human medicine is remarkable due to its reemergence in the 21st century. In 1884, Karl Koller was keen to anesthetize and operate on the cornea. Morphine and chloral bromide were tried unsuccessfully. When Koller and Joseph Gartner instilled a cocaine solution into the conjunctival sac of a frog, the cornea could be operated without "reflex action or defense" from the frog (Vandam 2000). When the cocaine solution was placed underneath their own eyelids, the investigators were able to touch their corneas with the head of a pen. The results were reported and demonstrated at the Ophthalmological Congress at Heidelberg in 1884. Although the anesthetic and stimulant effects of the leaves of the *Erythroxylin* coca bush were known to South Americans many years earlier (Covino 1986), the discovery was credited to Koller's mentor, Sigmund Freud (Vandam 2000).

> The actions of local anesthetics have been known for over 100 years!

Topical 1% morphine sulfate TID was recently used to provide analgesia in eyes of dogs (not frogs) with corneal ulcers (Stiles et al. 2003). Blepharospasm decreased in the eyes of dogs that were treated with topical morphine. The dogs tolerated more corneal pressure, measured as tactile sensitivity using an esthesiometer (rather than a pen head). Healing was not affected by morphine. In a normal eye, morphine is not effective, which explains why Koller judged morphine an unsuccessful corneal analgesic in 1884. Stiles and others (2003) presented their findings in dogs at the American College of Veterinary Ophthalmologists in 2002. Similar results were obtained in rabbits and humans treated with topical morphine a few years earlier (Peyman et al. 1994).

Although peripheral opioids are not yet extensively used in local anesthetic techniques in veterinary medicine, they do offer some advantages over local anesthetics. Topical local anesthetics such as proparacaine are used extensively in ophthalmology to desensitize the cornea for diagnostics and surgery (e.g., debridement of corneal wounds) but are very epitheliotoxic. With chronic use, proparacaine will result in a nonhealing corneal ulcer. Importantly, topical morphine provided analgesia without impacting healing in dogs, rabbits, and humans (Peyman et al. 1994; Stiles et al. 2003). The use of opioids as single agents or to enhance analgesia from local anesthetics is discussed subsequently.

LOCAL ANESTHETICS

Local anesthetics generally have an aromatic ring (lipophilic) and an amide group (hydrophilic) connected by a hydrocarbon chain. If an ester link attaches the aromatic ring to the intermediate chain, the local anesthetic is an "amino ester" (e.g., procaine, chloroprocaine); if an amide links the aromatic ring and the intermediate chain, the local anesthetic is an "amino amide" (e.g., lidocaine, bupivacaine). Esters are less stable than amides. Esters are hydrolyzed by plasma cholinesterase and produce *para*-aminobenzoic acid (antigen responsible for some allergic reactions); amides are degraded in the liver and rarely result in allergic reactions. Lipid solubility, pK_a, and protein binding influence local anesthetic activity. The addition of epinephrine to a local anesthetic prolongs the duration of action. Because epinephrine also delays uptake, the local activity is enhanced and the potential for systemic toxicity is decreased. Local anesthetics with epinephrine should not be used in distal limbs or areas in which circulation may be compromised or in patients that may not tolerate epinephrine. An acidic pH is necessary for local anesthetics containing epinephrine since epinephrine is unstable in alkaline pH.

Due to compromise in circulation, local anesthetics with epinephrine should not be used in:
- Distal limbs, ears, or tails
- Areas with compromised circulation
- Patients that may not tolerate epinephrine

Alkalinization of local anesthetic solutions will shorten the onset, increase the amount of drug that is lipid soluble (available), increase the epidural spread of local anesthetics, and enhance the depth of sensory and motor blockade. Due to the low pH, administration of local anesthetics can be quite painful. The pain on injection is particularly important when dealing with young or aggressive patients.

Mixing sodium bicarbonate with local anesthetics was proposed in 1892 (Milner et al. 2000). The addition of sodium bicarbonate should make the injection more acceptable by normalizing the pH. With renewed interest and use of local anesthetics, alkalinizing the solutions is gaining popularity. Several different concentration ratios of sodium bicarbonate to local anesthetic are published; the dilution for cats and dogs is extrapolated from human medicine. For lidocaine, a 1 : 10 dilution of sodium bicarbonate (1 mEq/ml) to lidocaine (10 ml 1% or 2%) increases comfort without precipitation; 0.1 mEq/ml sodium bicarbonate to 20 ml of bupivacaine (0.5%) or 1 mEq/ml sodium bicarbonate to 29 ml of bupivacaine (0.25%) does not precipitate.

Alkalinization would be more easily accomplished and more readily accepted by practitioners if a standard dilution could be relied on to decrease the sting of local anesthetics without precipitation. To that end, seven local anesthetics (19 ml each of bupivacaine 0.5%, bupivacaine 0.25%, bupivacaine 0.125%, bupivacaine 0.5% plus 1 : 200,000 epinephrine, bupivacaine 0.25% plus 1 : 200,000 epinephrine, lidocaine 2% plus 1 : 200,000 epinephrine) were successfully mixed with 1 ml of sodium bicarbonate (Milner et al. 2000). Ropivacaine (the S-enantiomer of bupivacaine) solutions precipitated at both concentrations studied (0.75% and 1%).

One milliliter of sodium bicarbonate can be mixed with 19 ml of most common local anesthetics (e.g., 0.125% to 0.5% bupivacaine, 1% to 2% lidocaine) without precipitation to reduce sting and increase duration of action.

Due to the increase in pH, the addition of sodium bicarbonate to local anesthetics decreases the shelf-life. The stability of epinephrine in local anesthetics is dependent on an acidic pH, so the addition of sodium bicarbonate to local anesthetics containing epinephrine should be cautiously undertaken. The addition of sodium bicarbonate to commercial local anesthetic and epinephrine solutions has not been examined.

Lidocaine and bupivacaine solutions, the most commonly used local anesthetics in small animal medicine, are also commercially available as slow-release liposomes that prolong duration of action and decrease toxicity. The liposomes are vesicles with bilayers of phospholipids around an aqueous phase. These liposome preparations are being investigated to extend the duration of local anesthetic blocks in veterinary patients (Dodam et al. 2002), including epidural administration (Mashimo et al. 1992), and to increase compliance for intravenous catheterization (Flecknell et al. 1990; Fransson et al. 2002).

INDICATIONS FOR LOCAL ANESTHETIC OR ANALGESIC TECHNIQUES

As described earlier, local anesthesia results from administration of local anesthetics (e.g., lidocaine, bupivacaine) and refers to both afferent and efferent blockade. In conjunction with neuroleptic analgesia (e.g., fentanyl plus droperidol), local anesthesia may be sufficient for surgery. Local analgesia that results from the administration of many different analgesics (e.g., morphine, buprenorphine) refers to a decrease or loss of sensation without impacting motor function. Diminution of the sensory component of pain increases the pain threshold but is insufficient for surgery.

Local anesthesia and analgesia decrease the minimum alveolar concentration (MAC) of an inhalant and minimize the amount of injectable analgesic required. Local anesthetic and analgesic techniques are important components of balanced anesthesia and multimodal analgesia. The minimum local anesthetic concentration needed to produce nervous impulse blockade is the "Cm" (also referred to as "Cmin"). Each local anesthetic has its own Cm. A thorough discussion of various local anesthetics and a complete discussion of local anesthetic mode of operation are available for the interested reader (Stoelting and Hillier 2006; Berde and Strichartz 2000).

> Local anesthetic techniques decrease the MAC of inhalants and additional drugs needed for anesthesia and provide postoperative analgesia.

Local anesthetics decrease the intensity of postoperative pain beyond the expected duration of the local anesthetic. This probably occurs through the suppression of the hyperexcitable state of the nerve (e.g., windup), which may be responsible for maintaining a degree of postoperative pain. Opioids obtund windup, *N*-methyl-D-aspartic acid (NMDA) receptor antagonists (e.g., ketamine) reverse windup, and local anesthetics prevent windup.

> Local anesthetics decrease the intensity of postoperative pain beyond the expected duration of the local anesthetic.

GENERAL PRECAUTIONS

Although rare, complications specific to a particular local anesthetic technique will be covered with the technique. Some difficulties may be avoided by always calculating and never exceeding the maximum local anesthetic dose.

> Always calculate and never exceed the maximum local anesthetic dose.

Regardless of the technique or agent used, there are some cautions when contemplating using local anesthesia. For example, there is a certain failure rate (up to 20%) in a local anesthetic technique when everything is done correctly. Even experienced anesthetists should ensure analgesia is being provided by the technique because some local anesthetic techniques will fail. Local anesthetics are not efficacious in infected wounds.

> There is up to a 20% failure with local anesthetic techniques even when everything is done correctly.

Local anesthetics share CNS and cardiovascular (CV) toxicity. When local anesthetics are combined, the toxicity is additive. Local anesthetics that cross the placenta (e.g., lidocaine, bupivacaine) may precipitate "ion trapping" in a fetus with acidosis (prolonged labor).

Local anesthetics prevent nerve impulse transmission by inhibiting sodium ion passage through nonselective sodium channels in nerve membranes.

The rate of transmission is slowed such that threshold potential is not reached and the action potential is not propagated. At low concentrations, the sodium channel blockade likely contributes to the antiarrhythmic properties of local anesthetics. At higher plasma concentrations, cardiac impulses are slowed and automaticity is depressed; profound hypotension and negative inotropy may occur (Stoelting and Hillier 2006).

Accidental intravenous injection of bupivacaine may result in hypotension, arrhythmias, and atrioventricular block. Conditions that may increase toxicity of bupivacaine include pregnancy, concomitant therapy with β-adrenergic blockers, calcium channel blockers, digitalis, epinephrine, and phenylephrine. Cardiotoxicity of bupivacaine is enhanced in acidosis, hypoxemia, and hypercarbia (Stoelting and Hillier 2006).

Local Anesthetic Toxicity

In a classic study, Chadwick (1985) demonstrated the mean convulsive dose of lidocaine to be 11.7 ± 4.6 mg/kg IV and that of bupivacaine to be 3.8 ± 1.0 mg/kg IV in cats; the mean cardiotoxic dose was higher, although electrocardiographic changes occurred before EEG changes in both groups (only rarely in lidocaine group). The CV toxicity–to–CNS (CV/CNS) toxicity ratio in cats was 4.0 for lidocaine and 4.8 for bupivacaine. The resuscitation time was similar for both local anesthetics. Lidocaine may be used perineurally at 3 to 4 mg/kg in cats and 6 to 8 mg/kg in dogs; bupivacaine may be used perineurally at 0.5 to 1 mg/kg in cats and 1 to 2 mg/kg in dogs.

Acute CV toxicity (e.g., profound hypotension, decreased cardiac output and stroke volume) occurred in pentobarbital-anesthetized dogs receiving bupivacaine (10 mg/kg IV). Only moderate CV toxicity occurred in dogs receiving lidocaine (10 mg/kg IV). In dogs, the cumulative lethal dose of bupivacaine (20 mg/kg IV) and lidocaine (80 mg/kg IV) is proportional to their potency, indicating little difference in therapeutic ratio between the two (Liu et al. 1982).

> The *maximum* perineural dose of lidocaine that may be used is 3 to 4 mg/kg in cats and 6 to 8 mg/kg in dogs.

> The *maximum* perineural dose of bupivacaine which may be used is 0.5 to 1 mg/kg in cats and 1 to 2 mg/kg in dogs.

Most clinicians are familiar with the use of topical lidocaine to desensitize the larynx. Lidocaine is preferred over Cetacaine, which can cause methemoglobinemia in cats. The use of a eutectic mixture of local anesthetics (EMLA) cream consists of a mixture of lidocaine and prilocaine together with an emulsifier. The use of EMLA cream in cats has been reported (Flecknell et al. 1990). Although the EMLA cream substantially decreased pain and discomfort in cats in response to venipuncture, the cats did not care for the restraint or bandaging involved in its application. There is also concern that cats might be sensitive to prilocaine with a resulting methemoglobinemia. Transdermal liposome-encapsulated lidocaine contains only lidocaine as an active ingredient. After topical application of 15 mg/kg liposome-encapsulated lidocaine to healthy adult cats, maximum plasma concentrations were substantially below the toxic plasma concentrations for cats; therapeutic plasma concentrations were not reached but analgesia was not tested (Fransson et al. 2002). Plasma concentrations were variable and the median time to maximum concentration was 2 hours (Fransson et al. 2002). Bandaging will continue to be necessary to avoid oral and buccal absorption. Further clinical studies are needed before it can be recommended in cats.

AGENTS

Local Anesthetics

In addition to perineural use of lidocaine in cats and dogs, lidocaine may be given intravenously and is used as a constant rate infusion (CRI) for analgesia and to decrease MAC (20 to 30 μg/kg/min IV) and to treat arrhythmias (50 to 75 μg/kg/min IV) in dogs. Significant CV depression occurs in isoflurane-anesthetized cats administered a lidocaine CRI similar to that used in dogs. The use of lidocaine infusion to decrease MAC is not recommended in cats (Pypendop and Ilkiw 2005).

Intravenous regional anesthesia (IVRA) with lidocaine is useful for digit amputations, biopsies, and minor lacerations in the dog. This technique is appropriate for procedures below the hock in the hind limb and below the elbow in the forelimb. A tourniquet is applied to occlude arterial blood flow. Venipuncture (25-gauge needle or catheter) should be above the lesion and below the tourniquet. Ten minutes should be allowed before beginning surgery. The tourniquet should be slowly released, while observing an electrocardiogram for arrhythmias after release of the tourniquet. Potential complications include swelling and edema of the limb and peripheral nerve damage.

IVRA with lidocaine in isoflurane-anesthetized cats was recently investigated (Kushner et al. 2002). Leakage of lidocaine into the circulation occurred in four of six cats before tourniquet removal, but no adverse hemodynamic events occurred at the dose and tourniquet time studied. The temperament of cats does not allow IVRA without general anesthesia, which removes the primary advantage of IVRA (i.e., doing surgery without general anesthesia). Due to potential for toxicity and limited indications for IVRA in cats, routine use of IVRA in cats is not recommended.

Bupivacaine has more selectivity for afferent than efferent nerves and is believed to cause less motor dysfunction than many of the local anesthetics. Bupivacaine is available as a $50:50$ racemic mixture. Ropivacaine, the *S*-enantiomer of bupivacaine, was suspected to have less toxicity, which has not proved to be true. However, under no circumstances should bupivacaine or its isomers be given intravenously. Bupivacaine in larger than 1 mg/kg IV doses causes seizures and cardiac arrest. Resuscitation is difficult and prolonged and in animal studies only responded to massive amounts of epinephrine.

> Bupivacaine should not be administered IV!

Recently, mixing local anesthetics for administration has become popular. The rationale is that mixing a short- and a long-acting local anesthetic will provide the fast onset of the short-acting local anesthetic (e.g., lidocaine) and the duration of the long-acting local anesthetic (e.g., bupivacaine). Clinically, there does not appear to be an indication for this practice (Stoelting and Hillier 2006; Berde and Strichartz 2000).

As indicated earlier, several different drugs may be used in local anesthetic techniques. The class of drug (e.g., local anesthetic versus opioid) chosen will determine the effect of the technique (e.g., afferent and efferent blockade versus afferent only); the specific agent (e.g., lidocaine versus bupivacaine) will determine the onset and duration of effects. The indications, limitations, onset and duration, and side effects are agent-dependent. Bupivacaine is generally chosen for perioperative analgesia due to its long duration of action (about 6 hours) but requires at least 20 minutes of contact time. Lidocaine is chosen when a short duration of action (about 1 to 1.5 hours) is needed with a speedy onset (less than 5 minutes).

Procaine is an aminoester with intermediate onset (10 to 15 minutes) and a shorter duration of action (30 to 60 minutes) than lidocaine. Mepivacaine, etidocaine, and ropivacaine are amino amides with similar onset of activity to each other (5 to 10 minutes) but shorter than bupivacaine (10 to 20 minutes). Mepicavaine has a similar duration to lidocaine (90 to 180 minutes), whereas the duration of action of etidocaine and ropivacaine is similar to that of bupivacaine (180 to 300 minutes). There is no compelling evidence to change from lidocaine and bupivacaine at this time.

Analgesics

Opioids are the most commonly used analgesics in local analgesic techniques. Systemic and CNS effects result from epidural administration of opioids. The use of opioids in peripheral local anesthetic techniques is successful only if peripheral opioid receptors are present in the tissue. There are a few tissue beds in which opioid receptors have been demonstrated—synovium of the joint capsule and cornea; receptors have not been demonstrated in the abdominal or thoracic pleura. Opioid receptors may increase in inflammation, resulting in successful analgesic techniques using opioids in disease but perhaps not in health.

Some of the opioids used in local analgesic techniques (e.g., preservative-free morphine) have had the typical preservatives removed (in the case of morphine, formaldehyde, and formalin) in order to decrease tissue damage.[1] There are other preservatives that have not been implicated in tissue damage (e.g., methylparaben, propylparaben used in oxymorphone). There are some drugs that come in multidose vials preserved with methylparaben (e.g., hydromorphone) as well as preservative-free ampules. Depending on the concentration of the drug being administered, it may need to be diluted in order to increase the volume for good coverage.

LOCAL ANESTHETIC/ANALGESIC TECHNIQUES

Epidural Administration

Indications for epidurals include intraoperative management of high-risk patients, perioperative analgesia, cesarean section, caudal anesthesia/analgesia (perineum, hind limbs, tail, abdomen), and, depending on the agent chosen, thoracotomy and forelimb amputation. Specific contraindications for spinal/epidural drug administration include sepsis and hemorrhagic diathesis. If local anesthetics are used, volume depletion is a contraindication (pretreatment with fluids may improve response). There are some situations that require variations in the dose of local anesthetic drug administered epidurally. The dose of local anesthetic or opioid should be decreased in pregnancy, in geriatric patients, in obesity, and in patients with space-occupying lesions; the dose of local anesthetic or opioid should be halved if CSF fluid is encountered when performing an epidural.

> Decrease the dose of local anesthetic or opioid by half if CSF fluid is encountered when performing an epidural.

Avoid a head-down position when using a local anesthetic for an epidural. Remember, migration of local anesthetics follows gravity! A local anesthetic block to T1 leads to intercostal nerve paralysis and a block to C5–7 leads to phrenic nerve paralysis. Place the affected side down for several minutes after the epidural. General guidelines for volume of drug administered are that 0.3 ml/kg should not be exceeded. In the cat, 1.5 ml/cat, and in the dog, 6 ml/dog, are empiric volume guidelines.

> Volume depletion is a contraindication for a local anesthetic epidural; pretreatment with fluids may protect against peripheral pooling.

Infection and hemorrhage are potential complications of epidural technique (Table 8.1). The

Table 8.1. Potential side effects of epidural drug administration.

Side effects	Local anesthetics	Opioids
Central nervous system	Seizures only if toxic	Seizures unlikely unless over dose
Analgesia	Sensory and motor block	Sensory block
Cardiovascular	Only if toxic collapse; blood pressure due to sympathetic blockade	Bradycardia
Blood pressure	Hypotension; postural hypotension	Unlikely change
Pulmonary	If intercostal and phrenic nerve paralysis due to cranial migration	Respiratory depression (early due to systemic absorption and late due to cranial migration)
Drug-related side effects	Urinary retention (or rarely incontinence), hypotension, numbness, motor weakness, tachyphylaxis, systemic toxicity	Urinary retention, nausea, vomiting, pruritis, sedation
Treatment	Supportive until metabolized (see Table 8.3)	Antagonize with naloxone
Procedural side effects	Encephalitis, meningitis, hemorrhage; lack of hair regrowth; failure of the technique; paresthesia	

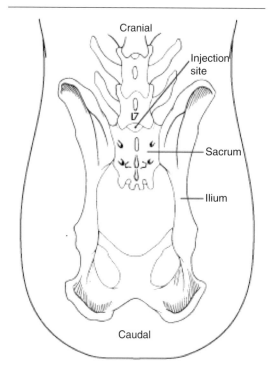

Figure 8.1. The dorsal view of the dog, with palpable landmarks: wings of the ilium, spinous process of L7, and the median sacral crest. (From Carroll, G.L. 1998. Performing selected regional techniques. In *Small Animal Pain Management*, pp. 103–112, Lakewood: AAHA Press.)

patient's hair may grow back slowly (8 of 72 dogs; Troncy et al. 2002). Also, the technique may fail, resulting in inadequate analgesia or anesthesia. Epidural administration of a local anesthetic can result in decreased heart rate, cardiac output, and blood pressure; postural hypotension can be expected. Local anesthetic administration at appropriate doses usually does not impair the respiratory system unless there is CV collapse. Local anesthetic administration results in sensory and motor blockade, while opioid administration results in only sensory blockade. Local anesthetic administration produces no or mild sedation; there can be convulsions with a toxic dose. There is a low incidence of nausea and vomiting, but there may be bladder dysfunction.

Minimal change in heart rate, cardiac output, or blood pressure can be expected from opioid administration at appropriate doses; the vasoconstrictor response is intact. Opioid administration may result in early respiratory depression due to systemic absorption. Late respiratory depression is due to opioid migration to the brain (6 to 24 hours) for opioids that are not lipid soluble. Opioid administration may cause marked sedation, nausea, vomiting, urinary retention, and pruritis. The side effects may be antagonized (e.g., naloxone).

EPIDURAL TECHNIQUE

Neuroleptanalgesia or general anesthesia is usually required to perform an epidural. Needed supplies include the following:

- Spinal needle (22 or 20 gauge, 1.5 to 3 in)
- Sterile gloves
- Appropriate dose and volume of epidural drug in a syringe
- Air and saline syringe (3 ml); glass offers the least resistance
- 3-ml syringe for 1 ml of 2% lidocaine and a 23-gauge needle to desensitize the skin (if patient is conscious)
- Fenestrated drape (eye drape)

The landmarks (i.e., the right and left cranial dorsal iliac spines, the spinous process of L7, and the median sacral crest) for performing an epidural are palpable (Fig. 8.1).

When performing an epidural in the conscious patient, after clipping and aseptic preparation of the skin, it is helpful to place a skin block with lidocaine (2%) in the subcutaneous tissues immediately dorsal to the lumbosacral space. The patient may be placed in lateral or sternal recumbency, but my preference is that the patient be in sternal recumbency with the rear limbs flexed and pulled cranially (opens the lumbosacral space). The needle should be inserted with the bevel directed appropriately (in the direction you want the drug to travel). Penetrate the skin on the dorsal midline, staying close to L7. Advance the needle through the subcutaneous tissues, the supraspinous ligament, the interspinous ligament, the ligamentum flavum, and into the epidural space. A "pop" or change in resistance to passage of the spinal needle is usually apparent as the ligamentum flavum is penetrated (Fig. 8.2).

Observe the hub of the needle for egress of blood or spinal fluid to check for correct needle placement. In the dog, the spinal cord variably ends at L6–7; the dural sac ends at L7–S1. In the cat, the cord and sac usually extend one vertebra more caudal (cord termination may be as caudal as S3), so dural punctures are more likely than in dogs. Gentle aspiration may be performed and no fluid should be detected if the needle is in the epidural space. There should be no resistance to an injection of air 0.5 ml or saline with a test syringe. If using a test syringe with air and saline, observe the meniscus for easy advancement of the liquid. The meniscus should not bounce (e.g., there should be no resistance). After the appropriate anesthetic or anal-

gesic is slowly injected, replace the stylet, remove the needle, and place the affected side down (for local anesthetics).

In large dogs, the hanging drop technique may also be used to perform an epidural. When performing the hanging drop technique, once the spinal needle has penetrated the skin, the stylet is removed. The hub of the needle is filled with saline and the needle advanced as described above. When the epidural space is penetrated, the saline in the needle hub will be drawn into the epidural space. If spinal fluid or blood is encountered, the saline will be spilled. Injection of the drug into the epidural space is similar to that described above.

There are several drugs currently used for epidural administration (Table 8.2). In general, the onset and duration of effect from epidurals is drug dependent.

Epidural Catheters

Prolonged analgesia may be accomplished by the use of epidural catheters. The risk from epidural catheter placement appears to be low. Commercial catheter trays are available. Skin preparation is similar to that for an epidural. A Touhy needle (Fig. 8.3) is used to facilitate catheter placement.

Once the positioning of the Toughy needle is confirmed by standard methods used for epidurals, the catheter may be placed through the needle. The desired length of catheter is estimated. The catheter should never be withdrawn through the needle! The catheter may be secured to the skin by suturing. Before each injection into the catheter, the catheter should be inspected for blood and CSF; gentle aspiration will guard against inadvertent intravenous or spinal injection. A filter should be used for injecting the contents of a glass vial into the catheter. A test dose, using a small amount of local anesthetic, is mandatory before each reinjection.

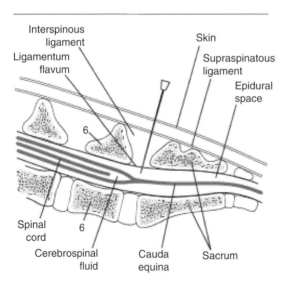

Figure 8.2. Layers of penetration for epidural administration: (1) skin, (2) supraspinatous ligament, (3) interspinous ligament, (4) ligamentum flavum, (5) epidural space, (6) intervertebral disc, (7) spinal cord, (8) cerebrospinal fluid, and (9) cauda equina. The needle should enter perpendicular to the skin. (From Carroll, G.L. 1998. Performing selected regional techniques. In *Small Animal Pain Management,* pp. 103–112, Lakewood: AAHA Press.)

An epidural catheter should never be withdrawn through the needle! Always inspect the catheter. Use a filter when injecting contents of a glass vial into an epidural catheter.

Table 8.2. Drug dosages for epidural* analgesia or anesthesia in dogs and cats.

Drug class	Drug	Dose†	Onset (min)‡	Duration (hr)‡
Opioid	Morphine§	Dog and cat: 0.1 mg/kg	20	20
	Hydromorphone§	Dog: 0.2 mg/kg; Cat: 0.1 mg/kg	15	10
	Fentanyl	Dog: 0.006 mg/kg; Cat: 0.004 mg/kg	15	6
	Oxymorphone‖	Dog and cat: 0.05–0.1 mg/kg	15	10
	Buprenorphine	Dog: 0.005 mg/kg	30	18
	Butorphanol	Dog and cat: 0.25 mg/kg	10	2–4
α_2-Agonists	Medetomidine	Dog and cat: 0.01 mg/kg	15	4
Local anesthetics	Lidocaine 2%¶	Dog: 1 ml/3.4 kg (T5); 1 ml/4.5 kg (L2)	10	1–1.5
		Cat: 1 ml/4.5 kg (T5)	2–10	0.75–1
	Bupivacaine 0.5%¶	Dog: 1 ml/4.5 kg	20–30	4.5–6
		Cat: 1 ml/7 kg	15–20	3–6

*Decrease the dose by half for spinal administration of local anesthetics; decrease the epidural dose in geriatric, obese, and pregnant animals, and animals with space occupying lesions of the spinal cord or conditions in which venous engorgement is expected.

†Volume should be below 0.3 ml/kg; do not exceed 6 ml/dog or 1.5 ml/cat (there are other volume recommendations; the author uses these).

‡When specific onset and duration of action are not known for veterinary patients, they are extrapolated from human literature or from the onset and duration of parenterally administered drugs.

§Preservative-free morphine (for example, Duramorph) should be used for epidural or spinal administration of morphine.

‖Oxymorphone is variably available.

¶Avoid head-down positioning of the patient after epidurals; a block to T_1 leads to intercostal paralysis, a block to C_5–C_7 leads to phrenic nerve paralysis.

Table modified from Carroll (1998).

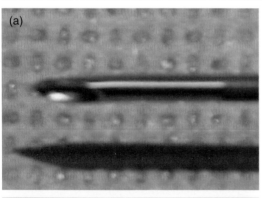

(a)

(b)

Figure 8.3. The Touhy needle is designed with a curved bevel (A) to direct the epidural catheter cranially. Similar to all epidural needles, the locking mechanism of the needle and stylet are on the same side as the bevel of the needle (B). The location of the bevel may be determined once you can no longer see the bevel (i.e., bevel is buried in tissue) by looking at the locking mechanism.

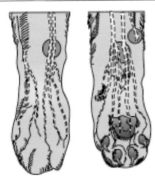

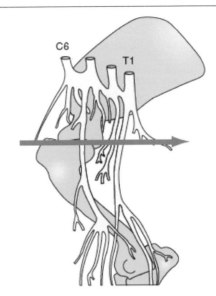

Figure 8.4. Three-point landmarks for onychectomy: The median and palmer branches of the ulnar nerve are blocked medial to the accessory carpal pad; the dorsal branch of the ulnar nerve is blocked lateral and proximal to the accessory carpal pad; and the superficial radial nerve branches are blocked at the dorsomedial aspect of the proximal carpus. (Reprinted from Carroll, G.L. 2007. Perioperative multimodal analgesic therapy. In *Essentials in Small Animal Surgery,* edited by T.W. Fossum, 3rd ed., pp. 130–145, New York: Elsevier Inc., with permission from Elsevier Inc.)

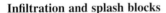

Figure 8.5. A brachial plexus block is accomplished by inserting a spinal needle at the point of the shoulder into the axillary area medial to the shoulder joint and lateral to the ribs. Direct the needle toward the costochondral junction and parallel to the vertebral column. (Reprinted from Carroll, G.L. 2007. Perioperative multimodal analgesic therapy. In *Essentials in Small Animal Surgery* edited by T.W. Fossum, 3rd ed., pp. 130–145, New York: Elsevier Inc., with permission from Elsevier Inc.)

Infiltration and splash blocks

Wound perfusion/infiltration are probably the simplest technique for providing wound analgesia. There is poor efficacy in infected wounds. Effective local infiltration can be used for incisional pain, nerve pain (amputation), onychectomy, and ear ablation. For example, a ring block, a splash block, or a more difficult distal block of the forepaw may be used for onychectomy.

ONYCHECTOMY

A ring block, in which the local anesthetic is instilled around the forelimb at the level of the carpus, is the easiest block to accomplish. A distal block of the forepaw involves blocking the distal radial, median, and dorsal and palmar branches of the ulnar nerve. Landmarks for accomplishing a three-point local anesthetic block for an onychectomy are illustrated in Figure 8.4. A splash block, one drop per toe of 0.5% bupivacaine delivered from a tuberculin syringe without a needle, admin-

istered prior to bandaging is probably the least reliable due to insufficient contact time.

Brachial Plexus and Related Nerve Blocks

Brachial plexus anesthesia is effective below the elbow region (radial, median, ulnar, musculocutaneous, and axillary nerves). To accomplish a brachial plexus block, insert a 22-gauge, 3-inch needle medial to the shoulder joint toward the costochondral junctions and parallel to the vertebral column. Aspirate and inject the local anesthetic as the needle is withdrawn (Fig. 8.5). A nerve stimulator may be used to find the brachial plexus but does not appear to be necessary for successful blockade. Bilateral simultaneous brachial plexus blocks will prohibit the patient from walking and is not recommended.

In patients undergoing amputation, the nerve may be directly visualized and injected with local anesthetic prior to incision. If both brachial plexus block (preemptive analgesia) and nerve stump injection (added analgesia) are performed, the dose of each should be adjusted to stay below the maximum dose.

MUMR Block

A modification of the brachial nerve block, a median, ulnar, musculocutaneous, and radial (MUMR) nerve block may also be used to desensitize the area below the elbow. These nerves can generally be palpated. The median, ulnar, and musculocutaneous nerves are blocked by injecting proximal to the medial epicondyle of the humerus between the biceps and the triceps (Fig. 8.6); the brachial artery can be palpated and the nerves are in proximity to the artery. Aspirate before injecting to avoid the brachial artery. The radial nerve is proximal to the lateral epicondyle between the brachialis and the triceps; inject below the triceps at approximately the same level injected for the other nerves (Fig. 8.6).

Nerve Blocks for Thoracotomy Pain

Management of thoracotomy pain can be accomplished with intercostal neural blockade and/or interpleural analgesia in addition to the use of systemic opioids. Patients undergoing thoracotomy, chest tube placement, or traumatic rib injury benefit from intercostal nerve blocks. Chest excursions increase and ventilation improves in thoracotomy patients as a result of pain control.

Intercostal Nerve Block Technique

For an intercostal block, the intercostal nerves supplying the incision site, two nerves cranial to the site, and two nerves caudal to the thoracotomy incision are selectively blocked (Fig. 8.7). Injections are made posterior to the ribs near the intervertebral foramen, being careful to avoid the artery and vein. Interpleural analgesia is an alternative to intercostal neural blockade for post-thoracotomy pain.

Interpleural Analgesia

Interpleural analgesia offers prolonged analgesia, without multiple needle sticks. Bupivacaine is

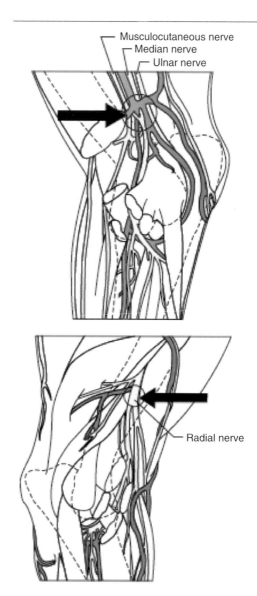

Figure 8.6. A median, ulnar, musculocutaneous, and radial (MUMR) nerve (n.) block. (*Top*) Medial aspect: The median, ulnar, and musculocutaneous n. are located by palpating proximal to the medial epicondyle of the humerus between the biceps and the triceps; the brachial artery can be palpated and the nerves are in proximity to the artery. (*Bottom*) Lateral view: To block the radial n., palpate proximal to the lateral epicondyle between the brachialis and the triceps at approximately the same level injected for the other nerves. (Reprinted from Carroll, G.L. 2007. Perioperative multimodal analgesic therapy. In *Essentials in Small Animal Surgery* edited by T. W. Fossum, 3rd ed., pp. 130–145, New York: Elsevier Inc., with permission from Elsevier Inc.)

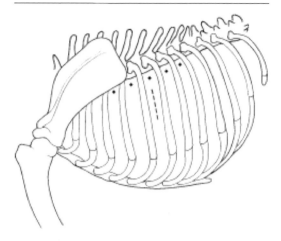

Figure 8.7. The intercostal nerve supplying the incision site, two nerves cranial to the site, and two nerves caudal to the thoracotomy incision are selectively blocked. (From Carroll, G.L. 1998. Treatment strategies for managing pain. In *Small Animal Pain Management*, pp. 31–52, Lakewood: AAHA Press.)

diluted with saline and instilled in the chest tube of the thoracotomy patient. The affected side is then placed down for 15 to 20 minutes. If the chest tube is left in place, additional bupivacaine can be placed postoperatively (every 6 to 8 hours). Remember that bupivacaine stings. Bupivacaine should only be administered through a chest tube to an awake patient (i.e., do not sneak up on a patient that is comfortably sleeping); interpleural injections should be made slowly. If the pericardium has been incised, the interpleural injection of local anesthetic should be avoided. If intercostal and interpleural blocks are both employed, the dose should be adjusted to stay below 2 mg/kg total dose. Potential complications of these techniques include pneumothorax, respiratory failure, and toxicity due to excessive drug administration.

Intra-articular Analgesia/Anesthesia

Intra-articular analgesia may be used instead of epidural analgesia for stifle surgery. Intra-articular morphine (0.1 mg/kg diluted with saline to 0.5 ml/kg of body weight) provides analgesia equivalent

to epidural morphine. Intra-articular bupivacaine (0.5% at 0.5 ml/kg) provides better analgesia than morphine in stifle surgery. Lower volumes (1 ml/4.5 kg) may be required. Sterile technique must be practiced.

Retrobulbar Nerve Block

Performing a retrobulbar nerve block prior to surgery of the globe will ensure that the eye position is appropriate without having to use paralytic agents or deepen the plane of anesthesia to a dangerous concentration.[2] An inferotemporal palpebral technique was described (Accola et al. 2006) and offers hope for surgeries in which neuromuscular blocking agents or appropriate monitoring equipment is not available.

Dental Nerve Blocks

Dental nerve blocks are indicated for patients undergoing tooth extraction, partial maxillectomy, or mandibulectomy. The most commonly used dental blocks include maxillary and mandibular blocks. A potential complication from local anesthetic dental blocks is self-mutilation due to loss of sensation to the tongue or lips. Avoiding bilateral blocks and using the smallest quantity (0.1 to 0.5 ml/site) of local anesthetic *may* help protect against damage.

INFRAORBITAL AND MAXILLARY TECHNIQUE

To perform an infraorbital nerve block, the landmark is the infraorbital foramen (Fig. 8.8). The nerves desensitized are the caudal maxillary alveolar nerve branch (caudal maxillary teeth), middle maxillary alveolar nerve (middle maxillary teeth), and rostral maxillary alveolar nerve (upper canine teeth and incisors). Be careful to avoid the infraorbital artery and vein. This block provides anesthesia to the ipsilateral canine teeth and incisors. In cats, the infraorbital foramen is not readily palpable. To locate the infraorbital nerve, the foramen is palpated between the dorsal border of the zygomatic process and the gingival of the canine tooth.

In order to desensitize the maxillary teeth without entering the infraorbital foramen, the area of the maxillary nerve may be injected before it enters the infraorbital foramen. To perform a maxillary nerve block, the landmarks are 1.5 cm caudal to the lateral

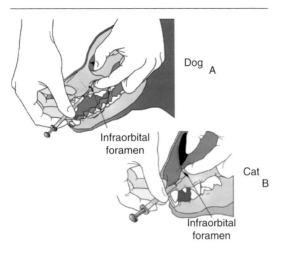

Figure 8.8. The infraorbital nerve (n.) may be palpated in the dog (*A*) by lifting the lip on the effected side and palpating the infraorbital foramen through the buccal mucosa above the upper third premolar. In cats (*B*), the infraorbital foramen is ventral to the eye at the junction of the zygomatic arch and maxilla; it is difficult to palpate. (Reprinted from Carroll, G.L. 2007. Perioperative multimodal analgesic therapy. In *Essentials in Small Animal Surgery* edited by T.W. Fossum, 3rd ed., pp. 130–145, New York: Elsevier Inc., with permission from Elsevier Inc.)

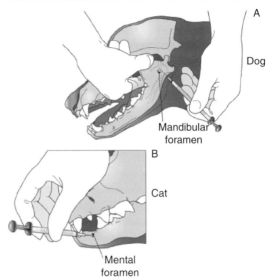

Figure 8.9. (*A*) Transcutaneous approach to the alveolar branch of the mandibular nerve (n.) is illustrated in a dog. The block may be accomplished by orally palpating the medial mandibular foramen with one hand and introducing the needle through the skin with the other. (*B*) The distal alveolar branch of the mandibular n. may be located by exposing the gum and inserting a needle rostral to the middle mental foramen, which is ventral to the first and second premolar teeth as demonstrated in a cat. (Reprinted from Carroll, G.L. 2007. Perioperative multimodal analgesic therapy. In *Essentials in Small Animal Surgery* edited by T.W. Fossum, 3rd ed., pp. 130–145, New York: Elsevier Inc., with permission from Elsevier Inc.)

cantus of the eye, ventral to the zygomatic arch, and rostral to the ramus. From 0.5 to 1 ml of local anesthetic (calculate maximum dose for each patient) may be injected after aspirating.

MANDIBULAR AND MENTAL NERVE BLOCKS

In order to perform a proximal block of the alveolar branch of the mandibular nerve (Fig. 8.9), the landmark that must be found is the mandibular foramen, which is on the medial aspect of the mandible just rostral to the angle of the mandible. It may be palpated inside the mouth caudal to the last molar. The cheek teeth, canine, incisors, skin, and lower lip are desensitized. The nerve may be blocked transorally or transcutaneously. In the cat, the needle is inserted percutaneously at the lower angle of the mandible approximately one cm rostral to the angular process. The needle is advanced along the medial surface of the mandible for about 0.5 cm. When contemplating a mandibular nerve block, a local splash block may be most satisfactory because

it will provide analgesia without self-mutilation (even though preemptive analgesia will not be provided).

To perform a distal alveolar branch of the mandibular nerve, palpate the middle mental foramen (Fig. 8.9). The lower lip and lower dental arcade are blocked. The middle mental foramen is ventral to the first and second premolar teeth.

MISCELLANEOUS TECHNIQUES

As described earlier, a unique local anesthetic technique in dogs with unremitting pain is a lidocaine infusion at $20 \mu g/kg/min$ IV in conjunction with other pain relief techniques. This technique is not recommended for cats.

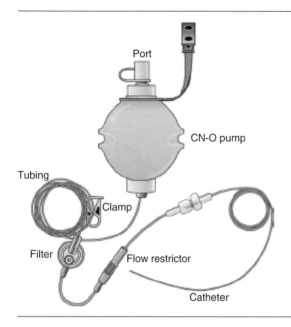

Port

CN-O pump

Tubing

Clamp

Filter

Flow restrictor

Catheter

Figure 8.10. PainBuster for intralesional administration of local anesthetic in orthopedic or soft tissue surgery. (Reprinted from Carroll, G.L. 2007. Perioperative multimodal analgesic therapy. In *Essentials in Small Animal Surgery,* edited by T. W. Fossum, 3rd ed., pp. 130–145, New York: Elsevier Inc., with permission from Elsevier Inc.)

Table 8.3. Drugs and dosages relevant for local anesthetic overdose.

Symptom	Drug	Dosage	Caution
Seizures	Diazepam	0.5–1 mg/kg IV	Monitor closely
	Phenobarbital sodium	6 mg/kg IV q 6–12 hr	
Arrhythmias: ventricular tachyarrhythmias	Bretylium	2–6 mg/kg IV	
	Procainamide	5–10 mg/kg IV, then 20–50 µg/ kg/min IV	May cause hypotension
Sinus bradyarrhythmia	Atropine	0.02–0.04 mg/kg IV	
	Glycopyrrolate	0.005–0.011 mg/kg IV	
Hypotension	Dobutamine	2–10 µg/kg/min IV	Monitor urine output
	Dopamine	2–10 µg/kg/min IV	
	Vasopressin	0.25–1.0 mU/kg/min IV	
Dyspnea	*N*-Acetylcysteine	140 mg/kg diluted to 5% in 5% dextrose or H_2O, PO then 70 mg/kg PO q 4 hr	
	Oxygen	See Chapter 3	
	Oxyglobin	10–15 ml/kg IV at 1–5 ml/kg/ hr IV	Low end of dose and rate for cats
Methemoglobinemia	Methylene blue	4 mg/kg, dog	Controversial in cats due to Heinz body formation
	Vitamin C	20 mg/kg IM or 125 mg PO BID	
Hypovolemia	Crystalloids, colloids	See Chapter 11	

From Welch (2000).

There are various continuous administration pumps available for local anesthetic administration. Intralesional and intraarticular infusion pumps (e.g., PainBuster; dj Orthopedics, LLC; Fig. 8.10) are systems providing continuous infusion of a local anesthetic directly into the surgical wound. Their effectiveness in veterinary patients has not yet been established. The main advantage to this system is that it can be used in outpatient surgery. When performing local anesthetic blocks, the maximum dose for each species should not be exceeded.

TREATMENT OF OVERDOSE

In case of an overdose, treat underlying CNS, CV problems (e.g., methemoglobinemia, seizures, dyspnea, hypotension, dysrhythmias, vomiting, cyanosis, tachypnea) (Table 8.3). If the symptoms are due to opioid or α_2-agonist overdose, consider antagonizing the opioid or α_2-agonist. If the patient is supported while the drugs are metabolized, recovery should occur. In humans, CV bypass is recommended if needed to allow sufficient time for recovery.

ENDNOTES

1 Not all anesthesiologists agree that preservative-free formulations are needed for epidural administration. Although clinically significant reactions are uncommon, the severity of CNS signs associated with pre-servative-induced changes is so great, this author prefers to use preservative free formulations.
2 Previously, methoxyflurane in oxygen was used for ocular surgeries due to the amount of muscle relaxation that resulted from methoxyflurane.

REFERENCES

Accola, P.J., Bentley, E., Smith, L.J., et al. 2006. Development of a retrobulbar injection technique for ocular surgery and analgesia in dogs. *J Am Vet Med Assoc* 229:220–226.

Berde, C.B., and Strichartz, C.R. 2000. Local anesthetics. In *Anesthesia,* edited by R.D. Miller, 5th ed., pp. 491–521. Philadelphia: Churchill Livingstone.

Chadwick, H.S. 1985. Toxicity and resuscitation in lidocaine- or bupivacaine-infused cats. *Anesthesiology* 63:385–390.

Covino, B.G. 1986. Pharmacology of local anaesthetic agents. *Br J Anaesth* 58:701–716.

Dodam, J.R., Boedeker, B., Gross, M., et al. 2002. Phospholipid-encapsulated bupivacaine and analgesia after onychectomy in cats. *Vet Anaesth Analg* 29(2):101.

Flecknell, P.A., Liles, J.H., and Williamson, H.A., 1990. The use of lignocaine-prilocaine local anesthetic cream for pain-free venepuncture in laboratory animals. *Lab Anim* 24:142–146.

Fransson, B.A., Peck, K.E., Smith, J.K., et al. 2002. Transdermal absorption of a liposome-encapsulated formulation of lidocaine following topical administration in cats. *Am J Vet Res* 63(9):1309–1312.

Kushner, L.I., Fan, B., and Shofer, F.S. 2002. Intravenous regional anesthesia in isoflurane anesthetized cats: Lidocaine plasma concentrations and cardiovascular effects. *Vet Anaes Anal* 29:140–149.

Liu, P., Feldman, H.S., Covino, B.M., et al. 1982. Acute cardiovascular toxicity of intravenous amide local anesthetics in anesthetized ventilated dogs. *Anesth Anal* 61:317–322.

Mashimo, T., Uchida, I., Pak, M., et al. 1992. Prolongation of canine epidural anesthesia by liposome encapsulation of lidocaine. *Anesth Anal* 74:827–834.

Milner, Q.J.W., Guard, B.C., and Allen, J.G. 2000. Alkalinization of amide local anesthetics by addition of 1% sodium bicarbonate solution. *Eur J Anaesth* 17:38–42.

Peyman, G.A., Rahimy, M.H., and Fernandes, M.L. 1994. Effects of morphine on corneal sensitivity and epithelial wound healing: Implications for topical ophthalmic analgesia. *Br J Ophthalmol* 78:138–141.

Pypendop, B.H., and Ilkiw, J.E. 2005. Assessment of the hemodynamic effects of lidocaine administered IV in isoflurane-anesthetized cats. *Am J Vet Res* 66:661–668.

Stiles, J., Honda, C.N., Krohne, S.G., et al. 2003. Effect of topical administration of 1% morphine sulfate solution on signs of pain and corneal wound healing in dogs. *Am J Vet Res* 64:813–818.

Stoelting, R.K., and Hillier, S.C. 2006. *Pharmacology and Physiology in Anesthetic Practice,* 4th ed. Philadelphia: Lippincott Williams & Wilkins.

Troncy, E., Keroack, S., Sammut, V., et al. 2002. Results of preemptive epidural administration of morphine with or without bupivacaine in dogs and cats undergoing surgery: 265 Cases (1997–1999). *J Am Vet Med Assoc* 221:662–672.

Vandam, L.D. 2000. History of anesthetic practice. In *Anesthesia,* edited by R.D. Miller, 5th ed., pp. 1–11. Philadelphia: Churchill Livingstone.

ADDITIONAL READING

Carroll, G.L. 2007. Perioperative multimodal analgesic therapy. In *Essentials in Small Animal Surgery* edited by T.W. Fossum, 3rd ed., pp. 130–145, New York: Elsevier.

Carroll, G.L. 1998a. Treatment strategies for managing pain. In *Small Animal Pain Management*, pp. 31–52, Lakewood: AAHA Press.

Carroll, G.L. 1998b. Performing selected regional techniques. In *Small Animal Pain Management*, pp. 103–112, Lakewood: AAHA Press.

Day, T.K., Pepper, W.T., Tobias, T.A., et al. 1995. Comparison of intra-articular and epidural morphine for analgesia following stifle arthrotomy in dogs. *Vet Surg* 24(6):522–530.

Welch, S.L. 2000. Local anesthetic toxicosis. *Vet Med* 95:670–673.

Chapter 9
Analgesia

Phillip Lerche and William Muir

Pain in animals can be defined as an aversive sensory and emotional experience (a perception) that elicits protective motor actions, results in learned avoidance, and may modify species-specific traits of behavior, including social behavior (Morton et al. 2005). Pain is thus a complex experience, which, although exhibiting stereotypical physiologic and behavioral responses within a species (predator versus prey), is different for every individual. The experience of pain includes detection of tissue injury by the nervous system (*nociception*), conscious perception of pain, behavior modification, and variable degrees of sickness and suffering in response to pain.

Pain serves an important role in the interaction between the individual animal and its environment in that it signals the potential for tissue damage and thus is protective in nature. This type of short-lived pain, where no or minimal tissue injury occurs, is referred to as *physiologic pain*. Pain that occurs following tissue injury is referred to as *pathologic pain*. Pathologic pain sensation may be also be experienced in the absence of a noxious stimulus (*spontaneous pain*), in response to a normally innocuous stimulus (*allodynia*), or as an exaggerated response to a noxious stimulus (*hyperalgesia*). Pathologic pain is somewhat arbitrarily divided based on duration into acute (hours) and chronic (days to years).

It is helpful to determine the mechanism, origin, and severity of pain, as this may help in determining treatment options. The mechanism of pain may be due to inflammation, nerve injury, cancer, or idiopathic. Pain may be *visceral* (organ pain, such as peritonitis) or *somatic* (superficial, such as skin laceration) or deep (e.g., tibia fracture). Some diseases or surgeries may result in more than one of these types of pain (e.g. ovariohysterectomy will have components of somatic and visceral pain).

PAIN PHYSIOLOGY

Nociception consists of *transduction* (transformation of noxious stimuli into electrical signals called action potentials), *transmission* (sensory impulses are conducted to the spinal cord), *modulation* (impulse amplification or suppression within the spinal cord), *projection* (impulses are transmitted to the brain), and *perception* (integration, processing and recognition of nociceptive information). In the absence of tissue damage, this process is somewhat "hard-wired" or static and is characterized by a basic stimulus-response pattern. If the stimulus is persistent or tissue injury occurs, this process becomes dynamic.

Transduction of noxious stimuli (mechanical, chemical, and thermal) is mediated by Aδ (myelinated) and C (unmyelinated) fibers peripherally. Aδ fibers mediate the fast onset sharp pain (*first pain*), whereas C fibers are responsible for longer-lasting, burning pain (*second pain*) that follows. Visceral nociceptors are more sensitive to distension, volvulus, and ischemic injury. NSAIDs, opioids, local anesthetics, and corticosteroids can inhibit transduction.

Transmission of painful stimuli from peripheral nociceptors to the spinal cord occurs via primary afferent sensory nerve fibers. The cell bodies of these afferents are located in the dorsal root ganglia of the spinal nerves; sensory axons extend from there to synapse with neurons in the dorsal horn of the grey matter of the spinal cord. Local anesthetics and α_2-agonists can block transmission of nociceptive impulses.

Modulation of impulses occurs in the spinal cord. Impulses can be amplified or suppressed by excitatory or inhibitory interneurons. Sensory neurons in the dorsal horn are either wide-dynamic-range neurons that receive input from all sensory nerves and are sensitive to low- and high-threshold sensory input or neurons that process high-threshold specific nociceptive information. Neurotransmitters that are important at this level of the nociceptive pathway include amino acids (glutamate, aspartate), prostaglandins (PGE_2), and peptides (substance P, neurokinin A). Local anesthetics, opioids, α_2-agonists, NSAIDs, *N*-methyl-D-aspartate receptor (NMDA) antagonists, tricyclic antidepressants, and anticonvulsants all inhibit modulation of nociceptive information.

Projection of impulses from the dorsal horn to the brain occurs via nerve tracts. The spinothalamic tract ascends to the thalamus. The spinoreticular tract projects to the reticular formation and thalamus. The spinomesencephalic tract terminates in the periaqueductal gray matter, limbic system, and hypothalamus of the midbrain; the spinohypothalamic tract ascends to the forebrain and hypothalamus.

Perception is the integration and processing of nociceptive information in the brain to produce a response via descending tracts in the spinal cord. Responses transmitted from the brain to inhibitory neurons in the dorsal horn of the spinal cord can stimulate inhibitory neurons. Removal of this descending inhibitory activity, or disinhibition, can increase pain via decreased endogenous opioid release.

The areas of the brain involved in perception are the periaqueductal gray matter, the reticular activating system, and the thalamus. Anesthetic agents, opioids, α_2-agonists, benzodiazepines, and phenothiazines may alter perception.

CONSEQUENCES OF UNTREATED PAIN

Pathologic pain has multiple consequences for the patient. These unwanted consequences include but are not limited to physiologic adaptations, sickness syndrome, the development of chronic pain and dynamic changes to the nervous system, undesirable neuroendocrine responses, stress, discomfort, debilitation, and suffering.

Tissue damage resulting in sustained noxious stimulation of the central nervous system (CNS) can dynamically and profoundly alter the function of neurons and pathways involved in pain. This alteration is known as CNS plasticity and can result in hypersensitivity in both acute and chronic pain.

Both peripheral and central neurons show plasticity. Tissue trauma results in release of cellular mediators (ATP, H+, K+, prostaglandins, leukotrienes) from damaged cells and also attracts inflammatory cells, which in turn release additional mediators (serotonin, histamine, cytokines). These and other mediators (nerve growth factor, substance P) form a "sensitizing soup" that increases the sensitivity (lowers the threshold) of nociceptors. Centrally, dorsal horn neurons that are stimulated by constant nociceptive input (*temporal summation*) become hyperexcitable and sensitive to low-intensity stimuli. This is partially mediated via unblocking of NMDA receptors and leads to CNS hypersensitivity, a phenomenon also referred to as "windup."

Pain also causes sympathetic stimulation leading to vasoconstriction, increased myocardial work, and increased myocardial oxygen consumption. Skeletal muscle blood flow tends to increase, whereas blood flow to the gastrointestinal and urinary tracts decreases.

Neurohumoral changes that occur in response to pain include but are not limited to release of ACTH, elevation in cortisol, norepinephrine and epinephrine, and decrease in insulin. This results in a catabolic state and signifies a strong stress response. This stress response is important for immediate survival but, if left unchecked, can lead to increased morbidity and mortality. Prolonged stress also leads to immunosuppression.

Distress is an extreme form of stress, and it occurs when stressors negatively affect the animal's physiology and behavior, which includes pain. By definition, an animal that is enduring pain is suffering. Additionally, painful patients may be reluctant or unable to eat with resultant wasting and may also suffer from insomnia. Many of these symptoms are also seen with the *sickness response*, the body's reaction to inflammation that is mediated by the immune system (Watkins and Maier 2000). Additional symptoms of this syndrome include fever and hyperalgesia. This exaggerated pain response is mediated by proinflammatory cytokines, which have been shown to alter nervous tissues at all stages involved in conveying pain information from the periphery to the brain.

The quality of an animal's life can be difficult to clearly define and is probably best expressed by the "five freedoms" (Table 9.1).

Veterinary professionals are in a unique position to improve the quality of their patients' lives in that they can alleviate animal pain and suffering, and this should be a goal when treating each individual patient.

RECOGNIZING THE PAINFUL PATIENT

Unlike adult people, animals cannot verbally express their pain. Recognition of animal pain therefore relies heavily on observation of behavior, which assumes an appropriate understanding of normal patient behavior both in and out of the hospital.

> Pets may not exhibit behavioral signs of pain in the presence of people.

Physiologic Response to Pain

Assessment of physiologic responses to pain is also important, with the understanding that some patients, especially those with chronic pain, will be painful and, aside from the endocrine system, will not show major changes in physiologic parameters (Table 9.2). Furthermore, they may not exhibit behavioral signs of pain in the presence of people.

Recognition of pain in animals may be very challenging as there is no single parameter that is a specific indicator of pain. Although it is important to avoid *anthropomorphizing* (projecting complex human emotions onto animals), pain perceptions in animals and people have common characteristics, so our own human experiences may guide us when determining whether a disease or procedure is likely to be painful.

Expectations

> Expectations may be used to provide preemptive analgesia but should not be used to deny analgesic therapy.

Many disease processes and surgical procedures are associated with moderate to severe pain (Table 9.3). Pain management may be initiated for these types of patients when they present (e.g., cancer pain) or prior to surgery. Preemptive analgesia, the administration of pain medication before pain occurs (e.g., prior to injury, surgery), reduces the requirement for analgesics and the duration of analgesic administration postoperatively. Preemptive analgesia also helps to prevent "windup" and central sensitization, which leads to pain that is chronic and more difficult to manage. Utilizing several drugs with different mechanisms of action, or multimodal therapy, also helps to prevent "windup."

> Multimodal analgesia provides pain relief using different classes of drugs in order to minimize the side effects of each.

Behavioral Responses

Behavioral responses to pain vary depending on species, age, breed, personality, and the nature,

Table 9.1. The five freedoms.

Freedom from hunger and thirst
Freedom from discomfort
Freedom from disease
Freedom from injury
Freedom from pain

Table 9.2. Physiologic changes associated with pain.

Cardiovascular	Hypertension
	Tachycardia
	Peripheral vasoconstriction
Respiratory	Tachypnea
	Shallow breathing (abdominal or thoracic guarding)
	Exaggerated abdominal component panting
	Open-mouth breathing
Ophthalmic	Mydriasis
Neuroendocrine	Elevated serum cortisol
	Elevated serum epinephrine and norepinephrine

Table 9.3. Some medical and surgical conditions that are known to be painful.

Painful medical conditions	Arthritis
	Otitis
	Cancer and metastasis
	Dermatitis
	Pancreatitis
	Peritonitis
	Cystitis
	Pleuritis
Painful surgical conditions	Cervical intervertebral disc disease
	Pancreatitis
	Fracture repair
	Total hip replacement
	Tibial plateau leveling osteotomy (TPLO)
	Total ear canal ablation
	Bulla surgery
	Rhinotomy
	Polytrauma with soft tissue (muscle) injury
	Corneal surgery
	Thoracotomy
	Gastric dilatation/volvulus

duration, and severity of pain. Younger patients are less likely to tolerate pain and more likely to vocalize, whereas older animals may be more stoic and are more likely to become aggressive. Certain breeds of dog appear to have lower pain thresholds (examples include toy breeds, Siberian Husky, Greyhound). Remember that certain individuals, regardless of breed or age, may be less tolerant of pain.

It may be useful to observe patient behavior when people are not present (e.g., via remote camera or one-way window), although this is more difficult to do in a busy hospital setting. Many animals change their behavior when a human observer is watching the patient, when a person interacts verbally with a patient, and, finally, when the patient undergoes physical examination. A thorough assessment of pain-related behavior can thus be time-consuming, although decreasing the time devoted to the assessment may result in subtle changes being overlooked. A complete history including owner observations of their pet's behavior is important when assessing subtle alterations in behavior associated with chronic pain. The short-term stress experienced by an animal during a visit to the veterinarian is often enough to mask overt as well as subtle signs of pain.

Changes in gait and locomotor activity such as limping, stiffness, and reluctance to move are all indicators of limb pain. A decrease in exercise tolerance may also indicate the presence of limb pain. Dogs that will not walk as far as their owners report they usually do may be suffering from arthritis. The most common symptom in cats with arthritis has been shown to be reluctance to jump as high or as often as before, rather than lameness, and this can lead to weight loss in cats fed on the counter (Clarke and Bennett 2006). A reluctance to lie down is an indicator of thoracic or abdominal pain. Patients may stand, sit, or adopt a prayer position rather than lie down, eventually becoming exhausted. Frequent changes in body position may indicate that an animal cannot find a comfortable position, which may be due to pain. Some animals will demonstrate "incident" pain. In other words, pain may not always be present (e.g., the patient is comfortable when lying down and does not exhibit pain-associated behaviors) but can be elicited by an event such as palpation or manipulation of a joint or being forced to walk or run.

Vocalization is frequently associated with pain. Dogs tend to whine, growl, whimper, and groan. They may snarl or bite if palpation is painful. Cats are more likely to groan, growl, and purr. They may also bite or hiss if direct manipulation causes pain. Vocalization is common in the immediate postoperative period and may be due to emergence delirium. Emergence delirium may be differentiated from pain by the fact that the vocalization is typically short-lived and responds to sedation.

Facial expressions, appearance, and attitude may all be altered in painful patients. Common facial expressions encountered in painful dogs are a glazed or fixed stare. Cats may squint and have a furrowed brow. Painful animals do not groom themselves, leading to an unkempt appearance. Hospitalized patients may sit staring at the back of the cage, oblivious to their surroundings and unwilling to interact or not interested in interacting. Painful cats will attempt to hide by moving as far from view as possible, a form of escape behavior, and will often become unresponsive to people. Aggression is most commonly observed with severe acute pain that is present on palpation or manipulation (Figs. 9.1 through 9.5 give examples expressions of pain by pets).

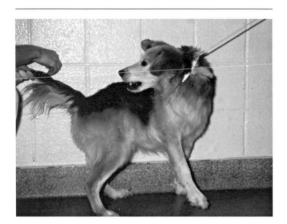

Figure 9.1. Aggressive behavior in response to touch. This dog was exquisitely sensitive (hyperalgesia) to light touch of the tail.

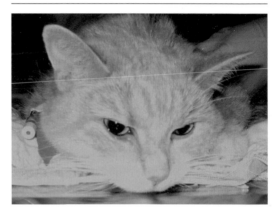

Figure 9.3. Fixed stare and glazed eyes with slight squint on one side. This cat was painful following resection of a fibrosarcoma that involved the dorsal spinous processes of several thoracic vertebrae.

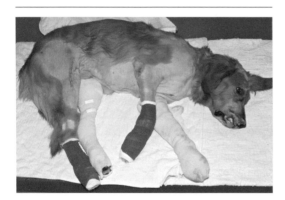

Figure 9.2. Reluctance to move and interact and dull facial expression. This dog was dragged behind a car and suffered injuries to all four limbs.

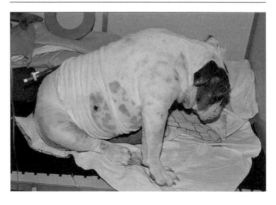

Figure 9.4. Reluctance to lie down, not interactive, and staring at cage wall. Post-thoracotomy (ventral midline approach), this dog would not lie down, eventually becoming exhausted from lack of sleep.

PAIN ASSESSMENT TOOLS

Several pain assessment tools have been developed for use in animals, including verbal rating scales, simple descriptive scales, numeric rating scales, and visual analogue scales.

Verbal rating and simple descriptive scales (Fig. 9.6) rate pain as absent, mild, moderate, or severe. In general, each one of these categories would imply a different approach to treatment. This type of scale is simple and easy to use, giving a rapid assessment. However, subtle changes may be missed.

Numeric rating scales assign point values in various categories, such as physiologic parameters, locomotor activity, vocalization, and so on. Due to the nature of pain-related changes in physiology and behavior, no scale of this type is ever inclusive, and in general they are simplified to make them useful.

A visual analogue scale consists of a ruler where the left side of the line equates to no pain, and the right end of the line, to worst pain imaginable (Fig. 9.9). An observer then places a mark on the ruler corresponding to the amount of pain he or she feels the animal is experiencing.

A more comprehensive tool to assess pain behavior in dogs is the Glasgow University Composite Pain Scale (Fig. 9.7) (Holton et al. 2001). This uses silent observation of, vocal interaction with, and, finally, palpation of the patient. This type of scale is more time consuming, and this particular scale does not produce a pain score.

The University of Melbourne Pain Scale also assesses behavioral changes and assigns scores to the various descriptors (Fig. 9.8) (Firth et al. 1999).

At The Ohio State University Veterinary Teaching Hospital, a one-page pain assessment form is used to categorize and evaluate patient pain (Fig. 9.9).

A questionnaire assessing quality of life for dogs in chronic pain (degenerative joint disease) has recently been validated (Wiseman-Orr et al. 2006). Dog owners selected from negative and positive descriptors in 13 domains: activity, comfort, appetite, extroversion-introversion, aggression, anxiety, alertness, dependence, contentment, consistency, agitation, posture-mobility, and compulsion. A questionnaire for evaluating quality of life in dogs with cancer-related pain has also been validated (Yazbek et al. 2005).

Pain scales generally produce a number, where a higher number indicates more pain. Suffice to say, each type of assessment has its limitations. For example, the least complex scales allow quicker assessment but may not be as effective at detecting subtle changes. However, they all share the common purpose of determining how painful the animal is as well as helping to assess response to treatment. Pain scales are also more accurate, and therefore

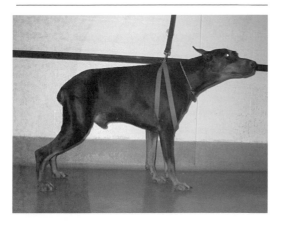

Figure 9.5. Abnormal neck and head posture. This dog's neck was extremely painful due to cervical intervertebral disc disease. Courtesy Dr. J. Dyce.

No pain	
Mild pain	
Moderate pain	
Severe pain	

Figure 9.6. Simple descriptive pain scale.

The questionnaire is made up of a number of sections each of which has several possible answers. Please tick the answers that you feel are appropriate to the dog you are assessing. If more than one answer is appropriate then tick all that apply. Approach the kennel, ensure you are not wearing a laboratory coat or surgical scrubs as the dog may associate these with stress and/or pain. While you approach the kennel look at the dog's behavior and reactions. From outside the dog's kennel look at the dog's behavior and answer the following questions.

Look at the dog's posture, does it seem...

    Rigid ☐
    Hunched or tense ☐
    Neither of these ☐

Does the dog seem to be...

    Restless ☐
    Comfortable ☐

If the dog is vocalizing is it...

    Crying or whimpering ☐
    Groaning ☐
    Screaming ☐
    Not vocalizing/none of these ☐

If the dog is paying attention to its wound is it...

    Chewing ☐
    Licking or looking or rubbing ☐
    Ignoring its wound ☐

Now approach the kennel door and call the dog's name. Then open the door and encourage the dog to come to you. From the dog's reaction to you and its behavior when you are watching it assess its character.

Does the dog seem to be...

    Aggressive ☐
    Depressed ☐
    Disinterested ☐
    Nervous or anxious or fearful ☐
    Quiet or indifferent ☐
    Happy and content ☐
    Happy and bouncy ☐

Now look at the dog's response to stimuli. If the mobility assessment is possible then open the kennel and put a lead on the dog. If the animal is sitting down encourage it to stand and then come out of the kennel. Walk slowly up and down the area outside the kennel. If the dog was standing up in the kennel and has undergone a procedure which may be painful in the perianal area, ask the animal to sit down.

During this procedure did the dog seem...

    Stiff ☐
    Slow or reluctant to rise or sit ☐
    Lame ☐
    None of these ☐
    Assessment not carried out ☐

Figure 9.7. Glasgow University Composite Pain Scale. From: Holton, L., Reid, J., Scott, E.M. et al. 2001. Development of a behaviour-based scale to measure acute pain in dogs. *Veterinary Record*, 148: 525–531.

Continued

The next procedure is to assess the dog's response to touch. If the animal has a wound, apply gentle pressure to the wound using two fingers in an area approximately 2 inches around it. If the wound is impossible to touch, then apply pressure to the closest point to the wound. If there is no wound then apply the same pressure to the stifle and surrounding area.

When touched did the dog…

Cry	☐
Flinch	☐
Snap	☐
Growl or guard wound	☐
None of these	☐

Figure 9.7. *Continued*

The pain scale includes 6 categories. Each category contains descriptors of various pain behaviors that are assigned numeric values. The assessor examines the descriptors in each category and decides whether a descriptor approximates the dog's behavior. If so, the value for that descriptor is added to the patient's pain score. Certain descriptors are mutually exclusive (e.g. a dog cannot be in sternal recumbency and standing up at the same time). These mutually exclusive descriptors are grouped together with the notation "choose only one." For category 4, mental status, the assessor must have completed a preprocedural assessment of the dog's dominant/aggressive behavior to establish a baseline score. The mental status score is the absolute difference between preprocedural and postprocedural scores. The minimum possible total pain score is 0 points, the maximum possible total pain score is 27 points.

Category	Descriptor	Score
Physiologic data		
a)	Physiologic data within reference range	0
b)	Dilated pupils	2
c) *choose only one*	Percentage increase in heart rate relative to preprocedural rate	
	>20%	1
	>50%	2
	>100%	3
d) *choose only one*	Percentage increase in respiratory rate relative to preprocedural rate	
	>20%	1
	>50%	2
	>100%	3
e)	Rectal temperature exceeds reference range	1
f)	Salivation	1
Response to palpation		
choose only one	No change from preprocedural behavior	0
	Guards/reacts when touched*	2
	Guards/reacts before touched*	3

Figure 9.8. University of Melbourne Pain Scale. From: Firth, A.M., Haldane, S.L. 1999. Development of a scale to evaluate postoperative pain in dogs. *Journal of the American Veterinary Medical Association*, 214(5):651–659.

Activity			
choose only one	At rest - sleeping	0	
	At rest - semiconscious	0	
	At rest - awake	1	
	Eating	0	
	Restless (pacing continuously, getting up and down)	2	
	Rolling/thrashing	3	
Mental status			
choose only one	Submissive	0	
	Overtly friendly	1	
	Wary	2	
	Aggressive	3	
Posture			
a)	Guarding or protecting affected area (includes fetal position)	2	
b) *choose only one*	Lateral recumbency	0	
	Sternal recumbency	1	
	Sitting or standing, head up	1	
	Standing, head hanging down	2	
	Moving	1	
	Abnormal posture (e.g. prayer position, hunched back)	2	
Vocalization**			
choose only one	Not vocalizing	0	
	Vocalizing when touched	2	
	Intermittent vocalization	2	
	Continuous vocalization	3	

*Includes turning head toward affected area; biting, licking, or scratching at the wound; snapping at the handler; or tense muscles and a protective (guarding) posture.
**Does not include alert barking.

Figure 9.8. *Continued*

useful, with training of observers, and with observer consistency. It is important to note that these tools are an adjunct to thorough exam and observation of the potentially painful patient, not a replacement.

RESPONSE TO THERAPY

Determining adequate response to therapy depends on the nature (severity and origin) and chronicity of pain. Animals undergoing major surgery may need to be assessed hourly in the immediate postoperative period, whereas patients with arthritis may require weekly or monthly evaluation.

When analgesic treatment is effective, patient behaviors associated with pain will gradually recede (Fig. 9.10). Hospitalized patients will be able to rest and sleep more easily and will assume normal body positions when doing so (Fig. 9.11), as well as when awake. Appetite will return to normal, and appearance will improve as grooming behaviors also return to normal. When awake, animals will be more likely to interact with caregivers rather than ignore them or try to escape. Owners will report that they feel their pet's quality of life has improved.

If pain assessment tools are being used to assist in determining response to therapy, the pain scores will decrease if analgesic therapy is effective. In many cases, it is almost impossible to remove all pain that an animal experiences, so the aim is a reduction in the pain score and a more comfortable patient rather than the production of a pain-free patient.

PAIN MANAGEMENT PLAN

PATIENT ID CARD

"Pain assessment is considered part of every patient evaluation, regardless of presenting complaint."

Date: _____ Department: _____

Pulse rate:	Temperature:	°C / °F	
Respiratory rate:	Weight:	lbs / kg	Attitude:

Is pain present upon admission? Y • N • Pain on palpation only? Y • N • Cause of pain:

Signs of pain (describe): | **Descriptors** (Please Circle):

Behavior:	Normal □	Depressed □	Excited □	Agitated □	Guarding □	Aggressive □
Vocalization:	None □	Occasional □	Continuous □	Other □		
Posture:	Normal □	Frozen □	Rigid □	Hunched □	Recumbent □	Reluctant to move □
Gait:	Sound □	Lame weight bearing □		Lame non-weight bearing □		Non-ambulatory □

Descriptors (Please Circle):
Restless — Not grooming
Agitated — Obtund
Trembling — Inappetant
Nervous — Biting or Licking area

Other signs of pain: | Previous Analgesic History:

Classification of pain: | **Anatomical location of pain** (circle):

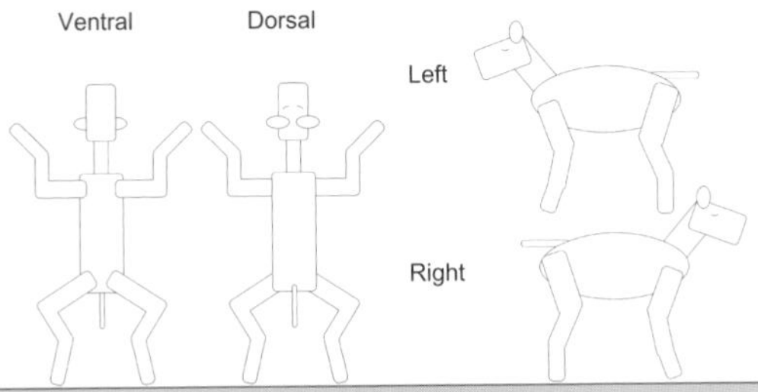

Classification	
Acute	□
Acute recurrent	□
Chronic (>weeks)	□
Chronic progressive	□
Superficial	□
Deep	□
Visceral	□
Inflammatory	□
Neuropathic	□
Both	□
Primary hyperalgesia	□
Secondary hyperalgesia	□
Central analgesia	□

Ventral   Dorsal   Left   Right   Comments:

VISUAL ANALOGUE SCALE

No Pain   Worst Possible Pain

Event	Time (HH:MM):	Date:	Comments:
1			
2			
3			
4			

PAIN THERAPY
(pharmacologic and alternative)

	Date	Dose/Route	Efficacy/Duration	Comments
Current				
Prescribed				

VISUAL ANALOGUE SCALE

No Analgesia   Complete Analgesia

Clinician: _____   Release date: _____

Figure 9.9. Pain assessment and management work sheet used at The Ohio State University Veterinary Teaching Hospital. Notice the visual analogue scale (VAS).

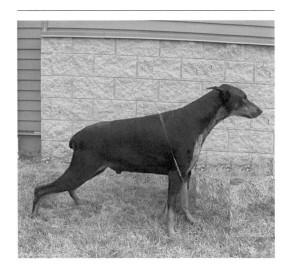

Figure 9.10. Note the normal neck and head position. This is the same dog from Figure 9.5 three days after surgery. Countesy Dr. J. Dyce.

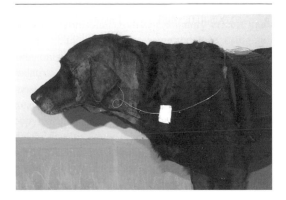

Figure 9.11. This dog was comfortable and adopted a normal head position following total ear canal ablation surgery with placement of a soaker catheter for local anesthetic instillation (PainBuster).

> Do not spend a great deal of time trying to determine if a patient is painful. Treat for pain and then determine the response to therapy. This approach helps to identify animals that have insidious subtle pain.

PERIOPERATIVE (ACUTE) PAIN

Key concepts of perioperative analgesia are preemptive analgesia and multimodal therapy. Many receptors and mechanisms have been identified that are responsible for nociception as well as peripheral and central sensitization. An analgesic plan can therefore be constructed that makes use of several drugs, each with a different mechanism of action. The additional benefit to practicing multimodal therapy for pain management is that each individual drug dose, and therefore risk of side effects, is reduced.

> Key concepts of perioperative analgesia are preemptive analgesia and multimodal therapy.

Management of perioperative pain begins in the preoperative period. Anesthetic premedication (see Chapter 5) offers an opportunity to administer analgesia prior to surgery, a concept known as preemptive analgesia. Analgesia can be administered as part of the anesthetic premedication if they also provide or enhance sedation (opioids, α_2-adrenoceptor agonists, ketamine). Another commonly used modality to provide preemptive analgesia is the application of a transdermal patch (fentanyl). NSAIDs (see Chapter 10) have not typically been administered preoperatively in the United States as injectable forms of drugs, although in Europe and Canada, this is more routine. With the increase in availability of injectable NSAIDs in the United States, this may change.

Opioids

Opioid analgesics (Table 9.4) are the mainstay of analgesia in the perioperative period. They are classified according to their receptor selectivity and activity at opioid receptors (see Chapter 5).

Opioid receptors in the central nervous system are concentrated in the brain and dorsal horn of the spinal cord. Opioid agonist drugs acting centrally inhibit perception (brain) and central sensitization (spinal cord). Agonism of opioid receptors inhibits pain transmission in the spinal cord and neurotransmitter release. Methadone has also been shown to be an NMDA receptor antagonist. Opioid receptors are also present in peripheral tissues. Efficacy of drug activity on peripheral sensitization may depend

Although sedation contributes to analgesia by decreasing perception of pain, it can make evaluation of a patient's level of pain difficult to impossible (masking). Excessive or unwanted sedation can be remedied by administering an α_2-antagonist (atipamezole, yohimbine), although rapid emergence from sedation may lead to excitement. Cardiorespiratory effects of this drug class occur even at low doses. Initially, α_2-agonists cause peripheral vasoconstriction, leading to increased blood pressure and reflex bradycardia or bradysrhythmias with a resultant decrease in cardiac output. This is followed by a centrally mediated decrease in sympathetic tone characterized by hypotension and decreased cardiac output. Respiratory depression is most likely to occur when α_2-agonists are administered with other drugs that also affect ventilation (e.g., opioids, general anesthetics). Other side effects include vomiting, ileus, increased urine output, decreased insulin, and hyperglycemia (see Table 9.5).

Local Anesthetics

Use of local anesthetics (see Chapter 8) as part of a multimodal approach to pain management in small animal practice has gained popularity in recent years (Table 9.6). Local anesthetics are unique among drugs used to provide analgesia in that they completely prevent nociceptive transmission and transduction through their sodium channel–blocking action. Local anesthetics also inhibit

Table 9.5. α_2-Adrenoceptor agonists used for analgesia.

Drug	Route	Dose (dog)	Dose (cat)	Notes
Xylazine	SC, IM	0.2–0.5 mg/kg	0.2–0.5 mg/kg	Lasts 30–40 minutes
	IV	0.1–0.2 mg/kg	0.1–0.3 mg/kg	Lasts 20–30 minutes
Medetomidine	SC, IM	10–40 µg/kg	20–80 µg/kg	Dose for premedication
	IV	1–5 µg/kg	1–5 µg/kg	Microdose intraoperatively or postoperatively
	Epidural	1–5 µg/kg	1–5 µg/kg	
Clonidine*	Transdermal patch			

*Analgesic dose not established.

Table 9.6. Local anesthetics commonly used for analgesia.

Drug	Route	Dose (dog)	Dose (cat)	Notes
Lidocaine	Local, nerve block, IA	Up to 12 mg/kg total dose	Up to 6 mg/kg total dose	Short onset, lasts 1–2 hours
	CRI	2 mg/kg bolus, then 50–75 µg/kg/min	Not recommended	Monitor BP
	Epidural	1 ml of 2% per 4.5 kg body weight	1 ml of 2% per 4.5 kg body weight	Motor function likely to decrease. Monitor BP
	Transdermal patch	Apply patch to area affected	—	
	Soaker system	0.5–5 ml/hr	—	Administer for up to 5 days
Bupivacaine	Local, nerve block, IA, epidural	Up to 2 mg/kg	Up to 1 mg/kg	Longer onset. Lasts 3–8 hours. Do not administer IV.

nociceptive input at the level of the spinal cord and prevent central sensitization. Local anesthetics can be administered topically, locally, intra-articularly, epidurally, and intravenously.

EMLA cream (eutectic mixture of local anesthetics) is a mixture of lidocaine and prilocaine that is used to desensitize the skin for procedures such as intravenous catheterization in children. It has also been used successfully in small animal practice, although the long onset time (30 to 60 minutes) and necessity for an occlusive dressing over the treated area must be taken into account. A newer topical local anesthetic product, ELA-Max, contains liposome-encapsulated lidocaine. It is characterized by a faster onset and does not need to be covered in order to be effective. A transdermal patch is also available (Lidoderm) and is effective locally.

Local anesthetics can also be injected via chest tubes to provide direct analgesia of the pleura following thoracotomy. An additional direct application of local anesthetics is via a continuous local application system. Tubing is placed directly at the site of injury and local anesthetic is administered at a constant rate by an infusion pump or elastomeric reservoir (PainBuster; see Figs. 8.10, 9.11) for up to 5 days. This technique is particularly useful for deep surgery such as total ear canal ablation, limb amputation, and joint surgery when peripheral nerve block is difficult or impossible. Local anesthetic can also be deposited directly into joints or surgical sites prior to closure of the surgical wound. "Splash" application of local anesthetic is particularly helpful when the area to be blocked is too large to anesthetize via specific nerve blocks (e.g., sternal approach for thoracotomy).

Many peripheral nerve blocks have been described for the head and limbs (see Chapter 8). Animals undergoing procedures including but not limited to rostral mandibulectomy, dental extraction, declaw, and toe amputation will benefit from application of a local anesthetic nerve block. Intercostal nerve block should be performed routinely for intrathoracic surgery when the approach is via lateral thoracotomy.

Epidural administration of local anesthetic blocks nerve transmission at the level of the spinal cord and is an effective technique to provide analgesia for hindlimb and abdominal surgery. Motor as well as sensory impulses are usually blocked, with motor function returning before pain sensation. Local anesthetics can be combined with opioids for epidural injection.

Recently, attention has been given to continuous intravenous administration (CRI) of lidocaine for analgesia, and a technique where lidocaine by itself or in combination with morphine and ketamine (MLK) is added to intravenous fluids has been described that is easy to use and is relatively inexpensive (see later in this chapter).

Side effects of local anesthetic administration are largely limited to the nervous and cardiovascular systems, with nervous system toxicity occurring before cardiovascular signs are seen. Nervous system side effects of sedation and reduction of anesthetic dose occur at non-toxic doses. Excitability of the nervous system occurs as the dose of local anesthetic increases due to inhibition of inhibitory neurons and manifests as seizures. Hypotension due to decreased sympathetic tone and vasodilation can occur at clinical doses and is seen with intravenous or epidural administration. Treatment consists of fluid support and vasopressors. At higher doses, local anesthetics will cause cardiac arrhythmias, decreased cardiac output, and even cardiac arrest. Bupivacaine has a lower margin of safety than lidocaine and should not be administered intravenously. Cats are more sensitive to the effects of systemically administered local anesthetics than dogs, so care should be taken to use the appropriate dose and route.

NMDA Antagonists

Ketamine (see Chapters 5 and 6), a dissociative injectable anesthetic agent, is also an NMDA receptor blocker. Antagonism of the NMDA receptor is important in preventing central sensitization (Pozzi et al. 2006). Much smaller doses of ketamine are needed to antagonize the receptors compared with the dose required to induce anesthesia. Ketamine can be administered as intravenous boluses (0.5 mg/kg) or as a CRI (10 to 15 µg/kg/hr). Ketamine is used as part of the MLK combination.

Low doses of ketamine rarely cause side effects, although it is possible that sympathetic stimulation may occur. If tachycardia and hypertension develop that are not related to breakthrough pain, turning off the ketamine infusion may result in resolution of the problem. Note that under anesthesia, there are many causes for tachycardia and hypertension (e.g., hypercarbia due to hypoventilation). These causes should be investigated before terminating analgesic infusions.

Orally administered NMDA antagonists include amantadine and dextromethorphan.

NSAIDs

NSAIDs provide analgesia both directly, by decreasing inflammation, and indirectly, through central activity in the spinal cord (see Chapter 10). This anti-inflammatory action occurs via inhibition of two of the isoenzymes of cyclooxygenase (COX-1 and COX-2). Current preference is to favor the use of NSAIDs with more COX-2 (the isoenzyme induced by inflammation) inhibitory activity, because the classic NSAID side effects (renal damage, gastrointestinal ulceration, decreased platelet function) are partially mediated via inhibition of constitutive COX-1. However, COX-2 is also expressed constitutively in some tissues (nervous system, kidney, and reproductive and gastrointestinal tracts), so complete inhibition of this isoenzyme may also be detrimental.

With the current increase in availability of injectable forms of NSAIDs (flunixin, phenylbutazone, carprofen, meloxicam, ketoprofen), their use in the perioperative period has increased (some off-label). They are generally given at the end of anesthesia and take effect within a few hours. NSAIDs are frequently given orally at home for several days to a few weeks after surgery, depending on the drug and level of postoperative pain anticipated. Starting therapy the day of surgery with an injectable NSAID will establish a therapeutic level prior to discharge from the hospital.

The injectable administration of NSAIDs avoids the issue of gastrointestinal irritation, but it is important to ensure that fluid therapy during and after anesthesia is appropriate in order to avoid renal toxicity.

Tramadol

Tramadol is a nonopiate drug with activity at the μ receptor that is given orally. It is thus useful as a postoperative alternative to opioids once a patient has resumed eating (usually 12 to 24 hours after surgery) and can be prescribed for continuation of analgesic therapy at home. An additional mechanism of action of tramadol is inhibition of norepinephrine and serotonin reuptake, which also promotes analgesia. Tramadol should not be administered with other norepinephrine and serotonin reuptake inhibitors (e.g., amitriptyline).

Drug Combinations

A multimodal technique (Table 9.7) in which MLK is added to intravenous fluids has been described that is easy to use and is relatively inexpensive (Muir et al. 2003). This combination also reduces the amount of inhalant anesthetic agent required for maintenance of anesthesia. Morphine can be replaced by the μ-opioid agonists hydromorphone or fentanyl. We have also added medetomidine to MLK.

Problems encountered with MLK include delayed recovery from anesthesia and accuracy of adminis-

Table 9.7. Formulae for preparing MLK and its variations.

Drug	Amount added to 1 L of crystalloid given at 10 ml/kg/hr	Amount added to 1 L of crystalloid given at 5 ml/kg/hr	Drug CRI
Morphine	24 mg	48 mg	0.24 mg/kg/hr
Hydromorphone* (replaces morphine)	2 mg	4 mg	0.02 mg/kg/hr
Lidocaine	300 mg	600 mg	3 mg/kg/hr
Ketamine	60 mg	120 mg	0.6 mg/kg/hr
±Medetomidine	100 μg	200 μg	1 μg/kg/hr

*Fentanyl may also be substituted for morphine.

tration, especially with smaller patients. Delayed recovery can be avoided by decreasing the infusion rate until the patient is awake. Use of infusion pumps or calibrated chambers (Buretrol) to deliver fluids with MLK added is recommended for smaller patients. Addition of medetomidine may result in moderate hypertension and marked respiratory sinus arrhythmia.

> Multimodal analgesic therapy contributes to patient comfort while decreasing the amount of each drug administered through additive or synergistic effects.

Environment

Nursing care in the perioperative period is very important. Care should be taken when positioning and moving patients under anesthesia for surgery and radiography. Postoperative provision of comfort includes appropriately padded, warm cages so that patients can lie down and sleep. If possible, a quiet, subdued light environment should be provided in order to decrease stress by disrupting sleep patterns as little as possible. A blanket or toy from home may provide some level of familiarity and security during the hospitalized part of the recovery period.

Dogs become anxious and distressed when they have full bladders or are forced to urinate in their cages. They should be taken outside to urinate if possible, and if the nature of the injury or surgery prevents this, an indwelling urinary catheter should be considered. Cats should have easy access to a clean litter tray.

Monitoring Pain Therapy After Surgery

> If a patient's pain is being adequately managed by administration of bolus injections of an opioid such as morphine every 3 to 4 hours, it is practical to assess pain 30 to 60 minutes before the next dose is scheduled.

Analgesic therapy should be monitored closely for the first 24 to 72 hours following surgery. An assessment of the degree of pain the patient is expe-riencing should be made every 1 to 2 hours for the first several hours. Once pain is under control, patient evaluations can be made at less-frequent intervals. If a patient's pain is being adequately managed by administration of bolus injections of an opioid such as morphine every 3 to 4 hours, it is practical to assess pain 30 to 60 minutes before the next dose is scheduled (Fig. 9.12).

Patients that have undergone major surgery that is associated with severe postoperative pain (e.g., thoracotomy, fracture repair, total ear canal ablation) may require frequent assessment and more aggressive therapy for 24 to 48 hours after anesthesia. Multimodal analgesic therapy for these types of surgeries is usually necessary to control the acute pain of surgery and to decrease the incidence of peripheral and central sensitization.

A transition is typically made after the first 24 to 48 hours from parenteral administration of analgesics (opioids and NSAIDs with or without adjuncts such as ketamine, lidocaine, and α_2-agonists) to oral drugs (NSAIDs, tramadol). Oral analgesics are usually continued at home for 3 to 14 days depending on drug selection, species, nature and severity of surgical pain, and the response of the individual.

Addition of low doses of sedatives to the analgesic plan may help reduce anxiety (e.g., acepromazine, α_2-agonists).

CHRONIC PAIN

NSAIDs form the mainstay of treatment of chronic pain (otitis, arthritis) (see Chapter 10). If NSAID therapy is not effective enough, consideration should be given to co-administration of other drug classes that will enhance analgesia through different mechanisms of action (multimodal analgesia). Although implementation of multimodal therapy is recommended, there are some patients that respond better to one specific NSAID over another. In the case that a change from one NSAID to another is warranted, a washout period of 7 days when doing so is advisable to avoid the risk of side effects.

In the case of otitis, corticosteroid administration may be a better alternative in some patients. Corticosteroids are potent anti-inflammatory drugs, acting to inhibit prostaglandin and leukotriene formation and thus inhibiting transmission of nociceptive impulses. This mechanism of action overlaps with that of NSAIDs, so they should not be co-

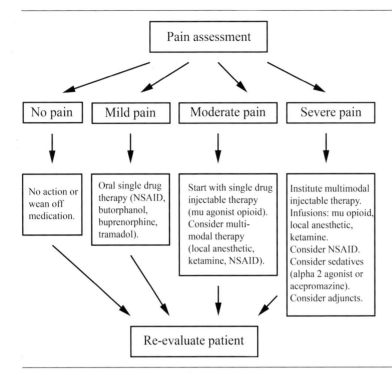

Figure 9.12. Flow chart for perioperative pain assessment and management.

administered. Side effects include gastric ulceration, immunosuppression, hyperadrenocorticism, hypoadrenocorticism, hepatopathy (dogs), polyphagia, and insulin resistance.

Patients with osteoarthritis may benefit from nutraceuticals (glucosamine, chondroitin), which are purported to improve joint cartilage growth. Injectable cartilage-promoting drugs are also available (polysulfated glycosaminoglycan, hyaluronic acid).

Chronic neurogenic or neuropathic pain results from inflammation or injury to the central nervous system (intervertebral disk disease, meningitis, nerve sheath, or root tumors). Neuropathic pain is generally poorly responsive to opioid analgesic therapy. Corticosteroids can be very effective in treatment of neuropathic pain, although long-term therapy increases the risk of side effects. Gabapentin, an antiepileptic with an incompletely understood mechanism of action, can also be effective for this type of pain and may have some activity as an NMDA-receptor antagonist.

Other drugs used as adjuncts for chronic pain include tramadol (see earlier), amantadine, dextromethorphan, and amitryptiline (Table 9.8). Amantidine and dextromethorphan are NMDA antagonists (see earlier discussion on ketamine) that are administered orally. Amitryptiline is a tricyclic antidepressant that inhibits norepinephrine and serotonin reuptake in the central nervous system.

Complementary Therapy

Several alternative (i.e., nonpharmacologic) therapies have been shown to provide analgesia such as stimulation of acupuncture points manually (traditional acupuncture) or electrically (electroacupuncture or percutaneous acupoint electrical stimulation). Dermatomes that are associated with individual sensory nerves can be stimulated transcutaneously (transcutaneous electrical nerve stimulation [TENS]) or percutaneously (percutaneous electrical nerve stimulation [PENS]). Laser therapy and pulsed magnetic field are also used to provide analgesia. These methodologies are generally used in conjunction with a pharmacologic approach to analgesia.

Physical rehabilitation, including range of motion exercises, hydrotherapy, and massage, plays an important role in treating both chronic and postsurgical pain in veterinary patients (see Chapter 14).

Table 9.8. Oral doses of drugs used as adjuncts in chronic pain therapy.

Drug	Mechanism	Dose	Notes
Amantadine	NMDA antagonism	D 3–5 mg/kg PO qd C 3 mg/kg PO qd	
Dextromethorphan	NMDA antagonism	D 0.5–2 mg/kg PO qd	
Amitriptyline	Reuptake inhibition	D 1–2 mg/kg PO qd or bid C 0.5–1 PO mg/kg bid	Do not use with Tramadol
Tramadol	μ agonist, reuptake inhibition	D 2–10 mg/kg PO qd or bid C 1–2 mg/kg PO bid	Do not use with Amitriptyline
Gabapentin	Unknown	D 3–5 mg/kg PO qd* C 1.25–5 mg/kg PO bid	Decrease dose slowly to avoid rebound seizures

D = dog; C = cat. Doses not well established. Used cautiously; watch curret literature for new recommendations. *Editor's note: more frequent dosing is used by some veterinarians.

Nutritional supplements may be appropriate for some chronically painful conditions (arthritis) (see Chapter 14).

Monitoring Chronic Pain Management

Establishing goals for management of chronically painful conditions is not as straightforward compared with monitoring the success of acute pain management. Important outcome measures will be determined by the nature of the disease process. For example, a goal for improvement in arthritis pain may be decreased limping. The overall goal should be to increase patient comfort and well-being; that is, the patient quality of life should be improved. Client input is very important: the client spends the most time with the patient and is most likely to notice subtle changes in activity, appetite, sleeping habits, and other behaviors that may be related to pain. The use of quality of life questionnaires/assessments may also be helpful to identify trends over time.

Patients with well-managed chronic pain may be evaluated as seldom as every 4 to 6 months. Episodes of breakthrough (more severe) pain may require much more frequent evaluations similar to acute pain. A change in medication, whether from one NSAID to another, or the decision to include additional drugs in the therapeutic plan will also require more frequent assessments in order to adjust dosages and monitor side effects.

REFERENCES

Clarke, S.P., and Bennett, D.D. 2006. Feline osteoarthritis: A prospective study of 28 cases. *J Small Anim Prac* 47:439–445.

Firth, A.M., and Haldane, S.L. 1999. Development of a scale to evaluate postoperative pain in dogs. *J Am Vet Med Assoc* 214(5):651–659.

Holton, L., Reid, J., Scott, E.M., et al. 2001. Development of a behaviour-based scale to measure acute pain in dogs. *Vet Rec* 148:525–531.

Morton, C.M., Reid, J., Scott, E.M., et al. 2005. Application of a scaling model to establish and validate an interval level pain scale for assessment of acute pain in dogs. *Am J Vet Res* 66(12):2154–2166.

Muir, W.W., Wiese, A.J., and March, P.A. 2003. Effects of morphine, lidocaine, ketamine, and morphine-lidocaine-ketamine drug combination on minimum alveolar concentration in dogs anesthetized with isoflurane. *Am J Vet Res* 64:1155–1160.

Pozzi, A., Muir, W.W., and Traverso, F. 2006. Prevention of central sensitization and pain by N-methyl-D-aspartate receptor antagonists. *J Am Vet Med Assoc* 228(1):53–60.

Watkins, L.R., and Maier, S.F. 2000. The pain of being sick: implications of immune-to-brain communication for understanding pain. *Annu Rev Psychol* 51:29–57.

Wiseman-Orr, M.L., Scott, E.M., Reid, J., et al. 2006. Validation of a structured questionnaire as an instrument to measure chronic pain in dogs on the basis of effects on health-related quality of life. *Am J Vet Res* 67(67):1826–1836.

Yazbek, K.V.B., and Fantoni, D.T. 2005. Validity of a health-related quality-of-life scale for dogs with signs of pain secondary to cancer. *J Am Vet Med Assoc* 226(8):1354–1358.

ADDITIONAL READING

Gaynor, J.S., and Muir, W.W. 2002. *Handbook of Veterinary Pain Management.* St Louis: Mosby.

Mathews, K.A. 2000. *Management of Pain, Veterinary Clinics of North America, Small Animal Practice.*

Muir, W.W., and Woolf, C.J. 2001. Mechanisms of pain and their therapeutic implications. *J Am Vet Med Assoc* 219(10):1346–1356.

Perkowski, S.Z., and Wetmore, L.A. 2006. The science and art of analgesia. In *Recent Advances in Veterinary Anesthesia and Analgesia: Companion Animals,* edited by R.D. Gleed and J.W. Ludders. Ithaca: International Veterinary Information Service (www.ivis.org), Document No. A1405.1006.

Wetmore, L.A. 2006. Options for analgesia in dogs. In *Recent Advances in Veterinary Anesthesia and Analgesia: Companion Animals,* Edited by R.D. Gleed and J.W. Ludders. Ithaca: International Veterinary Information Service (www.ivis.org), Document No. A1404.0906.

Chapter 10
Nonsteroidal
Anti-inflammatory Drugs

Steven M. Fox

Nonsteroidal anti-inflammatory drugs (NSAIDs) are the fastest growing class of drugs in both human and veterinary medicine. This reflects their broad use as anti-inflammatories, analgesics, and anti-pyretics. As with antibiotics, NSAIDs can be considered to have been introduced in successive generations to date: (1) first generation (i.e., aspirin, phenylbutazone, meclofenamic acid), (2) second generation (i.e., carprofen, etodolac, meloxicam), and (3) third generation (i.e., tepoxalin, deracoxib, firicoxib). However, unlike the logic of "saving the big gun antibiotic" for last so as to avoid microbial superinfections, logic would dictate using the optimal NSAID at the earliest opportunity so as to avoid the physiologic complication of "windup" (see Chapter 9).

HISTORY

In most respects, NSAIDs can be characterized as a class, whereas there are molecule-specific characteristics. NSAIDs manifest their mode of action in the arachidonic acid (AA) cascade (Fig. 10.1). Arachidonic acid is a ubiquitous substrate derived from the continual degradation of cell membranes. Corticosteroids act at this step. Arachidonic acid is thereafter metabolized to prostanoids via the cyclooxygenase pathway to prostaglandins or via the lipoxygenase pathway to leukotrienes. These end-product prostanoids are proinflammatory and generally enhance disease processes. At one time it was believed that blocking the cyclooxygenase pathway led to a buildup of arachidonic acid as a substrate, which would then lead to increased production of leukotrienes. The issue remains unresolved in vivo in veterinary species. Because corticosteroids have their mode of action at a location higher in the arachidonic acid cascade than do NSAIDs, it is redundant to use them concurrently, and doing so markedly increases the potential for adverse reactions.

Approximately 20 years following discovery of the arachidonic acid pathway as the mode of action for NSAIDs, it was discovered that the cyclooxygenase enzyme exists as at least two isoenzymes: cyclooxygenase (COX)-1 and COX-2 (Fig. 10.2). Early thinking was that COX-1–mediated prostaglandins were constitutively physiologic and should be retained, while COX-2–mediated prostaglandins were pathologic and to be eliminated for the control of inflammation. COX-2–selective NSAIDs were designed for this purpose—the selective suppression of COX-2–mediated prostaglandins.

NSAID SAFETY

The IC_{50} is defined as the concentration of drug (NSAID) needed to inhibit the activity of the enzyme (cyclooxygenase) by 50%. In keeping with the above logic, one would like to have a high concentration of NSAID before causing 50% inhibition of COX-1 (good guy) and a low concentration of NSAID to reach the IC_{50} for COX-2 (bad guy):

$$\frac{IC_{50} \text{ of COX-1 (good)}}{IC_{50} \text{ of COX-2 (bad)}} \quad \frac{\text{HIGH}}{\text{LOW}} \quad (10.1)$$

The higher the numerator and lower the denominator, the higher is the absolute value. Therefore, a greater COX-1/COX-2 ratio suggests (theoretically) the more optimal performing NSAID. With this in mind, pharmaceutical companies began designing

143

Cell injury

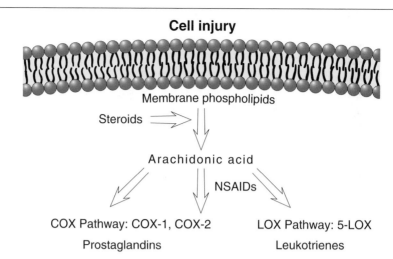

Membrane phospholipids

Steroids ⟹

Arachidonic acid

NSAIDs

COX Pathway: COX-1, COX-2

Prostaglandins

LOX Pathway: 5-LOX

Leukotrienes

Figure 10.1. Damaged cells release phospholipids which are the substrate for catalysis by phospholipase to arachidonic acid (AA). Arachidonic acid is thereafter metabolized to prostanoids via the cyclooxygenase (COX) pathway to prostaglandins or via the lipoxygenase (LOX) pathway to leukotrienes. Steroids act to block catalysis of phospholipids to AA. The nonsteroidal antiinflammatories (NSAIDs) block the catalysis of AA to inflammatory mediators. Illustrations by Mark M. Miller, Miller Medical Illustration & Design

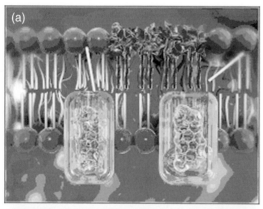

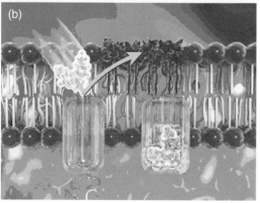

Figure 10.2a. The COX-1 receptor site (left) differs from the COX-2 receptor site (right) by only a couple of amino acids, however the COX-2 site has a larger entry port and a characteristic side-pocket. Small, traditional NSAIDs fit into both sites, blocking both COX-1- and COX-2-mediated prostaglandin production from arachidonic acid (white sticks), hence the term non-selective NSAIDs.

Figure 10.2b. Coxib-class NSAIDs were designed to be too large for the COX-1 receptor site (at labeled dose), however they fit hand-in-glove within the COX-2 receptor site. These drugs spare COX-1-mediated prostaglandin production and block COX-2-mediated prostaglandin production, i.e., they are COX-1-sparing and COX-2 selective.

Table 10.1. Theoretically, an NSAID for which it takes a low concentration to inhibit COX-2 (denominator) and a high concentration to inhibit COX-1 (numerator) will be optimal performers.

Drug	Ratio of IC_{50} COX-1/COX-2
Meloxicam	12.2
Carprofen	1.8
Ketoprofen	0.4

From Kay-Mungerford et al. (2000).

Drug	Ratio of IC_{50} COX-1/COX-2
Meloxicam	10
Carprofen	9
Ketoprofen	6.5

From Brideau et al. (2001).

Drug	Ratio of IC_{50} COX-1/COX-2
Meloxicam	2.7
Carprofen	16.8
Ketoprofen	0.2
Aspirin	0.4

From Streppa et al. (2002).

Drug	Ratio of IC_{50} COX-1/COX-2
Carprofen	5
Celecoxib	6.2
Deracoxib	36.5
Firicoxib	155

From Li et al. (2005).

NSAIDs for which it takes a low concentration to inhibit COX-2 but a high concentration to inhibit COX-1. More important than how COX-2 selective an NSAID might be is whether or not the NSAID is COX-1 sparing. COX-1/COX-2 ratios vary depending on laboratory techniques, and although finite ratios may vary among investigators, relative ratio standings provide insight into a drug's expected cyclooxygenase activity (Table 10.1).

> Selectivity nomenclature is used loosely, and comparative ranking has not been associated with clinical relevance.

Some suggest a COX-1/COX-2 ratio of less than 1 would be considered COX-1 selective, a ratio greater than 1 as COX-2 preferential, a ratio greater than 100 as COX-2 selective, and a ratio greater than 1000 as COX-2 specific. Selectivity nomenclature is used loosely, and comparative ranking has not been associated with clinical relevance.

We now know that the "good-guy-COX-1, bad guy COX-2" approach is naive, now recognizing that COX-2 is needed constitutively for reproduction, central nervous system nociception, renal function, and gastrointestinal lesion repair. In fact, the physiologic functions associated with cyclooxygenase activity overlap. Accordingly, there is surely a limit as to how COX-2 selective an NSAID can be without causing problems (e.g., inhibiting the repair of a gastric lesion). This limit is not known (Fig. 10.3). Further, it is logical to avoid a COX-1–selective NSAID (ratio less than 1) perioperatively so as not to enhance bleeding. In human studies the coxib-class NSAIDs, with their high COX ratio, have been shown to be associated with less risk for gastrointestinal complications (Singh and Fort 2006).

Coxib-class NSAIDs were designed to be more safe for the gastrointestinal tract, although any NSAID can be at risk for adverse reactions (adverse drug event).[1] Similar safety has not been investigated in the canine. Coxib-class NSAIDs were not designed to be safer for renal or hepatic function and they have been associated with potential cardiovascular risks in humans. Fortunately, companion animals are not at risk for coxib-class NSAID cardiovascular problems (e.g., atherosclerosis) (Liu et al. 1986), and it may well be that the canine is the optimal target species for this class of drugs. The label precaution regarding potential sulfonamide hypersensitivity is likely theoretical in dogs. Trepanier (2006) reported that drugs other than the antimicrobial sulfonamides do not produce the same hypersensitivity syndrome of similar pathogenesis in dogs.

Comparative safety of different NSAIDs in dogs is difficult to determine. Such a query compares the incidence of problems with one NSAID with that for a second NSAID. Incidence is a ratio consisting of the number of dogs with problems (numerator) over the number of dogs treated with that drug at a given point in time (denominator).

$$\text{Incidence of adverse event} = \frac{\#\text{ dogs with adverse events}}{\#\text{ dogs being treated at given time}} \quad (10.2)$$

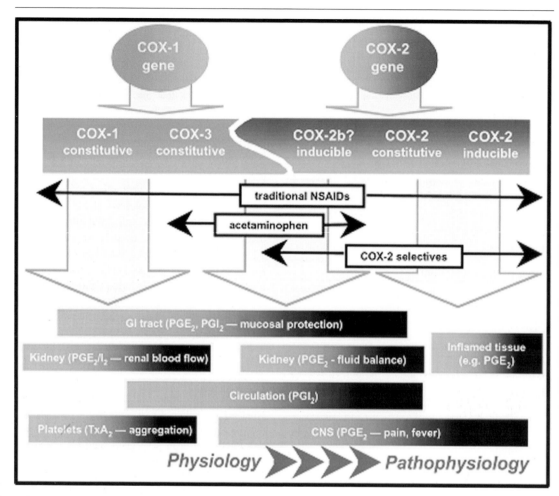

Figure 10.3. Two COX genes may be responsible for constitutive and inducible COX proteins with overlapping functions. The order of older NSAIDs, newer COX-2 selective NSAIDs, and acetaminophen in a COX continuum helps define their action. From: Warner, T.D., Mitchell, J.A. 2002. Cyclooxygenase-3 (COX-3): filling in the gaps toward a COX continuum? *P Natl Acad Sci* 99(21):13371–13373.

Not all adverse drug events are reported and not all reported events are directly causal; therefore, the numerator is unknown. The denominator is also unknown, because it is impossible to determine the number of dogs on a drug at any given time. For these reasons, accurate comparative data are unobtainable. Accordingly, most NSAID manufacturers can state with credibility that "no NSAID has been proved safer than (*fill in the blank*)." Nevertheless, all adverse drug events should be reported to the Food and Drug Administration (FDA) and drug manufacturer so that general trends can be tracked.

"No NSAID has been proved to be safer than (*fill in the blank*)."

Adverse drug event reports at the U.S. FDA Center for Veterinary Medicine provide some insights as to why adverse drug events from NSAID use might be so high (Hampshire et al. 2004):

• 23% of owners: veterinarian never discussed any adverse effects of the NSAID medication

- 22% of owners: veterinarian did not issue client information sheet provided by pharmaceutical company
- 14% of owners: veterinarian dispensed NSAID in other than original packaging
- 4% of owners: veterinarian did not perform pre-administration blood analyses

> All adverse drug events should be reported to the FDA and drug manufacturer . . . even if you know what and why it happened.

As a class of drug, NSAIDs are most commonly associated with adverse reactions to the gastrointestinal track, renal system, and liver, respectively. Gastrointestinal problems associated with NSAIDs can be as benign as regurgitation or as serious as gastric ulceration and perforation. Vomition has been identified as the most frequent clinical sign associated with gastric perforation (Lascelles et al. 2005). Pet owners should be informed that while taking an NSAID, if their pet experiences vomiting, the drug should be stopped and the patient should be rechecked (Table 10.2).

Gastric perforations are most frequently found near the gastric pylorus and have a poor prognosis

Table 10.2. Gastrointestinal adverse events (ADEs) reported in clinical trials for acute use.

Drug	Vomiting	Diarrhea
Carprofen	3.1% (3.8%)	3.1% (3.8%)
Etodolac	4.3% (1.7%)	2.6% (1.7%)
Deracoxib	2.9% (3.8%)	2.9% (1.9%)
Tepoxalin*	2.0% (4.8%)	4.0% (0%)
Meloxicam	25.5% (15.4%)	12.1% (7.4%)
Firocoxib	3.9% (6.6%)	0.8% (8.3%)

Values represent mean of test article (placebo). Data sourced from drug inserts. Caution should be used in comparing adverse events among different drugs because of differences in study populations, data collection methods, and reporting methods. According to the FDA-CVM, most ADEs are reported within 14 to 30 days of NSAID administration with a range of 3 to 90 days (Hampshire et al. 2004).
*Data for tepoxalin was collected at 28 days (19.6% vomiting and 21.5% diarrhea).

if not discovered early and treated aggressively. Risk factors identified with NSAID-associated gastric ulceration are most commonly seen with inappropriate use: (1) overdosing, (2) concurrent use of multiple NSAIDs, and (3) concurrent use of NSAIDs with corticosteroids (Lascelles et al. 2005).

Aspirin and Acetaminophen

Aspirin presents unique risk factors to the canine patient. Aspirin is both topically and systemically toxic (even at low doses of 5 mg/kg QD), chondro-destructive, causes irreversible platelet acetylation, and is associated with gastrointestinal bleeding of approximately 3 ml/day. The AMA reports that 16,500 people die each year associated with aspirin toxicity, yet pet owners often consider aspirin to be benign because it is available over-the-counter and the media suggests it is safe. Even low-dose aspirin has consistently been associated with gastrointestinal petechiation and hemorrhage. Aspirin does not have an FDA license for use in the dog. In theory, because aspirin causes gastrointestinal lesions, it would be inappropriate to sequentially progress from aspirin to a strongly COX-2–selective NSAID (which might restrict the COX-2 necessary for repair) without an adequate washout period following the aspirin. It is also dangerous to use aspirin together with another NSAID or corticosteroid.

> The American Medical Association reports that 16,500 people die each year associated with aspirin toxicity.

Development of gastric mucosal hemorrhage, erosion, and ulceration associated with administration of NSAIDs is largely attributed to reduction of prostaglandin E synthesis in the gastric mucosa. In addition, aspirin can cause direct cellular toxicosis, independent of the inhibition of PG synthesis. Standard formulations of buffered aspirin have been shown to provide insufficient buffering to neutralize gastric acid or to prevent mucosal injury. Enteric-coated aspirin causes less gastric injury in humans, compared with that from administration of unbuffered or buffered aspirin, but absorption is quite variable.

Salicylate toxicity in cats is well established. Cats present a unique susceptibility for NSAID toxicity because of slow clearance and dose-dependent elimination. Acetaminophen toxicity in cats results in methemaglobinemia, liver failure, and death. Cats are particularly susceptible to acetaminophen toxicity due, in part, to defective conjugation of the drug and conversion to a reactive electrolytic metabolite.

Gastric Protection

One goal of antiulcer treatment is to lower intragastric acidity to prevent further destruction of the gastrointestinal tract mucosa, enhancing ulcer repair. Cimetadine (Tagamet), a histamine, H_2-receptor blocker, is commonly used. Cimetidine requires dosing three to four times daily; however, it is not effective in preventing NSAID-induced gastric ulceration. Omeprazole (Prilosec) is a substituted benzimidazole that acts by inhibiting the hydrogen-potassium ATPase (proton pump inhibitor) that is responsible for production of hydrogen ions in the parietal cell. It is 5 to 10 times more potent than cimetadine for inhibiting gastric acid secretion and has a long duration of action, requiring once-a-day administration. Omeprazole may be useful in decreasing gastric hyperacidity but has minimal effect on ulcer healing. Misoprostol (Cytotec) is a synthetic prostaglandin E_1 analog used to prevent gastric ulceration. It decreases gastric acid secretion, increases bicarbonate and mucus secretion, increases epithelial cell turnover, and increases mucosal blood flow. Both cimetadine and misoprostol require dosing three to four times daily, and adverse reactions mimic those of gastritis and ulcerations.

Washout

Washout between NSAIDs is a poorly researched area of investigation. Theoretically, in a healthy patient, a washout period should not be required. Most agree that aspirin is an exception, due in part to the phenomena of aspirin triggering lipoxin[2] (Wallace and Fiorucci 2003). A 5- to 7-day washout following aspirin is probably adequate. One study has been conducted (Dowers et al., 2006) where injectable carprofen was followed at the next QD dosing with deracoxib. In this study of a limited number of healthy dogs, no difference was noted in following injectable carprofen with either oral carprofen or oral deracoxib. Pain relief during a washout period can be obtained by the use of other class drugs (e.g., tramadol, amantadine, gabapentin, or opioids).

> Appropriate washout periods between NASIDs are not established for most NSAIDs, with aspirin being the exception. Other analgesics (e.g., opioids) may be used during washout.

Adverse Drug Events and Good Medicine

Before placing a pet on NSAIDs, the owner should be informed of the potential for adverse drug events and to discontinue drug administration and contact their veterinarian promptly. Both verbal and written instructions should be given. Preadministrative urinalysis and blood chemistries are well advised for two reasons. First, the pet may be a poor candidate for any NSAID (i.e., it may be azotemic or have decreased liver function). These physiologic compromises may not preclude the use of NSAIDs, but such a determination must be justified. Second, a baseline status should be established for subsequent comparison, should the patient show clinical signs suggestive of drug intolerance.

> Minimal effective dose of NSAID should always be the therapeutic objective.

For the patient on a long-term NSAID protocol, the frequency of laboratory profiling should be determined by clinical signs and age. Minimal effective dose should always be the therapeutic objective, and routine examinations of the animal constitutes the practice of good medicine. Because ALT is more specific than SAP as a blood chemistry for liver status, an elevation three to four times laboratory normal should prompt a subsequent liver function test. Because the kidney expresses both COX isozymes constitutively, no one NSAID may be presumed safer than another for renal function.

> No one NSAID may be presumed safer than another for renal function.

Perioperative NSAID Use

NSAIDs play a major role in a perioperative protocol for healthy animals, due to their features as anti-inflammatories, analgesics, and antipyretics.

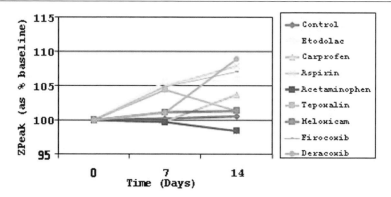

Figure 10.4. Force plate gait analysis has become the standard for analysis of dogs with osteoarthritis. From: Millis, D.L. 2006. Nonsteroidal anti-inflammatory drugs, disease modifying drugs, and osteoarthritis, in A Multimodal Approach to Treating Osteoarthritis Symposium. Novartis Animal Health, pp. 9–19. Peak Vertical Force of Dogs Treated for Stifle Osteoarthritis

NSAID inclusion helps prevent central nervous system "windup" (see Chapter 9) and shows a synergistic effect with opioids (Williams 1997). Surgery cannot be performed without resultant iatrogenic inflammation, and the best time to administer the anti-inflammatory drug is preemptively, before the surgery. It is imperative that surgical patients be sufficiently hydrated if NSAIDs are used perioperatively. Under the influence of inhalant anesthesia, renal tissue may suffer from underperfusion, at which point prostaglandins are recruited to assist with this perfusion. If the patient is under the influence of an antiprostaglandin (NSAID), acute renal function may be at risk.

It is difficult to differentiate NSAID efficacy in the perioperative setting, because most clinicians administer NSAIDs as part of a multimodal (balanced) analgesic protocol. Perioperative analgesia from an NSAID alone is rarely sufficient. Injectable carprofen was designed for perioperative use. For labeled intramuscular administration, the injectable drug has a different pharmacokinetic profile than the oral drug due to its mixed micelle formulation. Given IM, the C_{max} of the injectable (C_{max} of $8.0 \mu g/ml$ at 1.5 to 8 hours) is half that of the oral formulation (C_{max} of $16.9 \mu g/ml$ at 0.5 to 3 hours) and is reached later (Clark et al. 2003), suggesting that it be given several hours prior to surgery for maximal preemptive effect. There are few objective pain assessment models for soft tissue from which to compare NSAID efficacy.

In cats, meloxicam injection is approved for preemptive analgesia for soft tissue and orthopedic surgery in cats in the United States and other countries. The approved dose ($0.3 mg/kg$ SQ) may be reduced to $0.2 mg/kg$ SQ with good efficacy.

NSAID Treatment of Osteoarthritis

In contrast to soft tissue injury or surgery in which there are no standard pain evaluations, force plate gait analysis in an orthopedic model has become the standard for ranking NSAID efficacy on an objective basis. Millis et al. (2006) observed the force plate responses illustrated in Figure 10.4 to labeled dose administration of contemporary NSAIDs in the canine osteoarthritis model.

Dosing

Time of administration is a common question arising from QD-labeled NSAIDS: Should the drug be administered in the morning or in the evening? Some argue that morning administration is most logical, taking advantage of C_{max} during that time of the day when the dog might be most active. Others suggest the NSAID should be dosed so that C_{max} is reached to ensure maximal rest for the animal, proposing that the animal performs best following a good night's rest. There is no consensus.

Many of the contemporary NSAIDs are labeled for use either with or without food. Administration with food takes advantage of the increased production of gastric bicarbonate and associated buffering. Feeding an NSAID together with food may enhance acceptability in some dogs. Accurate dosing, particularly in small dogs and cats, is essential.

> NSAIDs are highly protein bound; the safety profile may be impacted by other highly protein bound drugs.

NSAIDs are highly protein bound and may compete with binding of other highly protein bound drugs, particularly in the hypoproteinimic animal, resulting in altered drug concentrations. Fortunately, the number of other highly protein bound drugs is minimal, excepting some anesthetic drugs. The following drugs and agents may be influenced by the concurrent administration of NSAIDs (Tables 10.3 and 10.4).

Role of NSAIDs in Cancer

Human studies have shown that patients with rheumatoid arthritis receiving long-term NSAID therapy have a reduced risk of colorectal cancer. Such observations have led to work examining the role of NSAIDs as a preventative measure against cancer development and as adjunctive antineoplastic therapy. Published data (Page et al. 2001) also suggest that control of oncologic pain can impact the course of cancer progression.

Prostaglandins play a major role in cancer development including inhibition of immune surveillance, promotion of angiogenesis, and inhibition of apoptosis. High levels of prostaglandins are found in tumors of many types that may exert effects in an autocrine or a paracrine fashion, and up-regulation of COX-2 has been directly associated with tumor aggression. Following is a list of veterinary tumor types demonstrating an up-regulation of COX-2:

- Transitional cell carcinoma
- Renal cell carcinoma
- Squamous cell carcinoma
- Prostate carcinoma
- Rectal polyps
- Nasal carcinoma
- Osteosarcoma
- Mammary carcinoma
- Intestinal adenocarcinoma
- Oral malignant melanoma

In addition to decreasing PG production via inhibition of COX-2, NSAIDs also have COX-

Table 10.3. Potential drug and NSAID interactions.

Drug	May increase the toxicity of	May decrease the efficacy of	Toxicity may be increased by
Classic NSAIDs (clinically significant COX-1 inhibition)	Warfarin, methotrexate, valproic acid, midazolam, furosemide, spironolactone, sulfonylureas, heparin	Furosemide, thiazide, ACE inhibitors, β-blockers	Aminoglycosides, furosemide, cyclosporine (renal), glucocorticoids (GI), heparin, gingko, garlic, ginger, ginseng (hemorrhage)
Coxibs and relatively COX-2 selective agents	Warfarin, methotrexate, valproic acid, midazolam, furosemide, spironolactone, sulfonylureas	Furosemide, thiazides, ACE inhibitors, β-blockers	Aminoglycosides, furosemide, cyclosporine (renal), glucocorticoids (GI)
Phenylbutazone, acetaminophen	Warfarin, sulfolureas		Phenobartital, alcohol, rifampin, metoclopramide

From Trepanier (2005).

Table 10.4. Potential herb–drug interactions.

Herb	Interacting drugs	Results
St. John's wort	Cyclosporine, fexofenadine, midazolam, digoxin, tacrolimus, amitriptyline, warfarin, theophylline	Decreased plasma drug concentrations
Ginko	Warfarin, heparin, NSAIDs, omeprazole	Bleeding, decreased plasma concentrations
Ginseng	Warfarin, heparin, NSAIDs, opioids	Bleeding, falsely elevated serum digoxin levels (laboratory test interaction with ginseng), decreased analgesic effect (laboratory test interaction with ginseng)
Garlic, chamomile, ginger	Warfarin, heparin, NSAIDs	Bleeding

From Goodman and Trepanier (2005).

independent anticancer mechanisms including activation or inhibition of cellular signaling pathways via up-regulation or inhibition of oncogenes. Preliminary results of a study involving deracoxib, a COX-2–selective inhibitor, as therapy for transitional cell carcinoma have demonstrated stable disease in nine of nine dogs (Boria et al. 2003). Many oncologists are now prescribing COX-2 inhibitors in conjunction with traditional modalities of surgery, radiation therapy, and chemotherapy for many tumors.

Because of its delivery form as an elixir, meloxicam is sometimes used preferentially in small dogs and cats. However, only one-time injectable dosing of meloxicam for perioperative pain is approved for use in the cat in the United States. Potentially causal gastric ulcerations have been observed (Runk et al. 1999; Lascelles et al. 2005; Enberg et al. 2006) with different NSAIDS and different formulations administered to dogs or cats. With any NSAID, accurate dosing of small dogs and cats is imperative.

NSAIDs are the fastest growing class of drugs in both human and veterinary medicine (Table 10.5) because of their relatively safe resolution of a wide range of pathological conditions. Based on current understanding of their mode of action, future NSAIDs will likely not be developed to be "stronger-longer" (i.e., supremely COX-2 selective), with a very long half-life. Instead, NSAID development may well offer species- and/or disease-specific molecules, increased safety profiles, and augmenting benefits such as nitric oxide inhibition. At present, this class of drug offers immense benefits, constrained most often only by issues of safe, responsible use.

The following guidelines provide minimal risk factors for NSAID adverse drug events:

1. Provide proper dosing.
2. Administer minimal effective dose.
3. Dispense in approved packaging together with owner information sheets.
4. Avoid concurrent use of multiple NSAIDs and NSAIDs with corticosteroids.
5. Refrain from use of aspirin.
6. Provide pet owners with both oral and written instructions for responsible NSAID use.
7. Conduct appropriate patient chemistry/urine profiling.
8. Conduct routine checkups and chemistry profiles for patients on chronic NSAID regimens. Do not fill NSAID prescriptions without conducting patient examinations.
9. Caution pet owners regarding supplementation with over-the-counter NSAIDs.
10. Administer gastrointestinal protectants for high at-risk patients on NSAIDs.
11. Avoid NSAID administration in puppies and pregnant animals.

Table 10.5. Commercially available NSAIDs* approved for use in the United States.

	Deramaxx	EtoGesic	Metacam	Previcox	Rimadyl	Zubrin
Company Active Ingredient Formulation	Novartis Deracoxib 25-, 75-, 100-mg scored chewable tablets	Fort Dodge Etodolac 150-, 300-mg scored tablets	Boehringer-Ingelheim Meloxicam Liquid suspension: to be squirted on food (0.5-, 1.5 mg/ml) Injectable: 5 mg/ml, SQ or IV	Merial Firocoxib Chewable tablets containing 57 or 227 mg	Pfizer Carprofen Caplets/chewable tablets: 25-, 75-, 100-mg scored caplets or scored chewable tablets SQ injectable: 50 mg carprofen/ml (refrigerate)	Schering-Plough Tepoxalin Rapidly disintegrating tablets of 30, 50, 100, or 200 mg
Dosage	For the control of pain and inflammation associated with orthopedic surgery in dogs: 3–4 mg/kg. Give prior to surgery for postoperative pain. For the control of pain and inflammation associated with OA in dogs: 1–2 mg/kg daily	10–15 mg/kg once daily (4.5–6.8 mg/lb) Adjust dose until a satisfactory clinical response is obtained reduced to minimum (maintain or minimum) effective dose	0.2 mg/kg injectable once or oral once: followed by 0.1 mg/kg oral suspension daily. Cats: 0.3 mg/kg SQ presurgical one-time dose (contraindicated to follow in cats w/another NSAID or Metacam)	5 mg/kg oral once daily. Tablets are scored and dosage should be calculated in ½-tablet increments.	Oral and injectable: 2 mg/lb daily: may be administered once daily or divided as 1 mg/lb twice daily. For postoperative pain, administer 2 hours before the procedure.	10 mg/kg orally or 20 mg/kg on the initial day of treatment, followed by a daily maintenance dose of 10 mg/kg

152

Indications	For the control of pain and inflammation associated with orthopedic surgery in dogs weighing >4lb For the control of pain and inflammation associated with OA	For the management of pain and inflammation associated with osteoarthritis in dogs	Control of pain and inflammation associated with osteoarthritis in dogs; postoperative pain and inflammation associated with orthopedic surgery, ovariohysterectomy and castration in cats when administered prior to surgery	For the control of pain and inflammation associated with osteoarthritis in dogs	For the relief of pain and inflammation associated with osteoarthritis in dogs and the control of postoperative pain in soft tissue and orthopedic surgeries in dogs	Control of pain and inflammation associated with osteoarthritis in dogs
Mechanism of action	A coxib class drug that uniquely targets COX-2 while sparing COX-1	Inhibition of COX activity; inhibits macrophage chemotaxis	MOA not on label; oxicam class NSAID	Inhibition of COX activity; in vitro studies show it to be highly selective for COX-2 in canine blood	Inhibition of COX enzyme; in vitro selective against COX-2	COX and LOX inhibitor: dual pathway inhibitor of arachidonic acid metabolism
Maximum Concentration (Tmax)	2 hours	1.08–1.6 hours	Dogs: 2.5 hours (inj) and 7.5 hours (oral) Cats: 1.5 hours postinjection		Oral: Cmax of 16.9 μg/ml at 0.5–3 hours Injectable: Cmax of 8.0 μg/ml at 1.5–8 hours	2.3 ± 1.4 hours
Half-life ($T_{1/2}$)	3 hours	7.6–12 hours	Dogs: 24 hours Cats: 15 hours after inj	7.8 hours in the dog	8 hours in dog	2.0 ± 1.2 hours converts to active with long $T_{1/2}$

Continued

Table 10.5. *Continued.*

	Deramaxx	EtoGesic	Metacam	Previcox	Rimadyl	Zubrin
Metabolism and Excretion	Metabolism primarily liver; excretion to GI to feces is 75%, urine excretion is 20%	Primarily hepatic metabolism and fecal excretion; enterohepatic recirculation	Not on label	Primarily hepatic metabolism and fecal excretion	Liver biotransformation: 70–80% in feces and 10–20% in urine. Some enterohepatic circulation	Primarily hepatic with excretion through feces 99%, minor urine
Side Effects within licensing studies **Serious adverse reactions associated with this drug class can occur without warning and in rare situations result in death**	Vomiting, incisional lesions	Weight loss, fecal abnormalities, hypoproteinemia, small intestine erosions	Vomiting, soft stools, diarrhea, inappetance, epiphora, autoimmune hemolytic anemia, thrombocytopenia, polyarthritis, pyoderma	Vomiting, diarrhea, decreased appetite. (Use of this product at doses above the recommended 5 mg/kg in puppies less than 7 months of age has been associated with serious ADEs, including death)	Black or tarry stools, hypoalbuminemia, dermatologic changes, increased liver enzyme levels, idiosyncratic hepatotoxicosis	Vomiting, diarrhea, gastric lesions, decrease in total protein, albumin and calcium, death
Packaging	30, 90 count	7, 30, and 90 count	Oral: 0.5 mg/ml: 15-, 30-ml dropper bottles Inj: 5 mg/ml in a 10-ml vial	10- and 30-count blister packs, 60-count bottles	14, 60, 150 count 20-ml bottle of injectable	Boxes containing 10 foil blisters each
Marketing status	By prescription only	By prescription only	By prescription only	By prescription only	By prescription only	By prescription only
Protein binding	>90%	>99%	>99%	>96%	>99%	>98%
Bioavailability	>90%	Nearly 100%	Nearly 100%	101%	>90%	

154

	Concurrent use statement	Pre-Rx advisement	Miscellaneous
Concomitant use with any other anti-inflammatory drugs, such as other NSAIDs and corticosteroids, should be avoided or closely monitored		Thorough history and physical exam; appropriate laboratory tests	In vitro: showed more COX-2 inhibition than COX-1
Concomitant use with any other anti-inflammatory drugs, such as other NSAIDs and corticosteroids, should be avoided or closely monitored		Thorough history and physical exam; appropriate laboratory tests	Not evaluated for IM injection
Concurrent use with potentially nephrotoxic drugs should be carefully approached. Concomitant use with other anti-inflammatory drugs, such as NSAIDs and corticosteroids, should be avoided or closely monitored		Thorough history and physical exam; appropriate laboratory tests	In vitro: showed more COX-2 inhibition than COX-1
Concomitant use with any other anti-inflammatory drugs, such as other NSAIDs and corticosteroids, should be avoided or closely monitored		Thorough history and physical exam; appropriate laboratory tests	IM comment? See metacam
Concomitant use with any other anti-inflammatory drugs, such as other NSAIDs and corticosteroids, should be avoided or closely monitored		Geriatric examination; appropriate laboratory tests	Give with a meal to enhance absorption

*A very fluid market that changes frequently.
Information contained in Table 10.5 is collected from the Freedom of Information (FOI) for each drug and the information contained in the drug insert. The information will necessarily vary.

155

12. NSAIDs may decrease the action of angiotensin-converting enzyme inhibitors and furosemide, a consideration for patients being treated for cardiovascular disease.

13. Geriatric animals are more likely to be treated with NSAIDs on a chronic schedule; therefore, their "polypharmacy" protocols and potentially compromised drug clearance should be considered.

14. Provide sufficient hydration to surgery patients that are administered NSAIDs.

15. Carefully consider risk/benefit in any volume-depleted patient such as patients with heart failure or kidney or liver failure.

16. Report adverse drug events to the product manufacturers and FDA Center for Veterinary Medicine.

ENDNOTES

1 Adverse drug experience may be reported to the FDA Center for Veterinary Medicine (CVM) at http://www.fda.gov/cvm/.

2 Aspirin-triggering lipoxin: Acetylation of cyclooxygenase (COX)-2 by aspirin can trigger the formation of $15(R)$-epilipoxin A_4 or aspirin-triggered lipoxin (ATL). ATL exerts protective effects in the stomach. Selective COX-2 inhibitors block ATL synthesis and exacerbate aspirin-induced gastric damage (Wallace et al. 2004).

REFERENCES

Boria, P.A., Biolsi, S.A., Greenberg, C.B., et al. 2003. Preliminary evaluation of deracoxib in canine transitional cell carcinoma of the urinary bladder. *Vet Cancer Soc Proc* 17.

Brideau, C., Van Staden, C., and Chan, C.C. 2001. In vitro effects of cyclooxygenase inhibitors in whole blood of horses, dogs, and cats. *Am J Vet Res* 62(11):1755–1780.

Clark, T.P., Chieffo, C., Huhn, J.C., et al. 2003. The steady-stage pharmacokinetics and bioequivalence of carprofen administered orally and subcutaneously in dogs. *J Vet Pharmacol Therap* 26:187–192.

Dowers, K.L., Rayroux, S., Hellyer, P.W., et al. 2006. Effect of short-term sequential administration of nonsteroidal anti-inflammatory drugs on the stomach and proximal portion of the duodenum in healthy dogs. Am *J Vet Res* 67(10):1794–1801.

Enberg, T.B., Braun, L.D., and Kuzma, A.B. 2006. Gastrointestinal perforation in five dogs associated with the administration of meloxicam. *J Vet Emerg Crit Care* 16(1):34–43.

Goodman, L., and Trepanier, L. 2005. Potential drug interaction with dietary supplements. Comp Cont Educ Pract Vet 27(10):780–789.

Hampshire, V.A., Doddy, F.M., Post, L.O., et al. 2004. Adverse drug events report at the United States Food and Drug Administration Center for Veterinary Medicine. *J Am Vet Med Assoc* 225(4):533–536.

Kay-Mugford, P., Benn, S.J., LaMarre, J., et al. 2000. In vitro effects of nonsteroidal anti-inflammatory drugs on cyclooxygenase activity in dogs. *Am J Vet Res* 61(7):802–810.

Lascelles, B.D.X., Blikslager, A.T., Fox, S.M., et al. 2005. Gastrointestinal tract perforations in dogs treated with a selective cyclooxygenase-2 inhibitor: 29 cases (2002–2003). *J Am Vet Med Assoc* 227(7):1112–1117.

Li, J., Lynch, M.P., Demello, K.L., et al. 2005; Mar 1. In vitro and in vivo profile of 2-(3-di-fluoromethyl-5-phenylpyrazol-1-yl)-5-methanesulfonylpyridine, a potent, selective, and orally active canine COX-2 inhibitor. *Bioorg Med Chem* 13(5):1805–1809.

Liu, S.K., Tilley, L.P., Tappe, J.P., et al. 1986. Clinical and pathologic findings in dogs with atherosclerosis: 21 cases (1970–1983) *J Am Vet Med Assoc* 189(2):227–232.

Millis, D.L. 2006. Nonsteroidal anti-inflammatory drugs, disease modifying drugs, and osteoarthritis, in *A Multimodal Approach to Treating Osteoarthritis Symposium.* Novartis Animal Health, pp. 9–19.

Page, G.G., Blakely, W.P., and Ben-Eliyahu, S. 2001. Evidence that postoperative pain is a mediator of the tumor-promoting effects of surgery in rats. *Pain* 90(1–2):191–199.

Runk, A., Kyles, A.E., and Downs, M.O. 1999. Duodenal perforation in a cat following the administration of nonsteroidal anti-inflammatory medication. *J Am Anim Hosp Assoc* 35:52–55.

Singh, G., and Fort, J.G. 2006. Celecoxib versus naproxen and diclofenac in osteoarthritis patients: SUCCESS-I Study. *Am J Med* 119:255–288.

Streppa, H.K., Jones, C.J., and Budsberg, S.C. 2002. Cyclooxygenase selectivity of nonsteroidal anti-inflammatory drugs in canine blood. *Am J Vet Res* 63(1):91–94.

Trepanier, L.A. 2005. Potential interactions between non-steroidal anti-inflammatory drugs and other drugs. *J Vet Emerg Crit Care* 15(4):248–253.

Trepanier, L.A. 2004. Idiosyncratic toxicity associated with potentiated sulfonamides in the dog. *J Vet Pharmacol Therap* 27:129–138.

Wallace, J.L., and Fiorucci, S. 2003. A magic bullet for mucosal protection . . . and aspirin is the trigger! *Trends Pharmacol Sci* 24(7):323–326.

Wallace, J.L., Zamuner, S.R., McKnight, W., et al. 2004. Aspirin, but not NO-releasing aspirin (NCX-4016), interacts with selective COX-2 inhibitors to aggravate gastric damage and inflammation. *Am J Physiol Gastrointest Liver Physiol* 286:G76–G81.

Warner, T.D., and Mitchell, J.A. 2002. Cyclooxygenase-3 (COX-3): Filling in the gaps toward a COX continuum? *Proc Natl Acad Sci* 99(21):13371–13373.

Williams, J.T. 1997. The painless synergism of aspirin and opium. *Nature USA* 390:557–559.

Chapter 11
Support

Alonso G.P. Guedes

Anesthesia is associated with variable and unwanted disruption of the homeostasis of many organs. Virtually all anesthetic agents depress the cardiovascular and respiratory functions. The result can be disastrous if proper monitoring and support are not provided intraoperatively and perioperatively, especially when anesthesia involves an already homeostatically unstable patient. Provision of supportive measures to compensate for anesthesia-related changes in the function of the major organ systems is vital for the success of an anesthetic procedure.

CARDIOVASCULAR SUPPORT

To adequately provide cardiovascular support in the anesthetized patient, it is necessary to understand the basic factors underlying the heart's ability to pump an adequate amount of blood to peripheral tissues (e.g., cardiac output). The physiologic determinants of cardiac output are preload, afterload, contractility, and heart rate. Cardiovascular "leaks" and cardiac hypertrophy are two additional factors that should be considered in the presence of cardiovascular disease (Kittleson and Kienle 1998). However, cardiac output is not routinely measured during anesthesia of clinical patients. Instead, measurement of systemic blood pressure (BP) is more commonly practiced. It is important to acknowledge that while BP does not necessarily correlate with blood flow or tissue perfusion, low BP is likely to result in hypoperfusion to organs and tissues. Hence, assurance of adequate BP is the first step in maintaining blood flow to tissues in patients under anesthesia.

Hypotension is the most common anesthetic complication in dogs and cats (Gaynor et al. 1999). It is difficult to determine adequacy of BP simply by pulse palpation since pulse quality reflects the difference between systolic and diastolic BPs (e.g., pulse pressure), and not their absolute values. A variety of BP monitoring devices is available for use in veterinary patients (Henik et al. 2005). Vital organs such as brain, heart, and kidneys have intrinsic mechanisms that maintain blood flow relatively constant within a range of BPs. This autoregulatory capacity becomes impaired in the healthy kidney when mean arterial blood pressure (MAP) falls below approximately 80 mm Hg, and below approximately 90 mm Hg in the face of renovascular disease. In the healthy myocardium, blood flow starts to decrease significantly when MAP falls below approximately 50 mm Hg, whereas in the hypertrophic heart flow starts to decrease when MAP falls below 70 mm Hg (Bellomo and Giatomasso 2001). Based on this, the MAP should be ideally maintained above 70 mm Hg (or systolic greater than 90 mm Hg) in anesthetized patients to minimize significant impairment of the perfusion pressure to these vital organs.

Because cardiac output is the most important determinant of tissue perfusion, but BP is the most widely measured cardiovascular parameter, it becomes important to understand how these two parameters are integrated (Fig. 11.1). Blood pressure result from the interplay between cardiac output (CO) and systemic vascular resistance (SVR), such that $BP = CO \times SVR$. Because CO is determined by stroke volume (SV) and heart rate (HR), it follows that $BP = SV \times HR \times SVR$. Hence, the therapy to correct BP abnormalities should be directed at restoring the component(s) most likely affected. For example, a hypotensive patient due to low heart rate may benefit from anticholinergic (atropine, glycopyrrolate) administration. Conversely, a hypotensive patient due to blood loss

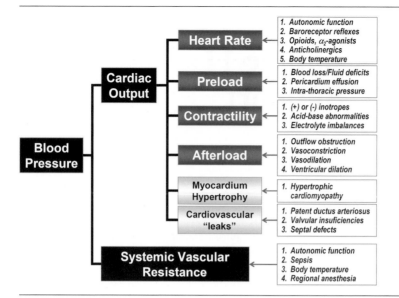

Figure 11.1. Flow chart illustrating the determinants of blood pressure and the factors that may influence each component. See text for details.

(reduced preload) will benefit from fluid replacement. Both patients will benefit from reducing the amount of drugs that depress myocardium contractility (e.g., negative inotropes) such as the inhalants, propofol or thiopental. Even better, cardiovascular alterations should be anticipated and preventive measures promptly instituted. As such, the factors that may underlie changes in BP need to be well known and quickly recognized (Fig. 11.1).

Heart Rate

Many are the anesthesia-related situations that can produce changes in heart rate. Heart rate below 50 beats per minute (bpm) in dogs and 100 bpm in cats can be considered bradycardia, but these numbers may vary because normal heart rate is related to the species, breed, size, and the overall hemodynamic status of each patient. Drugs such as opioids and α_2-adrenergic agonists are well known for their ability to reduce heart rate. As such, anticholinergic agents (e.g., atropine, glycopyrrolate) are commonly used with these drugs to prevent bradycardia. It should be recognized, however, that despite the effects on heart rate, opioids interfere only minimally with cardiac output and BP when used at clinically relevant doses (Pugsley 2002). Anticholinergic-induced sinus tachycardia increases myocardium metabolic demands and oxygen consumption that may not be well tolerated by cardiac patients. If the reduction in heart rate is negatively affecting BP, anticholinergic administration is warranted.

The bradycardia may initially and transiently be accentuated by the anticholinergic due to presynaptic muscarinic receptor inhibition leading to facilitation of acetylcholine release in vagus nerve terminals. The heart rate should increase once postsynaptic muscarinic receptors are blocked.

The bradycardia induced by potent α_2-adrenergic agonists such as medetomidine and romifidine is partly a reflex response due to increased systemic vascular resistance and BP. In this instance, administering an anticholinergic to increase heart rate may produce hypertension and impose undue stress on the myocardium (Sinclair et al. 2003). Therefore, anticholinergics should be used judiciously with α_2-adrenergic agonists. An alternative therapy if heart rate becomes dangerously low is to administer an α_2-antagonist such as atipamezole. The effects on heart rate will be reversed, as will the sedative and analgesic actions. Therefore, the administration of an antagonist may not be feasible when sedation and analgesia are to remain (e.g., sedation for diagnostic procedures such as radiographs, joint taps, wound cleaning, etc). Similarly, it may be more difficult to maintain a steady anesthetic depth during an invasive surgical procedure once the α_2-adrenergic has been antagonized, and the anesthetic requirement may be increased, potentially affecting homeostasis.

Some medical or surgical procedures are more likely to cause bradycardia. The classic example is bradycardia due to the oculocardiac reflex during ophthalmic manipulations. Endoscopic evaluation of the upper gastrointestinal system may cause gastric dilation that may be sufficient to trigger vagally mediated bradycardia. Similar phenomenon may be seen upon distension of the urinary bladder, such as during lithotripsy, through stimulation of sacral parasympathetic afferent neurons. It is important to be vigilant and have an anticholinergic readily available should bradycardia occur during these procedures. Elevated intracranial pressure may result in elevated systemic BP (a physiologic response to restore cerebral perfusion pressure) and baroreceptor-mediated bradycardia (late phase of the Cushing reflex) (Heymans 1928). Hence, bradycardia may be protective in preventing extreme hypertension and further increase in intracranial pressure such that anticholinergic use is contraindicated. The primary cause (elevated intracranial pressure) should be treated instead. Bradycardia is also present in patients with sick sinus syndrome and third-degree atrioventricular (AV) block. Mobitz type II second-degree AV block can progress without warning to third-degree AV block with a resultant slow and unstable idioventricular rhythm. These patients may not be anticholinergic responsive and a pacemaker may be the best treatment. Catecholamine infusion (e.g., isoproterenol, dobutamine) may be used in an attempt to increase heart rate until pacing is established. However, isoproterenol may cause significant vasodilation and hypotension at high doses, so pacing should not be delayed. Never treat third-degree AV block or ventricular escape beats with lidocaine.

Sinus tachycardia may also occur in the perioperative and intraoperative period and should be treated adequately. As with bradycardia, many factors determine the normal heart rate in each patient. As a general guideline, heart rates greater than 160 bpm in the dog and 180 bpm in the cat can be considered tachycardia. Inappropriate increases in heart rate may impair myocardium perfusion while oxygen demand is increased, dangerously compromising cardiac performance. Excessive sinus tachycardia may reduce diastolic time and ventricular filling, thus reducing cardiac output. When sinus tachycardia is present, the possible causes should be investigated promptly. Superficial anesthetic depth, autonomic response to nociception, blood loss, hyperthermia, hypercapnia, hypoxemia, drugs (ketamine, barbiturates, catecholamines), hyperthyroidism, and acute anaphylactoid reactions can all lead to increases in heart rate. Excessive anesthetic depth may also induce tachycardia (together with hypotension) as a physiologic response aimed at increasing cardiac output and restore BP. Eventually, the profound anesthetic depth may cause bradycardia due to myocardial hypoxia and cardiac arrest is likely the next event. The specific treatment for tachycardia should be directed towards the causative factor.

Stroke Volume

If heart rate is within normal limits for the patient but hypotension is present, a reduced stroke volume may be the likely underlying cause. Stroke volume is the amount of blood ejected from the ventricle (right or left) with each contraction, and its determinants include preload, contractility, and afterload. Preload is primarily represented by the end-diastolic volume and, as such, is dependent on circulating volume and venous return. Preload can be decreased by any factor that reduces venous return including fluid deficits (e.g., dehydration), blood loss, elevated intrathoracic pressure (e.g., positive-pressure ventilation, pneumothorax), elevated intra-abdominal pressure (e.g., gastric dilation, gravid uterus, pneumoperitoneum, large intra-abdominal tumors), surgery-related compression of thoracic or abdominal vena cava, reduced venous tone (e.g., septic shock, locoregional anesthesia), and atrial contraction (e.g., atrial standstill, atrial fibrillation). Ensuring adequate venous return is paramount for maintenance of adequate cardiac output and BP. The therapy should be directed to the cause(s) and may include fluid administration, reduction of intrathoracic or intra-abdominal pressure, adjustment of positive-pressure ventilation settings, and/or using vasopressors.

Contractility is another determinant of stroke volume and cardiac output. It is the intrinsic ability of the myocardium to contract and produce work from a given end-diastolic fiber length (e.g., end-diastolic volume), being closely related to the availability of intracellular calcium. Clinically useful indexes of contractility are ejection fraction (EF; normal 65% to 70%) and fractional shortening (SF; normal 30% to 40%). These parameters are very informative of the ventricular function, especially in patients with preexisting heart disease. A change in contractility is considered to be a change in myocardial contractile force in the presence of unchanged diastolic volume and pressure. Contractility is negatively and dose-dependently affected by virtually all general anesthetics with the exception of etomidate. Balanced anesthesia minimizes dose-related side effects of anesthetic drugs and is likely to contribute to better cardiovascular function (Ilkiw 1999). For example, the addition of the μ-opioid receptor agonist alfentanil to reduce the required amount of isoflurane resulted in a 2-fold increase in MAP and cardiac output in one study in cats (Pascoe et al. 1997). Avoiding excessive anesthetic depth is another approach that minimizes anesthetic-induced depression of myocardium contractility. If instituting balanced anesthesia and reducing anesthetic delivery (and after addressing preload) are not sufficient to restore BP to within acceptable limits, then administration of a positive inotrope agent should be considered.

The catecholamines dobutamine and dopamine are the most commonly used positive inotropes in anesthetized patients to improve myocardium contractility and restore BP. Dobutamine is a racemic mixture of two isomers, both of which are β-adrenergic receptor (AR) agonists. Dobutamine is considered relatively selective $β_1$-AR agonist, although it is also a weak partial $β_2$-AR agonist, and has both $α_1$-AR agonist [(−)-isomer] and antagonist [(+)-isomer] activities (Vernon et al. 1992). The usual net effect is elevation of myocardium contractility and stroke volume, although it may also increase heart rate especially at higher doses (Pascoe et al. 2006). The effects on vascular smooth muscle function are complex, but a reduction in systemic vascular resistance is not uncommon, suggesting some degree of vasodilation in both dogs and cats (Dyson and Sinclair 2006; Pascoe et al. 2006; Vernon et al. 1992).

Dopamine, a precursor of norepinephrine and epinephrine, is also a neurotransmitter in both the central and peripheral nervous system. The clinical effects of dopamine are complex and dose dependent. It directly stimulates dopaminergic receptors, $β_1$-AR and $α_1$-AR. Low doses (less than 3 μg/kg/min) predominantly affect arterial dopaminergic receptors on organs such as the kidneys. This vascular effect together with reduced Na^+ absorption due to inhibition of aldosterone release and the Na^+/K^+-ATPase in tubular cells increases urine output and has been advocated for use in nephropathic patients. While no convincing data are currently available about dopamine effects on outcome of dogs and cats with renal disease, information from humans indicate that dopamine has no renoprotective effects despite increased urine output (Schenarts et al. 2006). Medium doses (3 to 10 μg/kg/min) produce primarily β-AR effects (e.g., positive inotrope) and high doses (greater than 10 μg/kg/min) produce primarily α-AR effects (e.g., vasopressor). Calcium ($CaCl_2$) is a mild positive inotrope and vasopressor that is useful when massive blood transfusion depress myocardium contractility (e.g., citrate toxicity), when calcium channel blocker overdose is suspected and in the presence of low plasma ionized calcium concentration. Otherwise, it should not be used as primary inotrope support.

Afterload is another determinant of cardiac output, and in the intact heart it is defined as the impedance to ejection or the ventricular wall stress. Afterload as defined by ventricular wall stress is described by Laplace's law where T = Pr/2h, in which T = left ventricular wall tension, P = pressure, r = radius, and h = wall thickness. From this perspective, afterload is primarily influenced by the systolic intraventricular pressure (or aortic pressure) and the volume and thickness of the left ventricle. A ventricle that is dilated (increased r) or hypertrophic (increased h) has a significantly increased afterload (T) and stroke volume is frequently reduced. Afterload is also significantly affected by systolic intraventricular pressure. Reducing or minimizing increased afterload is an important goal during anesthesia of patients with congestive heart failure.

The impedance to ejection involves aortic pressure, the aortic valve, vascular distensibility, and systemic vascular resistance (SVR). The SVR accounts for approximately 95% of the resistance to ejection, being a major determinant of afterload in healthy hearts. Clinically, drugs (e.g., $α_2$-AR agonists, vasopressors) or situations (e.g., inefficient use of analgesics to blunt sympathetic response to nociception) that increase SVR should be avoided in patients with excentric cardiomyopathy, congestive heart failure, or static ventricular outflow tract obstruction (e.g., pulmonic or aortic stenosis). In cats with left ventricular hypertrophy and dynamic left ventricular outflow tract obstruction, one study showed complete elimination of the obstruction and systolic anterior motion of the mitral valve after medetomidine-induced sedation (Lamont et al. 2002). That study also demonstrated no significant changes in ventricular wall stress, fractional short-ening, and left ventricular ejection fraction. However, the combined effect with general anesthetics is unknown at present.

Systemic Vascular Resistance

The main vasopressors used during anesthesia of small animal veterinary patients include norepinephrine, phenylephrine, ephedrine, and vasopressin. Increasing SVR is usually not the primary approach to restore BP in a hypotensive, anesthetized patient. The exception is when systemic vasodilation is suspected as the main causative factor; when hypotension is nonresponsive to improving preload (e.g., fluid administration) and contractility (e.g., balanced anesthesia, positive inotropes); or when a further increase in myocardium contractility may not be desirable (e.g., hypertrophic concentric cardiomyopathy). Common clinical situations that may be associated with reduced SVR and hypotension include vasodilatory shock (e.g., sepsis), regional sympathetic blockade (e.g., epidurals with local anesthetics), anaphylactic or anaphylactoid reactions, and α-AR antagonists (e.g., acepromazine). Increased SVR is a common finding in diseases such as pheochromocytoma, which may cause significant vasoconstriction and hypertension. In patients undergoing anesthesia for pheochromocytoma removal, vasodilators (e.g., sodium nitroprusside) may be necessary to maintain BP within normal limits. However, the control of BP in these patients may be especially challenging because the catecholamine release usually occurs in bursts instead of being constant, making BP fluctuate significantly and unpredictably. The inotropes and vasopressors most commonly used during anesthesia are presented in Table 11.1.

INTRAOPERATIVE FLUID THERAPY

The principles of perioperative fluid therapy were first developed approximately five decades ago (Moore 1949; Shires et al. 1961). It is now known that preservation of normal fluid and electrolyte homeostasis is an essential component of anesthesia. Anesthesia affects the normal turnover of body water and electrolytes, which may be especially important in neonates, geriatric patients, and critically ill patients. At minimum, the insensible fluid losses that occur through salivation, urine production, and gastrointestinal tract secretions and loss of water through evaporation both through the respiratory tract and exposed body cavities and viscera should be replaced. Ideally, fluid therapy should replace not only insensible losses but also the fluid loss associated with the disease and/or the procedure. Maintenance of microcirculatory organ perfusion and oxygen delivery essential for cellular metabolism is the primary goal of perioperative fluid therapy. In addition, many patients undergoing anesthesia have acid-base imbalance, electrolyte disorders, and colloid osmotic pressure changes that should be corrected to minimize impairment of vital cellular functions.

Oxygen delivery (Do_2) is dependent on cardiac output and arterial oxygen content (Cao_2) (Fig. 11.2). In the presence of stable arterial oxygen saturation and hemoglobin content, Do_2 depends exclusively on cardiac output. As discussed earlier, virtually all anesthetic agents have various dose-dependent hemodynamic effects, frequently reducing preload and myocardial contractility, directly affecting cardiac output. Perioperative fluid therapy is essential to support intravascular volume and minimize reductions in preload, thus optimizing cardiac output and oxygen delivery. Under normal hemodynamic and hematological conditions, hemoglobin content and oxygen saturation are the major determinants of Cao_2. Almost all of the Cao_2 (greater than 97%) is chemically bound to hemoglobin, and only a small amount (less than 3%) of the total Cao_2 is dissolved in plasma. The Cao_2 can be calculated using the following equation:

$$Cao_2 = [1.38 \times Hb \times Sao_2] + [Pao_2 \times 0.003] \quad (11.1)$$

As can be seen, the largest portion of the Cao_2 is not revealed by knowing the partial pressure of oxygen (Pao_2) or the hemoglobin saturation with oxygen (Sao_2) in arterial blood.

There are numerous choices of solutions for fluid therapy (Table 11.2). The use of a balanced crystalloid (Ringer's, lactated Ringer's solution, etc.), colloid (plasma, gelatins, hydroxyethyl starch preparations, etc.), and/or oxygen-carrying (packed red blood cells, whole blood, hemoglobin-based oxygen carriers, etc.) solutions may be necessary to prevent reductions in oxygen delivery.

Crystalloids are aqueous solutions containing small, osmotically active particles that can easily cross the capillary membrane. Crystalloids may be

Table 11.1. Summary of inotropes and vasopressors commonly used for cardiovascular support during anesthesia in veterinary patients.

Drug	Receptors activated	Cardiovascular effect	Side effects	Doses
Dobutamine	β_1 β_2	(+) Inotrope, (+) Chronotrope (high doses) ±Improved perfusion ↑ CO, ↑ BP, ↑ HR	Tachyarrhythmias Vasodilation peripheral pulmonary	CRI: 1–10 µg/kg/min
Dopamine	Dose dependent: dopaminergic β_1, β_2 α_1, α_2	(+) Chronotrope (+) Inotrope ↑ CO, ↑ BP, ↑ HR, ↑ SVR (high doses)	Tachyarrhythmias Vasoconstriction at high doses	Dopaminergic (renal) = 0.5–2 µg/kg/min β_1-Adrenergic agonist = 2–10 µg/kg/min α-Adrenergic agonist = >10 µg/kg/min
Ephedrine	β_1, β_2 α_1, α_2	(+) Inotrope vasoconstriction (primarily venous) ↑ CO, ↑ BP, ↑ SVR	CNS stimulation ("lighten-up") Tachyarrhythmias	0.1–0.2 mg/kg CRI not indicated; tachyphylaxis after 1–2 doses
Phenylephrine	α_1 α_2	Vasoconstriction ↑ BP ↑ SVR ± ↓ CO	Bradycardia Reflex response) ± ↓ perfusion	0.001–0.01 mg/kg (1–10 µg/kg) CRI: 0.1–3 µg/kg/min
Vasopressin	V1, V2, V3 Oxytocin receptors (OTR) Purinergic receptors (P2)	Vasoconstriction	Hypertension Reduced urine output	0.1 unit/kg loading dose, followed by CRI of 0.2 unit/kg/hr
Norepinephrine	Predominantly α_1, α_2 Slightly β_1	Vasoconstriction (primarily arterioles) ± (+) Inotrope ↑ SVR, ↑ BP, ± ↑ CO	Tachyarrhythmias Decreased perfusion?	CRI: 0.1–1.0 µg/kg/min

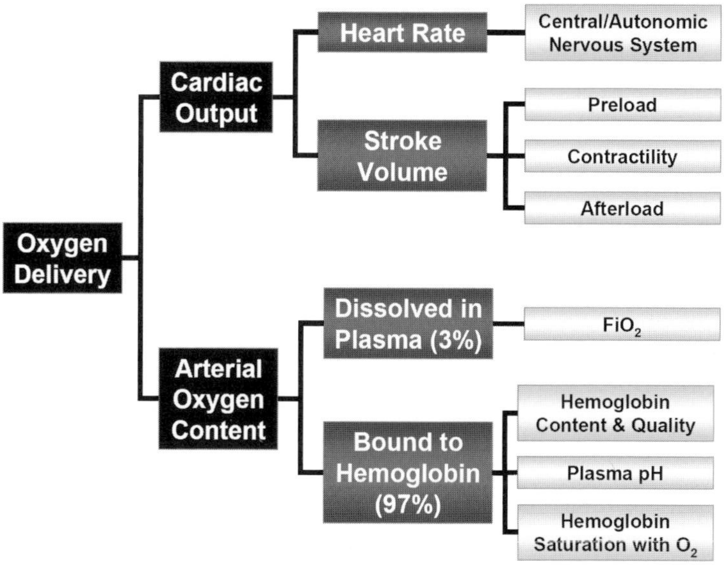

Figure 11.2. Flow chart illustrating the determinants of oxygen delivery with the factors that may influence each component. See text for details.

Table 11.2. Characteristics and electrolyte composition of commonly used crystalloid for fluid therapy during anesthesia.

	Electrolytes (mEq/L)								
Solution	Na^+	Cl^-	K^+	Ca^{2+}	Mg^{2+}	Buffer	pH	Osmolality (mOsm/L)	COP (mm Hg)
Ringer's lactated solution	130	109	4	3	—	Lactate	6.5	274	0
Ringer's solution	147	156	4	4	—	—	5.5	310	0
Normosol-R	140	98	5	—	3	Acetate	6.4	294	0
Plasma-Lyte A (Baxter)	140	98	5	—	3	Acetate gluconate	7.4	294	0
0.9% Saline	154	154	—	—	—	—	5.0	308	0
7.0% Saline	1197	1197	—	—	—	—	—	2396	
5% Dextrose	—	—	—	—	—	—	4.0	252	<1

classified into isotonic (e.g., lactated Ringer's solution), hypotonic (e.g., 5% dextrose in water), and hypertonic (eg, hypertonic saline) solutions. They can also be classified as replacement or maintenance solutions, where the primary difference is in electrolyte concentrations. A replacement crystalloid solution has electrolyte composition and tonicity similar to that of plasma (e.g., an isotonic balanced electrolyte solution) and is suitable for plasma volume expansion. The maintenance crystalloid fluids contain electrolytes in concentrations that are suitable for replacement of insensible and sensible electrolyte losses. Isotonic crystalloid fluids only expand the extracellular space because they have the same osmolality as that of the cells. Because the dextrose molecules are metabolized to free water, dextrose in water (5%) is considered a hypotonic solution. Hypotonic fluids are not appropriate for intravascular or interstitial volume replacement but can be used to replace free-water deficits. Administration of hypertonic fluids (e.g., hypertonic saline) improves intravascular hydrostatic pressure initially by pulling water down an osmotic gradient from the interstitial and intracellular fluid compartments into the intravascular space. It is important that isotonic crystalloids or colloids be administered after or concurrently with hypertonic saline solution to maintain the circulating volume. The reason is that the electrolytes (e.g., Na^+) will eventually move into the interstitial space, increasing the interstitial fluid tonicity, favoring movement of water away from the intravascular space which may cause further reduction of intravascular volume (Kudnig and Mama 2002; Rozanski and Rondeau 2002). Hypertonic saline (7% NaCl solution) can be administered at 4 to 6 ml/kg IV to treat severe hypotension. Hypernatremia, hyperchloremia, acidosis, and cardiac arrhythmias are potential side effects.

Isotonic replacement solutions are generally used during anesthesia, usually at a rate of 10 to 20 ml/kg/hr in most patients. This fluid rate may be changed depending on concurrent conditions (e.g., congestive heart failure, hypoproteinemia, pulmonary edema) or blood loss during surgery. Hypotonic solutions are not frequently used during anesthesia because the risk of developing hyponatremia and reduction in plasma osmolality. To prevent dilutional acidosis, replacement solutions may contain a buffer (e.g., lactate, acetate). Less than 25% of an infused balanced crystalloid solution, approximately, will remain into the intravascular space after 2 hours and less than 10% remains after 3 hours. Hence, crystalloid solutions should be administered at three to four times larger volumes to replace a given volume of blood that has been lost (Hein et al. 1988; Kudnig and Mama 2002; Muir and Wiese 2004). This may be limited because of dilution of plasma proteins and reduction of plasma osmotic pressure, thus increasing the risk of interstitial and intracellular edema. Hence, addition of colloids to maintain colloid osmotic pressure may be necessary (Hein et al. 1988; Kudnig and Mama 2002; Muir and Wiese 2004). Closely monitor packed cell volume and total proteins to assess hemodilution when administering large volumes of crystalloid solutions.

Colloids (Table 11.3) are solutions containing large molecules that do not readily escape the intravascular compartment. Plasma is a natural colloid, whereas hetastarch, dextrans, and pentastarch are synthetic or artificial colloids. Colloids exert their effect on plasma volume by acutely increasing colloid osmotic pressure within the vasculature. These solutions are indicated when crystalloids alone are insufficient to maintain osmotic pressure or in patients requiring large and rapid volume replacement. Administration of small volumes

Table 11.3. Characteristics and electrolyte composition of synthetic and natural colloids commonly used during anesthesia.

Solution	Electrolytes (mEq/L)					Mn* (×103)	Mw† (×103)	pH	Osmolality (mOsm/L)	COP (mmHg)
	Na^+	Cl^-	K^+	Ca^{2+}	Mg^{2+}					
Hetastarch	154	154	—	—	—	69	450	5.5	309	33
Dextran 40	154	154	—	—	—	26	40	3.5–7.0	311	40
Dextran 70	154	154	—	—	—	41	70	5.0	310	62
10% Pentastarch	154	154	—	—	—	63	264	5.0	326	40
Oxypolygelatin	145	100	—	2	—	23	30	—	200	45
Urea-linked gelatin	145	145	5.1	6.3		24.5	35	7.2	310	25–28
Plasma	145	105	5	5	3	—	—	7.4	300	17–28
Whole blood	140	100	4	—	—	—	—	—	300	~20
Oxyglobin	150	110	4	1	—	—	—	7.8	300	42

*Mn (number molecular weight) is a clinically significant term that refers to the total weight of all the molecules divided by the number of molecules, thus allowing recognition of smaller molecular weight particles in the solution. The colloid oncotic pressure (COP) exerted depends on the number of particles present, whereas the particles sizes determine the duration of action.

†Mw (molecular weight) is the average molecular weight of the solution and is significantly influenced by the larger particles in the solution.

results in rapid elevation in cardiac output and BP. Patients with increased capillary permeability (e.g., systemic inflammatory response syndrome [SIRS]), hypoproteinemic (total protein less than 3.5 g/dl or albumin less than 1.5 g/dl), hypovolemic shock, third space losses, and hypovolemia concurrent with cerebral or pulmonary edema may benefit from colloid administration. In patients with hypoproteinemia, colloids may be used as the sole maintenance solution (5 to 10 ml/kg/hr) or, more commonly, be combined with other crystalloid solutions (2 to 5 ml/kg/hr). The concurrent administration of a crystalloid solution helps replenish the interstitial and intracellular fluid compartments. The crystalloid dose should be reduced (40% to 60%) to minimize risks of fluid overload and interstitial edema. When colloids are used to quickly restore intravascular volume during anesthesia, a starting dose of 10 to 20 ml/kg/hr in dogs and 10 to 15 ml/kg/hr in cats may be used (Roznski and Rondeau 2002). Optionally, intravenous administration of small boluses (2 to 5 ml/kg) may be given to restore cardiac output and BP.

The goal of colloidal therapy is to maintain a colloid osmotic pressure (COP) close to physiologic to avoid interstitial and cellular edema. The adequacy of artificial colloid therapy is assessed by measuring COP since measurement of plasma protein levels with a refractometer will not reflect the osmotic force within the plasma. The duration of effect may vary depending on the situation and the colloid used. In an otherwise healthy patient, some volume expansion may remain for up to 24 hours following the initial dose, but this may be significantly shorter in patients with significant vascular leak or ongoing blood loss (Kudnig and Mama 2002). Ability to restore intravascular volume with smaller volumes thus minimizing hemodilution and a prolonged duration of action are known advantages of colloid therapy. Potential disadvantages of colloids include increased costs, volume overload, anaphylactoid reactions, coagulopathies, and hyperosmotic renal dysfunction. Synthetic colloids are contraindicated in patients with severe coagulopathy (Kozek-Langenecker 2005; Kudnig and Mama 2002). Colloids may affect coagulation by direct effects on platelets and the coagulation cascade or by hemodilution. Hetastarch-induced decrease in von Willebrand's factor has been reported to be ameliorated by administration of desmopressin (Kozek-Langenecker 2005; Lazarchick and Conroy 1995). Synthetic colloids should be used with caution in patients with oliguric or anuric renal failure, congestive heart failure, or pulmonary edema. Excessive colloid administration may increase COP to an extent that may reverse the Starling forces that govern glomerular filtration and result in oliguric acute renal failure (Kozek-Langenecker 2005; Rozich and Paul 1989).

Plasma is a natural colloid that can be used in cases of hypoalbuminemia, coagulopathies, disseminated intravascular coagulation, SIRS, and life-threatening thrombocytopenia. Although plasma is used primarily to provide plasma proteins, chiefly albumin, calculations indicate that 45 ml/kg would be required to increase serum albumin by 1 g/dl (Chiaramonte 2004; Wardrop 1997). The plasma proteins provide around 70% of the total COP, 80% of which is provided by albumin, with the remainder 20% coming from globulins and fibrinogen. The remaining 30% of the total COP is provided by the positively charged ions (mainly Na^+) that bind to the negatively charged plasma proteins (Donnan equilibrium effect). This causes the colloid osmotic pressure to be approximately 50% greater than that produced by the plasma proteins alone. Albumin also has other important functions in addition to exerting colloid osmotic forces, including binding and transport of drugs, hormones, metals and enzymes, free radical scavenging, and binding of inflammatory mediators. Fresh plasma or fresh frozen plasma (frozen at −20°C within 6 hours of collection) should be used instead of stored plasma in cases of thrombocytopenia or coagulopathies as a source of platelets and coagulation factors. Clotting factors maintain activity for up to 12 months in the fresh frozen plasma. Fresh frozen plasma may also be used as a source of albumin, α-macroblobulins, and immunoglobulins (Castellanos et al. 2004; Logan et al. 2001).

Adequate tissue oxygenation depends on the balance between tissue oxygen demand and tissue oxygen delivery. In patients with low hemoglobin content (anemia, hemorrhage), increases in cardiac output alone may not be sufficient to maintain oxygen delivery to sustain cellular metabolism. Hence, blood transfusion or use of blood substitutes becomes essential to restore oxygen-carrying capacity. The precise critical hematocrit or hemoglobin concentration (e.g., the hemoglobin concentration below which Do_2 becomes insufficient to meet oxygen demand in the anesthetized patient) in clinical patients is unclear. In experimental healthy dogs subjected to normovolemic hemodilution, the critical hemoglobin concentration was found to be between 3.5 and 4.0 g/dl (Van der Linden et al. 1998). While many factors may influence the decision to transfuse (e.g., chronicity anemia, presence of comorbidity, rate of ongoing losses, clinical signs, reduced organ perfusion, and anaerobic metabolism), patients with acute blood loss and hemoglobin concentrations below 5.0 g/dl (hematocrit below 15%) are in great risk of insufficient Do_2 for basal metabolism and should probably be transfused. In the clinical patient, blood transfusion should be instituted before the critical hemoglobin concentration is reached. As such, most patients with hemoglobin concentration less than 6 to 7 g/dl (hematocrit less than 18% to 21%) will benefit from blood transfusion or administration of hemoglobin-based oxygen carriers.

In practice, the blood volume can be estimated as 90 ml/kg in the dog and 60 ml/kg in the cat. Most healthy patients can tolerate a 10% loss of their blood volume before significant hemodynamic changes are evident. Losses between 20% and 30% of blood volume are often associated with reductions in BP and require immediate volume replacement. Losses greater than 30% of blood volume will likely cause signs of hemorrhagic shock and circulatory collapse may develop. Appropriate volume replacement with colloids or crystalloids must be provided. Blood loss in excess of 40% to 50% of blood volume may cause death, although depending on the initial hemoglobin concentration and presence of comorbidity and with the provision of adequate volume replacement, the patient may survive. Intra-operative blood loss can be estimated in different ways. It can be measured directly in the reservoir canister of the suctioning system if no lavage fluid has been used. If lavage fluid was used, the blood lost can be estimated with the following equation:

$$\text{Blood lost (ml)} = [\text{fluid's hematocrit/patient's preoperative hematocrit}] \times \text{volume of fluid} \quad (11.2)$$

The amount of blood soaked in sponges or drapes can be determined by weighing them and subtract-

ing the dry weight (1 g = 1 ml). When weighing is not practical or possible, it is useful to know that 5 to 10 ml of blood may be present in a 4×4-inch gauze sponge depending on the degree of saturation, 50 ml of blood may be present in a soaked laparotomy sponge, and that 100 ml of blood occupies the surface of a 12×12-inch floor tile. Equally important is to assess the rate of ongoing losses and the likelihood of timely control of the hemorrhage. The amount of red blood cells lost should ideally be replaced. If this is not feasible, then the objective should be to maintain hemoglobin concentration of at least 6 to 7 mg/dl (hematocrit greater than 18% to 21%). The patient should be blood-typed or crossmatched before transfusion whenever possible, especially cats (Klaser et al. 2005; Castellanos et al. 2004; Jutkowitz et al. 2002; Kudnig and Mama 2002). Although most cats (greater than 90%) in the United States have blood type A, many cats (less than 10%) have type B, and these include both mixed and purebred animals. A minority of cats have the AB blood type (Klaser et al. 2005; Castellanos et al. 2004). The amount of blood necessary can be calculated with the following equation:

$$\text{Blood requirement (ml)} = [\text{desired} - \text{recipient hematocrit}] \div \text{donor hematocrit} \times BW \times BV \quad (11.3)$$

where BW is body weight (kg) and BV is blood volume of recipient (90 ml/kg for dogs and 60 ml/kg for cats). A guide for the administration rate of different fluids during anesthesia is shown on Table 11.4.

VENTILATION, OXYGENATION, AND ACID-BASE BALANCE

Virtually all anesthetic drugs used in veterinary anesthesia are respiratory depressants. The increased awareness of preemptive and multimodal analgesia has increased the perioperative use of potent respiratory depressant drugs such as opioids and α_2-AR agonists. Similarly, the degree of sophistication of certain diagnostic and surgical procedures (e.g., endoscopies, minimally invasive surgeries, etc.) may have significant impact on the respiratory function. Finally, conditions that impose extra pressure over the diaphragm (e.g., large abdominal masses, gastric dilation volvulus, pregnant uterus, head-down positioning, etc.) will cause respiratory impairment requiring respiratory support.

Table 11.4. Crystalloid and colloid administration rates guidelines for fluid therapy during anesthesia (specific rates may vary depending on each clinical situation).

Fluid type	Rate of administration, IV
Crystalloids	10–20 ml/kg/h or 3 times the shed blood volume
Colloids	0.5–2 ml/kg/h to restore COP 10–20 ml/kg/h (dogs) or 10–15 ml/kg/h (cat) in hypovolemic shock, or equal to shed blood volume* 2–5 ml/kg boluses repeated until restoration of cardiac output or blood pressure
Hypertonic saline	4–6 ml/kg bolus
Fresh frozen plasma	6–10 ml/kg as a source of coagulation factors
Oxyglobin	10–30 ml/kg, not to exceed rates of 10 ml/kg/h**
Packed red blood cells	10 ml/kg will typically raise hematocrit by approximately 10%. Administration rate may vary depending on the severity of hemorrhage.

*Editors note: lower dose often used and lower dose for cats.

**Editors note: Editor uses these as daily doses and does not exceed 5 ml/kg/hr IV in dogs and 3 ml/kg/hr IV in cats. With high rates of colloids monitor central venous pressure (CVP).

Ventilation

The initial goal of ventilatory support during anesthesia is to provide adequate alveolar ventilation for optimum gas exchange. Because carbon dioxide (CO_2) production is relatively constant in most clinical settings, CO_2 elimination is proportional to alveolar ventilation. The normal $Paco_2$ varies between 35 and 45 mm Hg and hence $Paco_2$ less than 35 mm Hg (hypocapnia) implies hyperventilation, whereas $Paco_2$ greater than 45 mm Hg (hypercapnia) indicates hypoventilation. Controlled manual or mechanical ventilation is necessary to maintain normal alveolar ventilation in anesthetized animals experiencing hypoventilation. The alveolar minute ventilation (or minute volume) is determined by the respiratory rate and tidal volume (V_T) and both are under the control of groups of neurons within the medulla and pons—the respiratory center. The V_T is the movement of air "in" and "out" of the respiratory system during quite respiration and is composed of alveolar V_T and total physiologic dead space ($V_{D\ phys}$). The $V_{D\ phys}$ is partitioned into anatomic dead space ($V_{D\ ana}$; conducting airways not participating in gas exchange) and alveolar dead space ($V_{D\ alv}$; ventilated but not perfused alveoli).

When instituting intermittent positive-pressure ventilation (IPPV), the tidal volume is calculated in the range of 10 to 20 ml/kg in healthy animals. The respiratory rate is set to maintain normal $Paco_2$, usually between 8 and 12 breaths/min. Peak inspiratory pressures between 10 and 20 cm H_2O are normally generated during adequate lung inflation, and this is dependent on respiratory system compliance and tidal volume. Younger animals tend to have more compliant respiratory system and hence less pressure is generated for a given tidal volume compared to an older animal. Observation of chest wall expansion will provide a subjective but important assessment of lung inflation for the provision of adequate mechanical ventilation. The peak inspiratory pressure should be kept to a minimum in patients with lung trauma or pathology (e.g., bulla) to avoid further trauma and development of pneumothorax. The inspiratory time should be between 1 and 1.5 seconds during IPPV with inspiratory-to-expiratory (I:E) ratios between 1:2 and 1:4 to provide adequate ventilation while minimizing negative cardiovascular effects. The IPPV reduces preload, thus decreasing cardiac output and BP. The mean airway pressure is a more important determinant of the effects of IPPV on the cardiovascular system than the peak inspiratory pressure. Consider the following two ventilator settings as an example:

1. A respiratory rate of 10 breaths/min, with a 2.5-second inspiratory time and peak inspiratory

pressure of 15 cm H_2O will produce a mean airway pressure of 6.5 cm H_2O/min ($10 \times 2.5 \times 15 \div 60 = 6.5$).

2. A respiratory rate of 10 breaths/min, with a 1.5-second inspiratory time and peak inspiratory pressures of 15 cm H_2O will produce a mean airway pressure of 3.75 cm H_2O/min ($10 \times 1.5 \times 15 \div 60 = 3.75$).

The second scenario should produce less impact on the cardiovascular system and therefore is preferable from a cardiovascular standpoint.

Monitoring of $PaCO_2$ requires arterial blood sampling and capabilities to perform blood gas analysis. An alternative is to monitor the partial pressure of exhaled CO_2 ($ETCO_2$) with the use of capnography. In healthy animals, there is a good association between $PaCO_2$ and $ETCO_2$, the later being approximately 5 mm Hg lower than the former. Additional advantages of capnography include its noninvasiveness and the fact that it provides continuous measurement of $ETCO_2$. Furthermore, if a capnogram is also available, the analysis of the waveforms may provide very useful information (Anderson and Breen 2000; Thompson and Jaffe 2005). When used in combination with blood gas analysis, the $ETCO_2$ may be useful in calculating the percentage of alveolar dead space ventilation (V_D/V_T), as follows:

$$V_D/V_T = [PaCO_2 - ETCO_2] \div PaCO_2 \times 100 \quad (11.4)$$

Normally, the V_D/V_T is less than 10% in anesthetized healthy animals and results from lung regions with high alveolar ventilation–to–blood flow ratio. Greater values indicate that a larger portion of the tidal volume is being lost to dead space (Anderson and Breen 2000).

Oxygenation

Adequate oxygenation is dependent on factors, such as (1) fraction of inspired oxygen (FIO_2), (2) alveolar ventilation, (3) ventilation/perfusion ($\dot{V}/\dot{Q}$) mismatching, (4) right-to-left shunting, and (5) diffusion impairment. Tissue oxygenation also depends on hemoglobin concentration, quality and saturation, and cardiac output. The alveolar gas equation may be used to estimate the alveolar partial pressure of oxygen (PAO_2), as follows:

$$PAO_2 = [FIO_2 (P_B - P_{H_2O})] - (PaCO_2 \div R) \quad (11.5)$$

where P_B is barometric pressure in mm Hg (760 mm Hg at sea level), P_{H_2O} is water vapor pressure (47 mm Hg), and R is the respiratory quotient (0.8; the ratio between CO_2 production and O_2 consumption). The calculated PAO_2 at sea level of a healthy individual breathing room air ($FIO_2 = 0.21$) is 100 mm Hg, and the expected PaO_2 is 90 to 100 mm Hg (given that $\dot{V}/\dot{Q}$ matching and diffusion impairment are within normal physiologic limits). As can be noticed, the PaO_2 is approximately five times greater than the FIO_2. Hence, while the PaO_2 of a patient breathing room air is approximately 100 mm Hg, it will be approximately 500 mm Hg in a patient breathing 100% oxygen. The difference between the PAO_2 and the PaO_2 or alveolar-to-arterial (A-a) gradient can be used as an indicator of the degree of pulmonary disease or diffusion impairment present when the patient is breathing room air ($FIO_2 = 0.21$). This may be useful during the preoperative patient evaluation and preparation for anesthesia. At this FIO_2, an A-a gradient less than 10 mm Hg is considered normal. An A-a gradient between 10 and 20 mm Hg is considered mild, between 20 and 30 mm Hg is considered moderate, and greater than 30 is considered severe oxygenation impairment. The A-a gradient will be increased by right-to-left shunt, $\dot{V}/\dot{Q}$ mismatch, or diffusion impairment. The A-a gradient is not altered by hypoventilation (increased $PaCO_2$) but is profoundly affected by the FIO_2 (Herrick et al. 1990). Hence, the A-a gradient is of little utility in patients receiving higher FIO_2, although it may be useful to identify trends in pulmonary function changes.

Clinically, development of $\dot{V}/\dot{Q}$ mismatch and hypoventilation are the most common causes of hypoxemia in the anesthetized patient. In patients breathing high FIO_2, hypoventilation is usually not a cause of significant hypoxemia. However, reduced alveolar ventilation will cause hypoxemia in patients breathing lower FIO_2 as may occur during injectable anesthesia (if oxygen supplementation is not provided) or during anesthetic recovery. It is important that patients anesthetized with injectable anesthetics still be intubated (for airway protection) and receive oxygen supplementation to prevent hypoxemia. Similarly, many patients will benefit from oxygen supplementation during the anesthetic recovery period. Important causes for hypoventilation include anesthesia itself, neuromuscular disease, pleural space and chest wall diseases. The imbalance between ventilation and perfusion in various regions of the lung or $\dot{V}/\dot{Q}$ mismatching is an important cause of hypoxemia. $\dot{V}/\dot{Q}$ mismatching may result from all forms of pulmonary disease, and the resultant hypoxemia is responsive to oxygen therapy.

Shunts and diffusion impairment are less common causes of hypoxemia. Patent ductus arteriosus (PDA) and ventricular septal defect (VSD) are examples of extrapulmonary shunts, whereas intrapulmonary shunts develop in atelectasic or consolidated lung lobes and following pulmonary thromboembolism (e.g., heartworm disease). Clinically, shunt-induced hypoxemia varies in severity depending on the shunt fraction and is often not responsive to oxygen therapy. Nonetheless, a patient with shunt (e.g., PDA, VSD) undergoing anesthesia may still benefit from preoxygenation before induction of anesthesia, high F_{IO_2} during anesthesia, and oxygen supplementation during anesthetic recovery. These measures help minimize the effects of other causes of hypoxemia that may develop during the perianesthetic period. Diffusion impairment (e.g., lung fibrosis) represents a barrier for oxygen diffusion such that equilibration between the pulmonary capillary blood and the alveolar gas is compromised. It is relatively uncommon in veterinary patients and will usually respond to oxygen supplementation.

Clinically, hypoxemia may be considered mild if Pa_{O_2} is less than 80 mm Hg, moderate if Pa_{O_2} is less than 70 mm Hg, and severe if Pa_{O_2} is less than 60 mm Hg. The oxyhemoglobin dissociation curve is steep at Pa_{O_2} less than 60 mm Hg, meaning that hemoglobin saturation drops rapidly with small decrease in the Pa_{O_2} at this portion of the curve. Importantly, significant oxygenation deficiency may be present without evidence of hypoxemia in a patient breathing 100% oxygen. Even though the A-a gradient is not a very reliable measure of oxygenation impairment during high F_{IO_2} (Herrick et al. 1990), an A-a gradient greater than 200 in a patient breathing 100% oxygen is indicative of reduced ability of the lung to oxygenate blood (Haskins 1999). A continuous and noninvasive estimate of arterial oxygenation can be obtained by pulse oximetry in veterinary patients. Oxygen saturation obtained by pulse oximetry (Sp_{O_2}) appears to have good correlation with the oxygen saturation determined by arterial blood gas analysis in patients with saturation greater than 70% (Matthews et al.

2003; Nishimura et al. 1991; Sendak et al. 1988; Sidi et al. 1987). In anesthetized patients, the ideal Sp_{O_2} is greater than 98%, whereas the patient is experiencing hypoxemia at Sp_{O_2} less than 95%. The cause of the hypoxemia should be promptly identified and corrected.

Acid-Base Balance

Maintenance of plasma pH within the normal range (7.35 to 7.45) is critical for biological homeostasis. Respiratory, metabolic and mixed acid-base imbalances may be encountered in the anesthetized patient. Respiratory acidosis may result from hypoventilation during anesthesia, whereas overzealous ventilation may cause respiratory alkalosis. The arterial partial pressure of carbon dioxide (Pa_{CO_2}) should be maintained within the physiological range (35 to 45 mm Hg) to prevent respiratory acid-base abnormalities during anesthesia. Treatment for metabolic acidosis is accomplished by intravenous fluid therapy and removal of the inciting cause (DiBartola 2001a; Kudnig and Mama 2002). Diabetes, small bowel diarrhea, renal tubule acidosis (reduced bicarbonate reabsorption or defective acid excretion), and use of carbonic anhydrase inhibitors (e.g., acetazolamide) are common causes of metabolic acidosis. If acidemia is refractory to fluid therapy or it is severe (pH less than 7.2), bicarbonate administration is warranted (Kudnig and Mama 2002; Wathen et al. 1982). The following equation can be used to determine the amount of sodium bicarbonate to be administered:

$$\text{Bicarbonate required (mEq)} = \text{base deficit} \times \text{body weight (kg)} \times 0.3 \quad (11.6)$$

One-fourth to one-half of the calculated dose is administered initially during approximately 20 minutes and the acid-base status reassessed. Alternatively, 1 to 2 mEq of sodium bicarbonate/kg may be administered slowly intravenously if the base deficit is unknown. A diagram for rapid interpretation of acid-base balance and oxygenation of the patient under anesthesia is provided in Figure 11.3.

GLUCOSE AND ELECTROLYTES

Perioperative Glycemic Control

Both hypoglycemia and hyperglycemia should be avoided in anesthetized patients, and this may be an

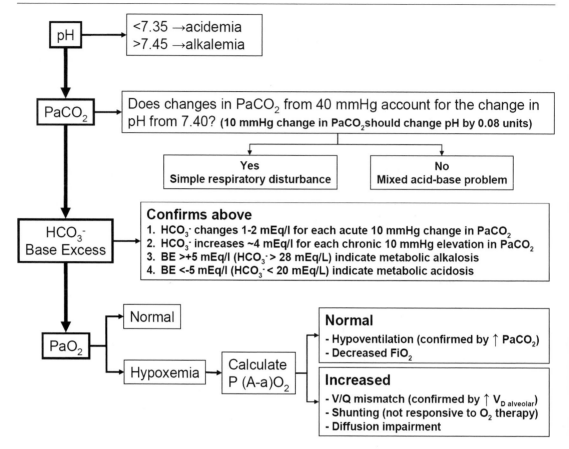

Figure 11.3. Flow chart illustrating the sequential steps for rapid interpretation of acid base balance and oxygenation during anesthesia.

especial challenge in certain patient populations such as neonates, pediatrics, geriatrics, diabetics, patients with insulinomas, and virtually all critically ill patients. Depending on the severity of hypoglycemia, dextrose may be added to a crystalloid solution to achieve a final concentration of 2.5% or 5% dextrose or may be given as an intravenous bolus injection. The following equation may be used to calculate the amount of 50% dextrose to be added to crystalloid solution to achieve the desired final dextrose concentration: $V_1 = (V_2 \times C_2)/C_1$ where V_1 is the unknown variable (e.g., the volume of concentrated dextrose solution to be added in the crystalloids), V_2 is the volume of the crystalloid solution where dextrose is to be added, C_2 is the final desired concentration of dextrose (e.g., 2.5% or 5%), and C_1 is the strength of the concentrated (e.g., 50%)

dextrose solution. An alternative is to administer an intravenous bolus of 1 to 2 ml/kg of 50% dextrose diluted with a crystalloid solution. Blood glucose concentration should be monitored periodically and maintained in the range of 70 to 120 mg/dl.

Electrolytes

Calcium is central in the maintenance of cellular function and physiologic homeostasis. It is essential for cardiac automaticity and contractility, smooth and skeletal muscle function, coagulation, synaptic transmission, hormone secretion, and mitotic division. Calcium is also a major intracellular signaling molecule (Aguilera and Vaughan 2000). Total serum calcium (8.0 to 11.5 mg/dl) is present as ionized (4.5 to 6.0 mg/dl) and protein bound, the former being the most important physiologically. Blood samples should be collected and handled anaerobically for accurate ionized calcium (iCa^{2+}) determination. Presence of heparin in blood samples may falsely reduce iCa^{2+} concentration. Calcium determination is also influenced by pH, in which higher values are measured during acidemia (Wang et al. 2002). In patients where serum calcium may be altered (e.g., lactation, parathyroid diseases), the iCa^{2+} should be determined because it is the biologically active form. Falsely low levels of calcium due to hypoalbuminemia should be excluded by measuring iCa^{2+} or the total serum calcium can be adjusted in adult animals with the following formula:

$$\text{Adjusted calcium (mg/dl)}$$
$$= \text{measured calcium (mg/dl)}$$
$$- \text{albumin (g/dl)} + 3.5 \qquad (11.7)$$

Perioperative hypocalcemia is more common than hypercalcemia. The threshold for developing symptoms of hypocalcemia is not very clear, but complications will likely occur when iCa^{2+} levels fall below 2 to 3 mg/dl. Hypocalcemia can cause hypotension due to loss of vascular tone, impaired cardiac contractility, and bradycardia. Changes in the electrocardiogram are inconsistent as it may be normal in appearance or may demonstrate QT and ST interval prolongation and T-wave inversion. Ventricular premature contractions, ventricular tachycardia, and ventricular fibrillation may develop during severe hypocalcemia. Weakness, lethargy, muscle tremors, and seizures may also occur in the perioperative period. Respiratory signs may include respiratory depression (secondary to muscle weakness) and bronchospasm. During anesthesia, hypocalcemia may develop as a result of rapid administration of fluids and citrated blood products (Jutkowitz et al. 2002; Kudnig and Mama 2002). Acute hypocalcemia can be treated with slow intravenous administration of 10% calcium gluconate (0.5 to 1.0 mg/kg) administered slowly over 15 to 20 minutes while monitoring the electrocardiogram. Repeat iCa^{2+} measurement and, if still low, a continuous intravenous infusion of 10% calcium gluconate (0.05 to 0.15 mg/kg/hr) may be instituted with continuous electrocardiogram monitoring. Importantly, the amount of elemental calcium contained in a 10% calcium chloride solution (2.72 mg/ml) is approximately three times greater than that

in 10% calcium gluconate solution (0.93 mg/ml). There is no evidence that one form is clinically superior to another, the only consideration being that the dose (in ml) of calcium chloride is a third lower than for calcium gluconate. Last, hypocalcemia can occur concurrently with hypomagnesemia, in which case the clinical signs are often refractory to treatment with calcium until correction of the magnesium deficiency (Aguilera and Vaughan 2000; Berkelhammer and Bear 1985).

Magnesium is the second most abundant intracellular cation after potassium and the fourth most abundant cation in the whole body. Magnesium is a frequently overlooked electrolyte, although it is involved in an incredibly large number of cellular processes and is essential for life. About half of the body's magnesium is located in bone and the rest is distributed in muscle and other soft tissues, with less than 1% present in the blood. Magnesium is central in maintaining cellular ionic balance through associations with sodium, potassium, and calcium (Gums 2004). Hypomagnesemia (serum magnesium less than 1.2 mg/dl) was frequently observed in association with hypokalemia, hypoalbuminemia, and cardiovascular diseases in hospitalized dogs (Khanna et al. 1998). In cats, magnesium abnormalities were associated with alteration in serum potassium, but not with sodium, calcium, or chloride (Toll et al. 2002). Concurrent magnesium and potassium deficiency is highly prevalent in critically ill patients (Dhupa and Proulx 1998). Through regulation of the Na^+/K^+-ATPase pump, magnesium controls the intracellular distribution of sodium and potassium ions. Magnesium blocks the outward flow of potassium from cardiac myocytes, controlling the resting membrane potential. Magnesium depletion decreases the intracellular potassium concentration, causing a reduction in the resting membrane potential, which increases myocardium excitability and predispose to cardiac arrhythmias (Gums 2004).

Critically ill dogs and cats, those with cardiovascular disease, and those with hypoalbuminemia may be susceptible to magnesium abnormalities, especially in the presence of other electrolyte (e.g., Ca^{2+}, K^+) abnormalities. In humans, magnesium infusion has been recommended to treat torsade de pointes, refractory ventricular tachycardia, refractory ventricular fibrillation, and supraventricular arrhythmias (Gums 2004). If hypomagnesemia is suspected as a cause for life-threatening ventricular arrhythmia, magnesium can be administered at 0.15 to 0.3 mEq/kg over a period of 10 to 15 minutes (Dhupa and Proulx 1998). In healthy dogs, a constant rate infusion of magnesium at 0.12 mEq/kg/min did not cause electrocardiographic and hemodynamic adverse effects up to cumulative doses of 1.0 to 2.0 mEq/kg. Prolonged PQ interval and hypotension were observed at higher cumulative dosages and dangerous arrhythmias occurred with cumulative dosages above 3.9 mEq/kg. Death occurred at cumulative infusions between 5.9 and 10.9 mEq/kg (Nakayama et al. 1999). Magnesium overdose may cause hypotension, atrioventricular and bundle-branch blocks, respiratory muscle weakness, and hypocalcemia. Calcium gluconate (50 mg/kg) is administered slowly intravenously over a period of 10 to 20 minutes to counteract magnesium toxicity. This may be followed by a constant rate infusion of 10 mg/kg/hr until signs of toxicity are resolved (Dhupa and Proulx 1998; Kudnig and Mama 2002).

Potassium abnormalities may also be seen in the perioperative period. Hyperkalemia is more common in patients with urinary tract disorders (urethral obstruction, ruptured bladder, anuric or oliguric renal failure), insulin deficiency in diabetic patients, hypoadrenocorticism, or metabolic acidosis (potassium translocation to the extracellular compartment in exchange for hydrogen ions being buffered intracellularly) (DiBartola 2001b; Parham et al. 2006). It may also occur in patients receiving potassium-sparing diuretics (spironolactone) or inadvertently during fluid therapy with potassium-supplemented fluids. Hypokalemia may occur due to decreased intake in critically ill patients, as a result of gastrointestinal losses (especially vomiting of stomach contents), and due to urinary loss (e.g., cats with chronic renal failure, distal renal tubular acidosis, loop or thiazide diuretic therapy, and post-obstructive diuresis following relief of urethral obstruction). Muscle weakness may develop during hyperkalemia (especially if serum potassium is in excess of 8 mEq/l) and also during hypokalemia when serum potassium falls below 2.5–3.0 mEq/L.

In experimental models, the progression of electrocardiographic changes induced by hyperkalemia are well defined (Fisch et al. 1963; Lanari et al. 1964). The appearance of narrow-based, peaked T waves at potassium concentrations greater than

5.5 mEq/L are the earliest electrocardiographic manifestation of hyperkalemia. Electromyographically, this may be caused by shortening of the myocyte action potential and an increase in the rate of repolarization. As hyperkalemia progresses to greater than 6.5 mEq/L, the rate of depolarization decreases, causing a longer action potential that is seen in the surface electrocardiogram as widened QRS complex and prolonged PR interval. As hyperkalemia worsens (K^+ greater than 8 to 9 mEq/l), the sinoatrial node, being less susceptible to hyperkalemia, continues to stimulate the ventricles in the absence of atrial activity, producing a sinoventricular rhythm. The electrocardiographic manifestation of this rhythm may be very similar to those of ventricular tachycardia, given the absence of P waves and a widened QRS complex. If hyperkalemia progresses further (K^+ greater than 10 mEq/L), sinoatrial conduction disappears and junctional pacemakers provide the electrical stimulation of the myocardium, which may be seen as an accelerated junctional rhythm. If hyperkalemia continues, the QRS complexes continue to widen and will eventually blend with the T waves, resulting in the classic sine-wave electrocardiogram, indicating that ventricular fibrillation and asystole are imminent. In clinical patients, electrocardiographic changes induced by hyperkalemia are inconsistent. Shortening of PR and QT intervals, sinus tachycardia and bradycardia, idioventricular rhythm, and atrioventricular conduction blocks may be seen with hyperkalemia in clinical patients. Electrocardiographic changes are also inconsistent during hypokalemia, but ventricular arrhythmias may be observed.

Potassium abnormalities should be corrected prior to anesthesia whenever possible. Hyperkalemia can be treated by removing potassium from the body through potassium-free fluid therapy (e.g., 0.9% NaCl, 5% dextrose) and diuresis, by antagonizing its effects on membrane electrical potential with calcium administration, and/or by promoting intracellular translocation with the use of bicarbonate, dextrose with or without insulin (DiBartola 2001b; Parham et al. 2006). Calcium (0.5 to 1.0 mg/kg) should be administered in emergency situations (e.g., potassium-induced life-threatening arrhythmias) to increase the threshold potential and restore the difference between resting and threshold membrane potentials. The onset of action occurs within minutes and will last less than 1 hour. Sodium bicar-

bonate (1 to 2 mEq/kg) is indicated if there is acidemia but may be of limited benefit if plasma pH
is within normal range. The onset of action occurs
within 1 hour, and the effects last a few hours.
Glucose (1 to 2 ml/kg of 50% dextrose) administration induces endogenous insulin secretion (DiBartola 2001b). Insulin stimulates the Na^+/K^+-ATPase
pump, which moves potassium intracellularly in
exchange for sodium in a 2 : 3 ratio, thus mediating
potassium translocation to the intracellular compartment. The insulin action is independent of its
effect on glucose metabolism (Parham et al. 2006).
Exogenous insulin may be necessary in severe
hyperkalemia and, in this case, glucose should
always be administered concomitantly to prevent
hypoglycemia.

PERIOPERATIVE TEMPERATURE REGULATION

Perioperative hypothermia is a common complication of anesthesia and surgery in veterinary patients.
It develops via several mechanisms, including
redistribution, convection, radiation, conduction,
and evaporation. Patients with larger ratio of body
surface area to body mass (e.g., neonatal, pediatrics,
poor nutrition) are more likely to develop perioperative hypothermia. The initial drop in core temperature is predominantly due to redistribution of heat
from the core to peripheral tissues. Normal thermo-
regulation through vasoconstriction and metabolism
is impaired during the perioperative period. Hypothermia interferes with the homeostasis of hepatic,
renal, cardiovascular, immune and central nervous
systems, potentially affecting infection rates, wound
healing, and return to function.

Decreased core temperature can slow intracardiac electrical conduction and predispose to
cardiac arrhythmias (Campbell and Day 2004;
Maisenbacher and Adin 2006). In the postoperative
period, hypothermia-induced shivering significantly
increases metabolic demand, oxygen consumption,
and cardiopulmonary work. Postoperative shivering
may increase oxygen consumption to more than
400% over basal levels and has been associated
with increased cardiac morbidity in humans (Alfonsi
2001). Hypothermia should be avoided by minimizing length of anesthesia, controlling operating room
temperature, covering exposed body regions with
blankets, reducing the amount of alcohol for surgical scrubbing, and using warmed lavage solutions.

In the hypothermic patient, active surface rewarming with heat sources such as forced warm air is
useful and effective (Armstrong et al. 2005). The
forced warm air blankets can be placed over the
patient (outside the surgical field) during surgery to
maintain body temperature or minimize its fall. It
is important, when using such devices, that body
temperature be continuously monitored because
hyperthermia may occur, especially in the smaller
patients.

Hyperthermia not related to the use of warming
devices may also occur in the perioperative period.
A recent retrospective study (Niedfeldt and Robertson 2006) has shown an association between postoperative hyperthermia and the perioperative use of
hydromorphone in cats. In that study, all cats had
decreased body temperature immediately at the end
of anesthesia with hyperthermia developing in the
following hours of recovery. This emphasizes the
importance of extended postoperative monitoring
of body temperature in this population of patients.
Malignant hyperthermia is an autosomal recessive
condition that most commonly occurs in pigs but
has occasionally occurred in dogs. Although halothane is the most potent trigger of malignant hyperthermia, it may be caused by virtually all commonly
used inhalant anesthetics at present. Hyperthermia,
independently of the cause, is potentially life threatening and should be treated promptly. Removal of
blankets and any heat source, placement of ice
packs in the cage floor, application of alcohol-con-
taining solution on feet and ears, improving ventilation with fans, and use of tranquilizers such as
acepromazine are measures that can be taken to
treat hyperthermic patients.

MISCELLANEOUS

Other perioperative support includes careful positioning and manipulation of animals under anesthesia. Patients with poor body condition benefit from
added padding to avoid development of pressure
sores or trauma to superficial nerves (e.g., radial
nerve). Geriatric patients frequently have arthritic
joints that may become very painful postoperatively
depending on body positioning during the procedure. This can be minimized by not applying excessive stress to the patient's articulations. For the
same reasons, patients should not be held solely
by the limbs when being moved from one table
or surface to another. Specific situations (e.g.,

fractured bones, intervertebral disc disease, vertebral luxation) require very careful manipulation of the patient to avoid worsening of the problem.

Eye lubrication is also important to avoid corneal damage during the procedure because the majority of anesthetic drugs decrease tear production. Applying moisture to the oral mucosa may add comfort to patients with dry mouth in the perioperative period. Similarly, a full urinary bladder may cause pain and discomfort to the patient; hence, palpating the urinary bladder and expressing it is important in the postoperative period. Patients that may benefit from expressing the bladder include virtually all patients receiving fluid therapy at anesthetic rates, patients receiving epidural morphine, and those that received α_2-adrenergic agonists as part of the anesthetic protocol. Adequate perioperative analgesia is another supportive measure in all patients undergoing potentially painful procedures, or any painful patient. Whenever possible, the patient should receive preemptive (e.g., before the painful insult) and multimodal (e.g., different drug combinations) analgesia such that perioperative pain is well controlled.

Adequate skeletal muscle relaxation is one of the three components of general anesthesia (along with unconsciousness and analgesia). Although most general anesthetics are good muscle relaxants, neuromuscular blocking drugs are occasionally required as anesthetic adjuncts to produce adequate muscle relaxation. Importantly, these drugs do not produce analgesia or unconsciousness and therefore cannot be used in isolation. Also, they produce respiratory paralysis, which require mechanical or manual ventilatory support. The most common situations where neuromuscular blocking drugs may be of benefit include facilitation of mechanical ventilation (usually not necessary), to provide centralization of the eye to facilitate intraocular procedures, and as an aid in fracture reduction in heavy-muscled animals. In veterinary medicine, intravenous administration of atracurium (0.05 to 0.2 mg/kg), cisatracurium (0.05 to 0.1 mg/kg), and pancuronium (0.04 to 0.1 mg/kg) (nondepolarizing neuromuscular blocking drugs) is most commonly used for peripheral muscle relaxation. Onset of action is fast (within minutes) and duration varies from approximately 20 to 30 minutes for atracurium and cisatracurium and 40 to 60 minutes for pancuronium. Atracurium undergoes Hoffman elimination, cisatracurium is metabolized by plasma esterases, and pancuronium undergoes primarily hepatic metabolism and renal elimination. Atracurium (but not cisatracurium) may produce histamine release in high doses, and pancuronium may produce sympathetic and vagolytic effects resulting in tachycardia and increased systemic arterial BP (Booij 1997a, 1997b; Fisher 1999; Kampe et al. 2003; Naguib and Magboul 1998).

Monitoring of the degree of muscle relaxation is done with the use of a nerve stimulator by observing the responses to supramaximal nerve stimulation. The electrodes are placed subcutaneously or over the skin on each side of the nerve (ulnar and peroneal nerves most commonly used). The train-of-four (TOF) pattern of stimulation is clinically useful to assess neuromuscular function. In this pattern, four sequential impulses are delivered (2-Hz frequency), each eliciting one twitch of equal strength if there is no neuromuscular blockade. The degree of neuromuscular blockade can be assessed by comparing the fourth to the first twitch in the TOF. Because the prerelaxation strengths of the fourth and first twitches are equal, the ratio is 1.0. This ratio decreases as the degree of relaxation deepens (e.g., fade). The fourth, third, second, and first twitches disappear in this sequence as the blockade becomes more profound. Clinically useful neuromuscular blockade is observed when one or two twitches (fourth and third) disappear. The twitches will gradually regain prerelaxation strengths as neuromuscular function is recovered, and a ratio greater than 0.7 correlates with clinically adequate recovery. The presence of strong palpebral reflex and the generation of inspiratory negative pressures between 10 and 20 cm H_2O are also indicators of adequate recovery. If needed, nondepolarizing neuromuscular blocking drugs can be reversed with anti-acetycholinesterase drugs such as neostigmine (0.04 mg/kg) or edrophonium (0.5 mg/kg) administered intravenously. Atropine (0.02 mg/kg) or glycopyrrolate (0.01 mg/kg) is normally used concomitantly to prevent the undesirable muscarinic effects of anti-acetylcholinesterase drugs (e.g., bradycardia, increased gastrointestinal motility, airway and salivary secretions) (Fisher 1999; Naguib and Magboul 1998).

REFERENCES

Aguilera, I.M., and Vaughan, R.S. 2000. Calcium and the anaesthetist. *Anaesthesia* 55:779–790.

Alfonsi, P. 2001. Postanaesthetic shivering: Epidemiology, pathophysiology, and approaches to prevention and management. *Drugs* 61:2193–2205.

Anderson, C.T., and Breen, P.H. 2000. Carbon dioxide kinetics and capnography during critical care. *Crit Care* 4:207–215.

Armstrong, S.R., Roberts, B.K., and Aronsohn, M. 2005. Perioperative hypothermia. *J Vet Emerg Crit Care* 15:32–37.

Bellomo, R., and Giantomasso, D.D. 2001. Noradrenaline and the kidney: Friends or foes? *Crit Care* 5:294–298.

Berkelhammer, C., and Bear, R.A. 1985. A clinical approach to common electrolyte problems: 4. Hypomagnesemia. *Can Med Assoc J* 132:360–368.

Booij, L.H. 1997a. Neuromuscular transmission and its pharmacological blockade. Part 1: Neuromuscular transmission and general aspects of its blockade. *Pharm World Sci* 19:1–12.

Booij, L.H. 1997b. Neuromuscular transmission and its pharmacological blockade. Part 2: Pharmacology of neuromuscular blocking agents. *Pharm World Sci* 19:13–34.

Campbell, S.A., and Day, T.K. 2004. Spontaneous resolution of hypothermia-induced atrial fibrilation in a dog. *J Vet Emerg Crit Care* 14:293–298.

Castellanos, I., Couto, C.G., and Gray, T.L. 2004. Clinical use of blood products in cats: A retrospective study (1997–2000). *J Vet Intern Med* 18:529–532.

Chiaramonte, D. 2004. Blood-component therapy: Selection, administration and monitoring. *Clin Tech Small Anim Pract* 19:63–67.

Dhupa, N., and Proulx, J. 1998. Hypocalcemia and hypomagnesemia. *Vet Clin North Am Small Anim Pract* 28:587–608.

DiBartola, S.P. 2001a. Interpretation of metabolic acid base disturbances using the routine serum biochemical profile. *J Feline Med Surg* 3:189–191.

DiBartola, S.P. 2001b. Management of hypokalaemia and hyperkalaemia. *J Feline Med Surg* 3:181–183.

Dyson, D.H., and Sinclair, M.D. 2006. Impact of dopamine or dobutamine infusions on cardiovascular variables after rapid blood loss and volume replacement during isoflurane-induced anesthesia in dogs. *J Am Vet Med Assoc* 229:234.

Fisch, C., Feigenbaum, H., and Bowers, J.A. 1963. The effect of potassium on atrioventricular conduction of normal dogs. *Am J Cardiol* 11:487–492.

Fisher, D.M. 1999. Clinical pharmacology of neuromuscular blocking agents. *Am J Health Syst Pharm* 56:S4–S9.

Gaynor, J.S., Dunlop, C.I., and Wagner, A.E., et al. 1999. Complications and mortality associated with anesthesia in dogs and cats. *J Am Anim Hosp Assoc* 35:13–17.

Gums, J.G. 2004. Magnesium in cardiovascular and other disorders. *Am J Health Syst Pharm* 61:1569–1576.

Haskins, S.C. 1999. Perioperative monitoring. In *Manual of small animal anesthesia*, edited by R.R. Paddleford, 2nd ed., pp. 123–146. Philadelphia: W. B. Saunders.

Hein, L.G., Albrecht, M., and Dworschak, M., et al. 1988. Long-term observation following traumatic-hemorrhagic shock in the dog: A comparison of crystalloid vs. colloidal fluids. *Circ Shock* 26:353–364.

Henik, R.A., Dolson, M.K., and Wenholz, L.J. 2005. How to obtain a blood pressure measurement. *Clin Tech Small Anim Pract* 20:144–150.

Herrick, I.A., Champion, L.K., and Froese, A.B. 1990. A clinical comparison of indices of pulmonary gas exchange with changes in the inspired oxygen concentration. *Can J Anaesth* 37:69–76.

Heymans, C. 1928. The control of heart rate consequent to changes in the cephalic blood pressure and in the intracranial pressure. *Am J Physiol* 85:498–505.

Ilkiw, J.E. 1999. Balanced anesthetic techniques in dogs and cats. *Clin Tech Small Anim Pract* 14:27–37.

Jutkowitz, L.A., Rozanski, E.A., Moreau, J.A., et al. 2002. Massive transfusion in dogs: 15 Cases (1997–2001). *J Am Vet Med Assoc* 220:1664–1669.

Kampe, S., Krombach, J.W., and Diefenbach, C. 2003. Muscle relaxants. *Best Pract Res Clin Anaesthesiol* 17:137–146.

Khanna, C., Lund, E.M., Raffe, M., et al. 1998. Hypomagnesemia in 188 dogs: A hospital population-based prevalence study. *J Vet Intern Med* 12:304–309.

Kittleson, M.D., and Kienle, R.D. 1998. Normal clinical cardiovascular physiology. In *Small animal cardiovascular medicine*, edited by M.D. Kittleson and R.D. Kienle, pp. 11–35. St Louis: Mosby.

Klaser, D.A., Reine, N.J., and Hohenhaus, A.E. 2005. Red blood cell transfusions in cats: 126 Cases (1999). *J Am Vet Med Assoc* 226:920–923.

Kozek-Langenecker, S.A. 2005. Effects of hydroxyethyl starch solutions on hemostasis. *Anesthesiology* 103:654–660.

Kudnig, S.T., and Mama, K. 2002. Perioperative fluid therapy. *J Am Vet Med Assoc* 221:1112–1121.

Lamont, L.A., Bulmer, B.J., Sisson, D.D., et al. 2002. Doppler echocardiographic effects of medetomidine on dynamic left ventricular outflow tract obstruction in cats. *J Am Vet Med Assoc* 221:1276–1281.

Lanari, A., Chait, L.O., and Capurro, C. 1964. Electrocardiographic effects of potassium. I. Perfusion through the coronary bed. *Am Heart J* 67:357–363.

Lazarchick, J., and Conroy, J.M. 1995. The effect of 6% hydroxyethyl starch and desmopressin infusion on von Willebrand factor: Ristocetin cofactor activity. *Ann Clin Lab Sci* 25:306–309.

Logan, J.C., Callan, M.B., Drew, K., et al. 2001. Clinical indications for use of fresh frozen plasma in dogs: 74 Dogs (October through December 1999). *J Am Vet Med Assoc* 218:1449–1455.

Maisenbacher, H.W., and Adin, D.B. 2006. ECG of the month. *J Am Vet Med Assoc* 229:40–42.

Matthews, N.S., Hartke, S., and Allen, J.C., Jr. 2003. An evaluation of pulse oximeters in dogs, cats and horses. *Vet Anaesth Analg* 30:3–14.

Moore, F.D. 1949. Adaptation of supportive treatment to needs of the surgical patient. *J Am Med Assoc* 141:646–653.

Muir, W.W., 3rd., and Wiese, A.J. 2004. Comparison of lactated Ringer's solution and a physiologically balanced 6% hetastarch plasma expander for the treatment of hypotension induced via blood withdrawal in isoflurane-anesthetized dogs. *Am J Vet Res* 65:1189–1194.

Naguib, M., and Magboul, M.M. 1998. Adverse effects of neuromuscular blockers and their antagonists. *Middle East J Anesthesiol* 14:341–373.

Nakayama, T., Nakayama, H., Miyamoto, M., et al. 1999. Hemodynamic and electrocardiographic effects of magnesium sulfate in healthy dogs. *J Vet Intern Med* 13:485–490.

Niedfeldt, R.L., and Robertson, S.A. 2006. Postanesthetic hyperthermia in cats: A retrospective comparison between hydromorphone and buprenorphine. *Vet Anaesth Analg* 33:381–389.

Nishimura, R., Kim, H., Matsunaga, S., et al. 1991. Evaluation of pulse oximetry in anesthetized dogs. *J Vet Med Sci* 53:1117–1118.

Parham, W.A., Mehdirad, A.A., Biermann, K.M., et al. 2006. Hyperkalemia revisited. *Tex Heart Inst J* 33:40–47.

Pascoe, P.J., Ilkiw, J.E., and Fisher, L.D. 1997. Cardiovascular effects of equipotent isoflurane and alfentanil/isoflurane minimum alveolar concentration multiple in cats. *Am J Vet Res* 58:1267–1273.

Pascoe, P.J., Ilkiw, J.E., and Pypendop, B.H. 2006. Effects of increasing infusion rates of dopamine, dobutamine, epinephrine, and phenylephrine in healthy anesthetized cats. *Am J Vet Res* 67:1491–1499.

Pugsley, M.K. 2002. The diverse molecular mechanisms responsible for the actions of opioids on the cardiovascular system. *Pharmacol Ther* 93:51–75.

Rozanski, E., and Rondeau, M. 2002. Choosing fluids in traumatic hypovolemic shock: The role of crystalloids, colloids, and hypertonic saline. *J Am Anim Hosp Assoc* 38:499–501.

Rozich, J.D., and Paul, R.V. 1989. Acute renal failure precipitated by elevated colloid osmotic pressure. *Am J Med* 87:359–360.

Schenarts, P.J., Sagraves, S.G., Bard, M.R., et al. 2006. Low-dose dopamine: A physiologically based review. *Curr Surg* 63:219–225.

Sendak, M.J., Harris, A.P., and Donham, R.T. 1988. Accuracy of pulse oximetry during arterial oxyhemoglobin desaturation in dogs. *Anesthesiology* 68:111–114.

Shires, T., Williams, J., and Brown, F. 1961. Acute change in extracellular fluids associated with major surgical procedures. *Ann Surg* 154:803–810.

Sidi, A., Rush, W., Gravenstein, N., et al. 1987. Pulse oximetry fails to accurately detect low levels of arterial hemoglobin oxygen saturation in dogs. *J Clin Monit* 3:257–262.

Sinclair, M.D., O'Grady, M.R., Kerr, C.L., et al. 2003. The echocardiographic effects of romifidine in dogs with and without prior or concurrent administration of glycopyrrolate. *Vet Anaesth Analg* 30:211–219.

Thompson, J.E., and Jaffe, M.B. 2005. Capnographic waveforms in the mechanically ventilated patient. *Respir Care* 50:100–108; discussion 108–109.

Toll, J., Erb, H., Birnbaum, N., et al. 2002. Prevalence and incidence of serum magnesium abnormalities in hospitalized cats. *J Vet Intern Med* 16:217–221.

Van der Linden, P., Schmartz, D., De Groote, F., et al. 1998. Critical haemoglobin concentration in anaesthetized dogs: Comparison of two plasma substitutes. *Br J Anaesth* 81:556–562.

Vernon, D.D., Garrett, J.S., Banner, W., Jr., et al. 1992. Hemodynamic effects of dobutamine in an intact animal model. *Crit Care Med* 20:1322–1329.

Wang, S., McDonnell, E.H., Sedor, F.A., et al. 2002. pH effects on measurements of ionized calcium and ionized magnesium in blood. *Arch Pathol Lab Med* 126:947–950.

Wardrop, K.J. 1997. Canine plasma therapy. *Vet Forum* 7:36–40.

Wathen, R.L., Ward, R.A., Harding, G.B., et al. 1982. Acid-base and metabolic responses to anion infusion in the anesthetized dog. *Kidney Int* 21:592–599.

Chapter 12
Cardiopulmonary Resuscitation

Maureen McMichael

Cardiopulmonary arrest (CPA) is the leading cause of death in people in the United States and Canada. The Centers for Disease Control and Prevention estimate the annual incidence of CPA to be approximately 0.55 per 1000 people in North America. The survival rate (overall survival to hospital discharge) of out-of-hospital CPA is less than 6.4% in people in the United States and Canada.

In veterinary medicine, the overall incidence of CPA is unknown, but the incidence of CPA associated with general anesthesia has been reported to occur at a rate of 0.5% in dogs and 0.4% in cats in one study (Kass and Haskins 1992). The overall survival rate has been reported to be 4% for dogs and cats in one study and 4.1% for dogs and 9.6% for cats in another study (Wingfield and Van Pelt 1992). Interestingly, in the latter study all of the animals that survived had received general anesthesia or drug administration prior to the arrest, suggesting that animals with CPA secondary to anesthesia have an improved chance of survival if CPR is initiated in an organized and prompt fashion (Wingfield and Van Pelt 1992).

In 2005, the new American Heart Association CPR guidelines were released and are available at no charge at www.circulationaha.org (American Heart Association 2005). Although they pertain to people, much of the data used are from experimental animals and may be applicable in veterinary medicine. This chapter addresses many of the changes in the guidelines under each individual section.

The most effective CPR is one that is anticipated and successfully prevented. This cannot be stressed enough in our anesthetized patients—a preanesthetic database (to include packed cell volume [PCV]/total solids [TS], electrolytes, creatinine, blood glucose, electrocardiogram [ECG], arterial blood pressure, and pulse oximetry or arterial blood gas), good monitoring and thorough evaluation of all equipment, excellent patient care, and a full knowledge of all current problems can help to avert many arrests. There are, however, unanticipated CPA patients despite the most vigilant preanesthetic work-up. For this and other reasons, it is essential to have a resuscitation code on all patients that are undergoing surgery. A simple system should be instituted, such as a red dot applied to the patient record for patients that are not to be resuscitated, a yellow dot for patients that are to be given closed-chest CPR, and a green dot for patients that are candidates for open-chest CPR. Although it is often a difficult conversation to have with an owner, it is invaluable to have this directive in place before the arrest. If there is an unexpected anesthetic death, the patient should be supported until the owner is reached.

The first part of this chapter covers the basics of CPR, including how to administer closed-chest CPR, what drugs to use, and the common arrhythmias seen during an arrest. The second part of this chapter covers, defibrillation, open-chest CPR, and postoperative care of the resuscitated patient.

RECOGNITION OF CARDIOPULMONARY ARREST

Before CPA, variations in respiratory rate or depth, bradycardia, hypotension, or hypothermia may be seen. Respiratory signs may be masked if the anesthetized patient is being ventilated. Gasping or agonal breaths and dilated, nonresponsive pupils are often seen a few seconds after an arrest. Capillary refill time and mucous membrane color may remain normal for several minutes after an arrest and cannot be used to assess the patient if they are normal. Cardiopulmonary arrest can be identified by absence of spontaneous ventilation, palpable pulses, and heart sounds. Check more than one peripheral pulse in case the patient has a saddle thrombus or ligated femoral artery.

Once an anesthetic arrest is confirmed, it is as bad as it gets; be aggressive in treatment.

TREATMENT OF ANESTHETIC

CARDIOPULMONARY ARREST

In an arrest, turn off the vaporizer!

The mnemonic ABCD (airway, breathing, circulation, drugs) has been changed in people to CABD (circulation, airway, breathing, drugs) to stress the importance of establishing a minimal circulation (with cardiac compressions or defibrillation) before ventilatory efforts are made. There are several justifications for this in people, including the lack of hypoxia before CPA in many people (sudden fibrillation is the most common arrhythmia in CPA in people) and the reluctance of bystanders to perform mouth to mouth resuscitation. In addition, the ventilation rate needed to maintain a normal ventilation-perfusion ($\dot{V}/\dot{Q}$) ratio is much smaller during CPR due to the significantly decreased pulmonary blood flow.

In contrast, in veterinary medicine, the majority of CPAs occur in animals hospitalized in intensive care units that are hypoxic before the arrest. In anesthetized patients that are intubated and being ventilated, this is not usually an issue. However, hypoxia in an underventilated patient during anesthesia can be a primary cause of CPA and should be averted. In veterinary medicine, ABCD is still the order of choice during CPA.

Airway

First establish an airway if not already done, with either a well-fitting, cuffed endotracheal (ET) tube or an emergency tracheotomy. Confirm placement of the ET tube either by visualization or palpation of the tube in the trachea. Although end-tidal capnography (ETCO₂) is often used to confirm tube placement in animals with adequate perfusion, this may not be reliable in patients with no perfusion (i.e., none of the CO_2 being generated in the tissues is making it to the lungs for elimination). In our experience, the ETCO₂ is near zero before starting

CPR in a CPA patient (see Chapters 2 and 11). Quickly place the animal in right lateral recumbency.

Breathing

Ventilate the patient with 100% oxygen using intermittent positive-pressure ventilation (IPPV). Confirm that the vaporizer and any anesthetic constant rate infusions (CRIs) are turned off. Give 2 breaths (approximately one ventilation per second) first and then evaluate if the patient begins to breathe spontaneously. If no spontaneous breaths occur within approximately 5 to 6 seconds, begin IPPV at a rate of 10 to 20 ventilations per minute (vpm). Be sure not to exceed airway pressures of 20 cm H_2O. Avoid excessive ventilation rates as positive-pressure ventilation decreases venous return and thereby cardiac output. If the patient has respiratory arrest only (the heart is still beating adequately and pulses can be palpated), consider acupuncture of the Jen Chung [Governing Vessel (GV) 26; Fig. 12.1] point (check state and AVMA guidelines[1] for use of acupuncture).

GV 26 has been shown to increase cardiopulmonary function in dogs (Clifford et al. 1983; Janssens et al. 1979). Place a 25-gauge, 1-inch needle in the nasal philtrum at the ventral nares and twirl it several times while checking for spontaneous ventilation. Also antagonize any drugs that have been given that are likely to cause apnea.

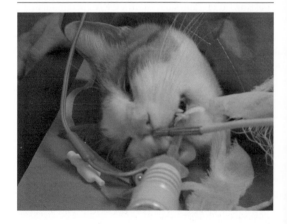

Figure 12.1. Governing Vessel 26 may be used in arrest to stimulate the cardiopulmonary system. Use a 25-gauge 1-inch needle to stimulate the nasal philtrum at the ventral nares and twirl it several times while checking for spontaneous ventilation.

Circulation

Auscultation of the heart using a stethoscope over the heart or an esophageal stethoscope and palpation of pulse (carotid or femoral) are done quickly, and if absent external cardiac compressions are begun. To determine if internal cardiac massage is indicated, see the section on open-chest CPR later in this chapter. Ideally, patients weighing less than 7 kg should have cardiac compressions done in lateral recumbency, while patients weighing more than 7 kg should be done in dorsal recumbency (with compressions applied on the distal sternum). However, performing adequate compressions in an animal in dorsal recumbency is very challenging. We currently perform compressions on all animals in lateral recumbency regardless of size (Fig. 12.2).

In small animals and pediatric patients, thoracic compressions can cause direct cardiac compression (cardiac pump theory). In larger patients, thoracic compression increases intrathoracic pressure and subsequently intravascular pressure, resulting in an arteriovenous pressure gradient for extrathoracic blood flow. During the relaxation phase, intrathoracic pressure falls, allowing blood to return to the heart and lungs (thoracic pump theory). Compressions should be done at a rate of 80 to 100 per minute with a 50% duty cycle (compression time should equal relaxation time).

> During CPR, minimize interruptions of compressions. Every time chest compressions stop, blood flow stops. Increased interruptions in chest compressions are associated with increased mortality in people.

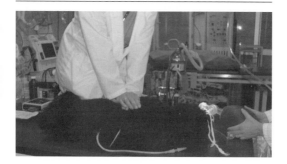

Figure 12.2. Appropriate positioning in right lateral recumbency for cardiopulmonary (CPR) resuscitation. Notice the Ambu bag.

During CPR in people, compressions occur less than 50% to 60% of the time due to interruptions for airway, intravenous access, rhythm checks, and drug administration. It is essential to minimize interruptions, as compressions are now thought to be the single most important aspect of successful CPR even with fibrillation. Assessment of effectiveness of compressions can be achieved by several methods. Palpation of peripheral pulses is the most common method used but may not be accurate because the lack of valves in the caudal vena cava may allow retrograde flow of blood into the venous system during compressions and may produce venous pulses that are mistaken for arterial pulses. A Doppler ultrasound transducer (see Chapter 2) can also be used to assess blood flow and can be applied to the lubricated cornea to estimate cerebral flow. Arterial blood gases are not an accurate reflection of tissue perfusion and acid base status during CPA due to markedly low perfusion (i.e., blood from the tissues is not getting to the lungs). Venous blood gases appear to be a more accurate reflection of tissue status during CPA. ETCO$_2$ is our preferred method of assessing cardiac output during CPR. ETCO$_2$ has been shown to be a good indicator of cardiac output when ventilation was controlled during CPR in people. Several case studies in people have correlated successful resuscitation with higher ETCO$_2$ levels during CPR. The ETCO$_2$ monitor is attached to the ET tube at the beginning of CPR and the monitor is assessed for an increase in ETCO$_2$. If the beginning ET number does not increase, the effectiveness of compressions must be improved. If the number begins to decrease after a period of increasing, it may be time to change out the person doing the compressions. The new guidelines in people suggest changing compressors every 2 minutes. If compressions are not effective, consider abdominal binding, increasing the force of compressions (if compressions are done correctly on a large dog, the person doing the compressions should fatigue after 5 minutes), or changing the position of the patient. Also reevaluate if this would be a good candidate for internal cardiac massage.

Drugs

Prior to anesthesia, a spreadsheet generated with software (e.g., Microsoft Excel) for your computer or personal digital assistant (PDA) may be used to

Table 12.1. Canine Emergency Drug Sheet. Veterinary Medical Teaching Hospital.

Patient Information
Patient: Generic Dog
Owner: Smith
Case #: 0000
Weight (kg): 10

Drug	Concentration	Dosage	Dosage in ml
Epinephrine first dose	1:1000	0.01 mg/kg	0.1 ml
Epinephrine subsequent dose	1:1000	0.1 mg/kg	1.0 ml
Atropine	0.5 mg/ml	0.04 mg/kg	0.8 ml
Calcium gluconate 10% IV over 20 minutes	100 mg/ml	100 mg/kg	10.0 ml
Lidocaine	20 mg/ml	2 mg/kg	1.0 ml
Naloxone	0.4 mg/ml	0.04 mg/kg	1.0 ml
Sodium bicarbonate[a]	1 mEq/ml	0.5 mEq/kg	5.0 ml
Diazepam	5 mg/ml	1 mg/kg	2.0 ml
Shock fluids	Isotonic crystalloids	90 ml/kg	900 ml

[a]after 10 min of arrest, then 8–10 min.

calculate emergency drugs for each patient based on their weight and species (Table 12.1).

Alternatively, a canine and feline CPR chart placed in a prominent place can be used (Tables 12.2 and 12.3). An algorithm for CPR (Fig. 12.3) with a job task list (Table 12.4) that directs people's actions may be also be posted. By following the order on the task list, no tasks will be overlooked.

The intracardiac route of drug administration is not indicated unless you can visualize the heart. Inadvertent administration of drugs into the myocardial muscle may lead to intractable arrhythmias. In people and animals, the intratracheal (IT) route of drug administration has been shown to result in lower drug concentrations than either the intravenous (IV) or intraosseous (IO; see Chapter 13) route. The lower drug concentrations of epinephrine given via the IT route have been shown to produce transient β-adrenergic effects, resulting in lowering of blood pressure and cerebral perfusion pressure in multiple animal studies (Efrati et al. 2003; Elizur et al. 2003; Vaknin et al. 2002). In people, the IV route was associated with a higher return of spontaneous circulation (ROSC) and survival than the IT route

in one study. If drugs must be delivered via the IT route, the dosage should be increased to 2.0 to 2.5 times the IV dosage and diluted in 5 to 10 ml of sterile water, which is associated with better drug absorption than saline (Naganobu et al. 2000). If sterile water is not available, 0.9% NaCl can be used. Drugs that can be given via the IT route include epinephrine, atropine, vasopressin, naloxone, and lidocaine. Sodium bicarbonate should never be given via the IT route as it has been shown to inactivate surfactant. Intravenous and IO are the preferred routes for delivery of drugs during CPR. If drugs are delivered via peripheral (versus central) vein, the injection should be followed by a bolus of 10 to 15 ml of 0.9% NaCl. Adrenergic drugs are inactivated in alkaline solutions (e.g., sodium bicarbonate) and should not be given in the same line.

> Intracardiac injections are not indicated unless the heart can be visualized.

Ideally, a minimum database (MDB) has been collected and analyzed while CPR is being per-

Table 12.2. Canine CPCR Drug Dosages in ml.

Body weight in kg (pounds)				1 (2.2#)	5 (11#)	10 (22#)	15 (33#)	20 (44#)	25 (55#)	30 (66#)	35 (77#)	40 (88#)	45 (99#)	50 (110#)	55 (121#)
Drug	Conc.	Dosage	Route						Dosage in ml						
Epinephrine (1st dose)	1:1000	0.01 mg/kg	IV	0.01	0.05	0.1	0.15	0.2	0.25	0.3	0.35	0.4	0.45	0.5	0.55
Epinephrine (subsequent doses)	1:1000	0.1 mg/kg	IV	0.1	0.5	1.0	1.5	2.0	2.5	3.0	3.5	4.0	4.5	5.0	5.5
Vasopressin	20 units/ml	0.8 unit/kg	IV	0.04	0.2	0.4	0.6	0.8	1.0	1.2	1.4	1.6	1.8	2.0	2.2
Atropine	0.5 mg/ml	0.04 mg/kg	IV	0.08	0.4	0.8	1.2	1.6	2.0	2.4	2.8	3.2	3.6	4.0	4.4
Calcium gluconate (Slow over 20 min)	100 mg/ml	100 mg/Kg	IV	1.0	5.0	10.0	10.0	10.0	10.0	10.0	10.0	10.0	10.0	10.0	10.0
Lidocaine	20 mg/ml	2 mg/kg	IV	0.1	0.5	1.0	1.5	2.0	2.5	3.0	3.5	4.0	4.5	5.0	5.5
Naloxone	0.4 mg/ml	0.04 mg/kg	IV	0.1	0.5	1.0	1.5	2.0	2.5	3.0	3.5	4.0	4.5	5.0	5.5
Sodium bicarbonate (after 10 min arrest, q 10 min)	1 mEq/ml	0.5 mEq/kg	IV	0.5	2.5	5.0	7.5	10.0	12.5	15.0	17.5	20.0	22.5	25.0	27.5
Diazepam	5 mg/ml	1.0 mg/kg	IV	0.2	1.0	2.0	3.0	4.0	5.0	6.0	7.0	8.0	9.0	10.0	11.0
Shock fluids	Isotonic crystalloids	90 ml/kg	IV	90 ml	450 ml	900 ml	1350 ml	1800 ml	2250 ml	2700 ml	3150 ml	3600 ml	4050 ml	4500 ml	4950 ml

Table 12.3. Feline Drug Dosages in ml.

Drug	Conc.	Dosage	Route	Body weight in Kg (pounds)									
				1 (2.2#)	2 (4.4#)	3 (6.6#)	4 (8.8#)	5 (11#)	6 (13.5#)	7 (15.7#)	8 (17.9#)	9 (19.8#)	10 (22#)
								Dosage in ml					
Epinephrine (1st dose)	1:1000	0.01 mg/kg	IV	0.01	0.02	0.03	0.04	0.05	0.06	0.07	0.08	0.09	0.10
Epinephrine (subsequent doses)	1:1000	0.1 mg/kg	IV	0.1	0.2	0.3	0.4	0.5	0.6	0.7	0.8	0.9	1.0
Atropine	0.5 mg/ml	0.04 mg/kg	IV	0.08	0.16	0.24	0.32	0.40	0.48	0.56	0.64	0.72	0.80
Calcium Gluconate (Slow over 20 mins)	100 mg/ml	100 mg/kg	IV	1.0	2.0	3.0	4.0	5.0	6.0	7.0	8.0	9.0	10.0
Lidocaine (caution in cats)	20 mg/ml	0.2 mg/kg	IV	0.01	0.02	0.03	0.04	0.05	0.06	0.07	0.08	0.09	0.1
Naloxone	0.4 mg/ml	0.04 mg/kg	IV	0.1	0.2	0.3	0.4	0.5	0.6	0.7	0.8	0.9	1.0
Sodium bicarbonate (after 10 min arrest, q 10 min)	1 mEq/ml	0.5 mEq/kg	IV	0.5	1.0	1.5	2.0	2.5	3.0	3.5	4.0	4.5	5.0
Diazepam	5 mg/ml	0.75 mg/kg	IV	0.15	0.3	0.45	0.6	0.75	0.9	1.05	1.2	1.35	1.5
Shock fluids*	Isotonic crystalloids	44 ml/kg	IV	44 ml	88 ml	132 ml	176 ml	220 ml	264 ml	308 ml	352 ml	396 ml	440 ml

*Patients receiving shock fluid doses must be carefully evaluated to avoid fluid overload.

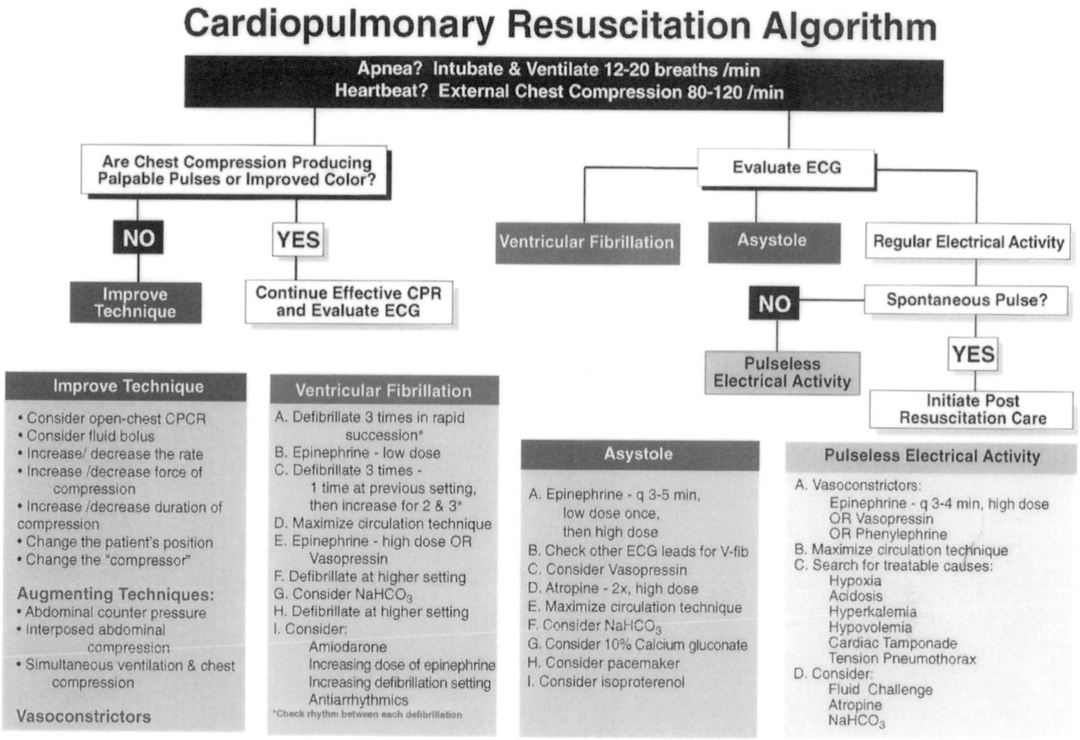

Cardiopulmonary Resuscitation Algorithm

Apnea? Intubate & Ventilate 12-20 breaths /min
Heartbeat? External Chest Compression 80-120 /min

Are Chest Compression Producing Palpable Pulses or Improved Color?

NO → Improve Technique

YES → Continue Effective CPR and Evaluate ECG

Evaluate ECG → Ventricular Fibrillation | Asystole | Regular Electrical Activity

Regular Electrical Activity → Spontaneous Pulse?

NO → Pulseless Electrical Activity

YES → Initiate Post Resuscitation Care

Improve Technique

- Consider open-chest CPCR
- Consider fluid bolus
- Increase/decrease the rate
- Increase/decrease force of compression
- Increase/decrease duration of compression
- Change the patient's position
- Change the "compressor"

Augmenting Techniques:
- Abdominal counter pressure
- Interposed abdominal compression
- Simultaneous ventilation & chest compression

Vasoconstrictors

Ventricular Fibrillation

A. Defibrillate 3 times in rapid succession*
B. Epinephrine - low dose
C. Defibrillate 3 times -
   1 time at previous setting, then increase for 2 & 3*
D. Maximize circulation technique
E. Epinephrine - high dose OR Vasopressin
F. Defibrillate at higher setting
G. Consider NaHCO₃
H. Defibrillate at higher setting
I. Consider:
   Amiodarone
   Increasing dose of epinephrine
   Increasing defibrillation setting
   Antiarrhythmics
*Check rhythm between each defibrillation

Asystole

A. Epinephrine - q 3-5 min, low dose once, then high dose
B. Check other ECG leads for V-fib
C. Consider Vasopressin
D. Atropine - 2x, high dose
E. Maximize circulation technique
F. Consider NaHCO₃
G. Consider 10% Calcium gluconate
H. Consider pacemaker
I. Consider isoproterenol

Pulseless Electrical Activity

A. Vasoconstrictors:
   Epinephrine - q 3-4 min, high dose
   OR Vasopressin
   OR Phenylephrine
B. Maximize circulation technique
C. Search for treatable causes:
   Hypoxia
   Acidosis
   Hyperkalemia
   Hypovolemia
   Cardiac Tamponade
   Tension Pneumothorax
D. Consider:
   Fluid Challenge
   Atropine
   NaHCO₃

Figure 12.3. An algorithm for cardiopulmonary resuscitation (CPR). Use in conjunction with the "CPR job task" list (see Table 12.4).

Table 12.4. CPR Job Task.

Start at the top of the list. Check if the task is being done, if not do it, if it is being done, move to next one.

- Check CPR code, proceed.
- Intubate; tie in tube; inflate cuff.
- Ventilate.
- Provide external chest compressions.
- Insert intravenous (intraosseous) catheter and start fluids.
- ECG (turn on machine and attach leads).
- Minimum database (PCV/TS, azo, BG, electrolytes, venous blood gas).
- Assess effectiveness of compression technique (pulse? Doppler? ETCO₂).
- Record all events and drug administrations, alert 1st clinician if not already done
- Draw up drugs:
  — Epinephrine and atropine and vasopressin (always have another dose ready).
- Turn on defibrillator; attach appropriate sized paddles; apply contact paste to paddles; do not precharge; if thoracotomy, attach appropriate sized internal paddles from bottom drawer.
- Set up suction select appropriate-sized tube.
- Monitor body temperature and provide warmth if necessary.
- Person to perform abdominal augmenting techniques or to relieve chest compressor
- Set out Doppler for attachment when return of spontaneous rhythm.

185

formed. This MDB should include a PCV, TS, azo stick, blood glucose, venous blood gas, lactate, ionized magnesium (if available), and electrolytes. The results of these tests will indicate if there are specific abnormalities that should be addressed (e.g., anemia, hypoglycemia, etc.).

ANTAGONISTS

All drugs given before or during anesthesia should be antagonized immediately when indicated. Current options include naloxone (μ-opioid antagonist: 0.02 to 0.04 mg/kg IV), flumazenil (benzodiazepine antagonist: 0.02 mg/kg IV), and yohimbine (α_2-adrenergic agonist: 0.1 to 0.2 mg/kg slow IV) or atipamazole (more specific α_2-adrenergic agonist: 0.15 to 0.3 mg/kg IM or 3.75 mg/m^2 IM). Antagonist agents may have to be dosed repeatedly because the drugs themselves may have longer-lasting effects than the antagonist agent.

EPINEPHRINE

Epinephrine is both an α- and β-agonist. β_1-Agonist effects include increased heart rate (HR), increased contractility, increased myocardial oxygen consumption, and increased automaticity. The β_2 effects include smooth muscle relaxation, which includes both dilation of peripheral vessels and bronchial smooth muscle (e.g., opens airways, easier to breathe). The α effects include peripheral vasoconstriction, which overrides the β_2 vasodilation. The α effects increase systemic vascular resistance and arterial blood pressure, shunting blood away from the periphery and toward the heart, lungs, and brain. Epinephrine is used during CPR primarily for its α-adrenergic effects (vasoconstrictor) which increases coronary and cerebral perfusion pressure during CPR.

There has been much controversy surrounding standard-dose (0.01 mg/kg IV) or high-dose (0.1 mg/kg IV) epinephrine. The high dose appears to be more efficacious in improving some parameters (aortic diastolic–right atrial gradient, maximizing cerebral blood flow) but does not improve survival. High-dose epinephrine is associated with a higher rate of refibrillation shortly after resuscitation, and in some studies, the 2-hour survival rates are less than those with the standard dose. The first dose of epinephrine is "low" (0.01 mg/kg IV); the second and subsequent doses are "high" (0.1 mg/kg IV).

Epinephrine may be administered every 3 to 5 minutes during CPR.

VASOPRESSIN

Vasopressin is a nonadrenergic peripheral vasoconstrictor that also causes renal and coronary vasoconstriction. It stimulates V_1 receptors in the vasculature to cause vasoconstriction when used at a pharmacologic dose. Most human and animal studies have shown no difference between epinephrine and vasopressin administration during CPR. In one study, significant improvement in survival to hospital discharge was seen in patients with asystole who were treated with vasopressin compared to epinephrine. Since the predominant CPA arrhythmia in companion animals is asystole, use in veterinary medicine is increasing. Vasopressin (0.8 unit/kg [0.2 ml/10 pounds] of the 20 unit/ml concentration) has been used at Texas A&M in the Small Animal ICU for approximately 2 years and seems to be more successful than epinephrine in the resuscitation of prolonged or refractory CPA. There are no data currently on repeat dosing.

ATROPINE

Atropine is a parasympatholytic (vagolytic) that reverses cholinergic mediated decreases in heart rate, systemic vascular resistance, and blood pressure. It increases atrioventricular (AV) node conduction and sinus node automaticity and is most helpful in treatment of asystole arising from vagal stimulation and pulseless electrical activity (PEA; previously electromechanical dissociation). The original atropine dose (0.04 mg/kg IV) is followed by a second dose within 3 minutes if no effect is seen. Lower doses can cause bradycardia and should not be used during CPA.

AMIODARONE

Amiodarone is a class III antiarrhythmic that causes prolongation of myocardial cell action potential duration and refractory period and noncompetitive α- and β-adrenergic inhibition. Numerous studies in people and experimental animals have documented consistent improvement in response to defibrillation with amiodarone compared to lidocaine for VF, and it is listed above lidocaine in the 2005 AHA guidelines. Vasodilation and hypotension, problems associated with the older formulation, are not seen with the new aqueous solution, which does not contain vasoactive solutes. Amiodarone (5 mg/kg IV) is given for refractory VF unresponsive to defibrillation, compressions, and vasopressor administration. It can be repeated one time at half the dosage (2.5 mg/kg IV).

LIDOCAINE

Lidocaine is a local anesthetic and antiarrhythmic agent that reduces automaticity and may increase the defibrillation threshold. It has been shown to be associated with more asystole after defibrillation than amiodarone, and a decreased ROSC was documented in three randomized human trials compared to amiodarone. Lidocaine (2 to 4 mg/kg IV followed by 50 to 75 μg/kg/min IV) may be useful after resuscitation for ventricular arrhythmias in the dog. In cats, a reduced bolus dose of lidocaine (0.2 mg/kg IV) may be administered.

MAGNESIUM

Magnesium (0.15 to 0.30 mEq/kg IV over 15 minutes) is recommended in refractory ventricular arrhythmias (including VF) that are associated with torsade de points.

SODIUM BICARBONATE

There are limited data to support therapy with buffers during a witnessed cardiac arrest. The metabolic acidosis from decreased perfusion and respiratory acidosis from decreased ventilation are best addressed by a strategy to maximize perfusion and ventilation.

> In an arrest, sodium bicarbonate is recommended for severe hyperkalemia, tricyclic antidepressant overdose, severe preexisting metabolic acidosis, or in an unobserved arrest (more than 10 minutes).

There are a wide variety of adverse affects associated with sodium bicarbonate administration during CPR including hypernatremia, hyperosmolality, reduced systemic vascular resistance, paradoxical central nervous system and intracellular acidosis, inhibition of oxygen release from hemoglobin (the extracellular alkalosis shifts the oxyhemoglobin curve to the left), and inactivation of catecholamines that are administered simultaneously. Sodium bicarbonate is recommended for

severe hyperkalemia, tricyclic antidepressant overdose, and severe preexisting metabolic acidosis. Sodium bicarbonate (0.5 mEq/kg IV) may be administered after 10 minutes of CPA. For every 10 minutes of arrest, additional sodium bicarbonate (0.5 mEq/kg IV) may be administered. If arterial blood gases have been done, the base deficit can be used to calculate the replacement bicarbonate dose using Equation 12.1.

$$\text{Sodium bicarbonate mEq/L} = 0.08 \times BW\ (kg) \times \text{base deficit (mEq/L)} \quad (12.1)$$

The replacement bicarbonate calculated from Equation 12.1 is similar to the previously discussed bicarbonate replacement equation (see Chapter 3, Equation 3.2). Only one half to one third of the deficit calculated from Equation 3.2 should be administered IV slowly (over 20 minutes). Otherwise, the previous formula overcorrects the metabolic acidosis in the entire extracellular fluid compartment and could cause alkalosis in the vascular space leading to severe hypotension and death if given as a rapid IV bolus.

> After 10 minutes of arrest, metabolic acidosis may be treated by administering sodium bicarbonate IV using the formula: $0.08 \times BW$ (kg) $\times$ base deficit (mEq/L).

Non–CO_2-generating buffers such as Carbicarb (an equimolar concentration of sodium bicarbonate and sodium carbonate), THAM (Trizma base; Sigma Chemical), or Tribonat have shown potential for minimizing the negative systemic effects of sodium bicarbonate administration. There is currently insufficient evidence to argue for their use during CPR.

CALCIUM

Although calcium is essential for myocardial contractility, retrospective and prospective studies have shown no benefit from calcium administration during CPR. Calcium gluconate 10% (0.5 to 1.5 ml/kg slow IV) is currently recommended for cases of calcium channel blocker toxicity, documented hypocalcemia, and hyperkalemia. Ionized calcium should be measured because total calcium does not correlate with ionized calcium in critically ill patients.

Glucose is not recommended for CPR except in instances of hypoglycemia. Hyperglycemia has been associated with a worse neurologic outcome following resuscitation, due to reperfusion injury. If the crystalloid being administered during anesthesia has glucose, it should be discontinued after arrest and replaced with a balanced electrolyte solution for resuscitation.

INTRAVENOUS FLUID THERAPY

There is limited evidence for the use of large-volume IV crystalloids during CPR. Volume loading during CPR increases right atrial pressure relative to aortic pressure, which may decrease cerebral perfusion pressure (CPP). In experimental CPR in dogs, the increased CPP produced by epinephrine is not augmented by an IV fluid bolus.

Current recommendations in veterinary medicine are to administer small-volume crystalloids (20 ml/kg IV bolus for dogs and 10 ml/kg IV bolus for cats) to patients that were euvolemic prior to arrest. If the patient was hypovolemic prior to arrest a shock dose of crystalloids (90 ml/kg IV for dogs; 45 ml/kg IV for cats) should be administered with a pressure bag. If the animal was hypovolemic from blood loss, a blood transfusion with whole blood or packed red blood cells and fresh frozen plasma should be initiated. Because packed red cells have essentially no colloid oncotic pressure, they should not be given alone for whole blood loss. Synthetic colloids should be given at 20 ml/kg/day IV (3 to 5 ml/kg/hr for dogs and 5 to 10 ml/kg/day IV in cats). In cats, one large bolus at 3 to 5 ml/kg/hr IV may be given, but afterward the rate should be decreased to 1 to 3 ml/kg/hr.

COMMON ARRHYTHMIAS DURING CPA

Rapid and accurate identification of the underlying cardiac rhythm is necessary to successfully treat CPA. The outcome of CPR may differ whether the patient has underlying cardiac disease or extracardiac disease (e.g., gastric dilation volvulus, pain, hypoxemia, hypercarbia, autonomic imbalance).[2]

Sinus Bradycardia

Sinus bradycardia in the anesthetized patient is defined as a normal sinus rhythm with a rate of less than 60 to 80 beats per minute (bpm) in dogs and less than 100 to 120 bpm in cats. Youngsters are rate dependent for their cardiac output, rather than contractility dependent, so higher rates are required in young patients. Hypothermia is a common cause of bradycardia, which responds poorly to anticholinergics. Increased vagal tone may result in several reflexes (e.g., oculocardiac reflex, carotid massage, micturition syncope) and may result from several drugs (e.g., opioids, α_2-agonists). Other causes include increased intracranial pressure (e.g., Cushing reflex), brachiocephaly, athletic fitness, hyperkalemia, and hypoxemia. Bradycardia may also be a precursor to CPA, especially in cats. Atropine is the drug of choice when increased vagal tone is suspected because it has a rapid onset of action. Repeated administration of medications should be avoided in hypothermia until the animal is warm to avoid toxicity.

Ventricular Tachycardia

Ventricular tachycardia is defined as a repetitive firing of ectopic foci in the ventricular myocardium or Purkinje system that can precipitate VF. It can be associated with hypoxia, electrolyte changes, trauma, sepsis, pancreatitis, gastric dilatation volvulus, ischemia, pain, primary cardiac disease, and other syndromes. After any underlying causes are treated, lidocaine is usually the first drug of choice. Several other options exist including procainamide. Administration of procainamide during anesthesia may result in hypotension.

Ventricular Fibrillation

VF is identified as a complete absence of P-QRS-T complexes with chaotic fibrillation waves, which may be either coarse (higher amplitude with more orderly appearance) or fine (lower amplitude and complete lack of organization). It may be easier to convert coarse VF to sinus rhythm than fine VF. VF is more responsive early and should be identified as early as possible during CPA. Epinephrine can improve the responsiveness of VF to defibrillation. The 2005 AHA guidelines stress the importance of compressions before and after defibrillation as multiple studies have documented increases in successful conversion when defibrillation was preceded by compressions. Refractory VF may occur due to lack of myocardial oxygen. New recommendations are to administer one shock immediately followed by compressions for 2 minutes before checking the rhythm. After VF is terminated, there is often a period of aystole or PEA that can last for several minutes and may be responsive to compressions. Fine VF can mimic asystole on the ECG, so check orthogonal leads (leads I and aVF, leads II and aVL) to verify the rhythm. The dose of joules (J) per kilogram body weight can be confusing. It is suggested that 7 J/kg be used for animals under 15 kg and 10 J/kg be used for animals over 15 kg for external defibrillation. One tenth of the dose calculated is used for internal defibrillation. Another suggestion is to use 50 J for small dogs, 100 J for medium dogs, and 200 J for large dogs for external defibrillation. Use conduction paste on paddles (NEVER ALCOHOL or ultrasound gel), place paddles on opposite sides of chest, applying pressure; when defibrillator is charged, call "Clear." No one can have contact with the animal or the table during defibrillation or they will get shocked. Defibrillate and immediately begin compressions for 2 minutes before checking the rhythm. If VF persists, deliver another shock of higher intensity. If defibrillation is unsuccessful after three cycles, consider amiodarone. Chemical defibrillation rarely works. The idea is to convert VF to asystole using KCl, which raises intracellular K^+, depolarizes myocardial cells, and ends VF. Then asystole is converted to sinus rhythm using epinephrine. Precordial thump will unlikely be successful but may be tried.

Asystole

> Atropine is indicated for treatment of asystole due to vagal stimulation; for asystole due to other causes, epinephrine or vasopressin should be administered.

Asystole is defined as the absence of QRS-T complexes on an ECG and is seen as a "flat line" on the ECG. It can be caused by increases in vagal tone (e.g., endotracheal intubation, airway suctioning) or it can be seen with disease. *Pulseless electrical activity* (PEA) is the term for a heterogeneous group of pulseless rhythms. Because of the similarity in causes and treatment of asystole and PEA, the two have been combined in the 2005 AHA guidelines. We will combine the treatment here for simplicity. If associated with vagal stimulation, the treatment is atropine; if it is associated with other diseases, epinephrine or vasopressin should be administered.

OPEN-CHEST CPR

Open-chest CPCR is indicated in large dogs and in cases of pneumothorax, chest trauma, pleural effusion, pericardial effusion, or diaphragmatic hernia, during surgery, or when there is no evidence of circulation (pulses) within 5 minutes of starting compressions.

At the left intercostal space 5–6, clip one strip of hair quickly, swab once with antiseptic, and make an incision midway between ribs down to pleura. Avoid the internal thoracic artery (1 cm lateral to sternum) and caudal rib vessels. Between ventilations, use blunt penetration into pleura with curved Mayo scissors, extend the incision dorsally and ventrally, open the pericardium, avoiding the phrenic nerve, and compress the heart from apex to base at a rate of 80 to 100 bpm. Small hearts can be compressed with one hand; larger hearts need both hands. Be careful not to rotate the heart and kink vessels. As compressions begin, feel the ventricle fill, and then compress again. Coordinate compressions with ventricular filling. Someone else should be evaluating perfusion. If the ventricle does not fill, add volume (e.g., fluids). If successful, because pericardial effusion is common post open-chest CPR, remove part of pericardium, being careful not to incise the phrenic nerve. Use warm sterile lavage of the thorax, place chest tube, close incision, and begin antibiotics and analgesia.

POSTOPERATIVE CARE OF THE RESUSCITATED PATIENT

After ROSC, the principal objective of CPR is to ensure optimal perfusion of essential organs. A common mnemonic in human medicine is to continually evaluate the Hs and Ts. The Hs stand for hypovolemia, hypoxia, hydrogen ion (acidosis), hyperkalemia/hypokalemia, hypoglycemia, and hypothermia, and the Ts stand for toxins, tamponade (cardiac), tension pneumothorax, thrombosis (coronary or pulmonary), and trauma.

The patient will need to be ventilated until spontaneous ventilation returns. It is essential to maintain $Paco_2$ between 35 and 40 mm Hg and Pao_2 greater than 80 mm Hg. Continuous monitoring of blood pressure keeping systolic blood pressure above 90 mm Hg, pulse oximetry, and ECG and frequent (hourly or more frequently) monitoring of pulses, mucous membrane color and refill time, lung sounds, body temperature, electrolytes, blood gases, urine output, analgesia (thoracotomy is extremely painful), glucose, PCV and TS, and neurologic function are essential. Lactate levels are also important post CPR to monitor tissue perfusion. Supplemental oxygen should be continued after spontaneous ventilations return. Some common post CPR abnormalities include reperfusion injury, coagulation abnormalities, cerebral edema, cardiac arrhythmias, hypoxemia, acute renal failure, and, of course, whatever disease process caused the arrest in the first place.

Specific Treatable Abnormalities

Treat specific abnormalities as they arise:

Ventricular arrhythmias: Lidocaine bolus (2 to 4 mg/kg IV) in dogs, followed by a constant rate infusion (CRI; 50 to 75 µg/kg/min IV) if lidocaine is successful in terminating or decreasing the ventricular ectopy. Some recommend using magnesium sulfate for ventricular premature complexes (VPCs) or ventricular tachycardia.

Hypotension: First make sure that the animal is fluid replete (urine output greater than 1 ml/kg/hr, CVP approximately 7 to 10 cm H_2O), not anemic, and total solids are above 5.0 g/dl on refractometer for adults and above 4.0 g/dl for puppies and kittens (caution if using synthetic colloids as they register at 4.5 g/dl on refractometer). Also rule out bradycardia, heart block, decreased cardiac contractility, and electrolyte abnormalities as causes of hypotension. Try colloid bolus (see earlier for dose for dogs and cats). If this fails to raise blood pressure, begin vasopressor treatment (vasopressin [0.5 milliunits/kg/min IV] or dopamine [5.0 µg/kg/min IV and raise by 1.0 µg/kg/min every 15 minutes to effect].

Neurologic abnormalities: Cerebral edema is common post CPR. If the patient is not overhydrated, anuric, hypernatremic, or has pulmonary edema, mannitol (0.25 to 0.5 g/kg IV over 20 minutes) may be administered.

Hypoxemia: Ventilate with 100% oxygen to start but wean them down to less than 60% as soon as possible (oxygen toxicity). You will most likely need to add PEEP.

CONCLUSION

The new 2005 AHA guidelines stress the importance of compressions during all events associated with CPR (airway establishment, intravenous access) and interruptions of compressions should be minimized wherever possible. Although the success rate of CPR is still quite low in both veterinary and human medicine, it is still highest in our anesthetized patients. Staff training, equipment check, continual vigilance and monitoring of anesthetized patients, and prompt recognition of pre-CPA signs are essential for a successful outcome.

ENDNOTES

1 AVMA guidelines may be found at http://www.vet-task-force.com/Guidelines.htm.
2 Autonomic imbalance is often used to explain unanticipated anesthetic death. "Anesthesia disease" might be used in its place because the balance between the sympathetic and parasympathetic nervous system may be altered by drugs used during anesthesia, resulting in altered reflexes. Editor's note.

REFERENCES

American Heart Association. 2005. Guidelines for cardiopulmonary resuscitation and emergency cardiovascular care. *Circulation* 112(Suppl I): IV-1–IV-203.

Clifford, D.H., Lee, D.C., and Lee, M.O. 1983. Effects of dimethyl and acupuncture on the cardiovascular system of dogs. *Ann NY Acad Sci* 411:83–84.

Efrati, O., Ben-Abraham, R., Barak, A., et al. 2003. Endobronchial adrenaline: Should it be reconsidered? Dose response and hemodynamic effect in dogs. *Resuscitation* 59:117–122.

Elizur, A., Ben-Abraham, R., Manisterski, Y., et al. 2003. Tracheal epinephrine or norepinephrine preceded by beta blockade in a dog model: Can beta blockade bestow any benefits? *Resuscitation* 59:271–276.

Janssens, L., Altman, S., and Rogers, P.A.M. 1979. Respiratory and cardiac arrest under general anesthesia: Treatment by acupuncture of the nasal philtrum. *Vet Rec* 105(12):273–276.

Kass, K.H., and Haskins, S.C. 1992. Survival following cardiopulmonary resuscitation in dogs and cats. *J Vet Emerg Crit Care* 2(2):57–65.

Naganobu, K., Hasebe, Y., Uchiyama, Y., et al. 2000. A comparison of distilled water and normal saline as diluents for endobronchial administration of epinephrine in the dog. *Anesth Analg* 91:317–321.

Vaknin, Z., Manisterski, Y., Ben-Abraham, R., et al. 2001. Is endotracheal adrenaline deleterious because of the beta adrenergic effect? *Anesth Analg* 92:1408–1412.

Wingfield, W.E., and Van Pelt, D.R. 1992. Respiratory and cardiopulmonary arrest in dogs and cats: 265 Cases (1986–91). *J Am Vet Med Assoc* 200(12): 1993–1996.

Chapter 13
Anesthesia for Patients With Special Concerns

Tamara L. Grubb

The patient population has changed fairly dramatically in the last 10 years as veterinarians' medical skills have progressed and veterinarians and their staff have become capable of supporting patients with advanced disease and advancing age. Furthermore, our surgical skills have improved, and surgery now is often complicated and long and may involve major blood loss and/or major physiologic manipulation. Anesthesia skills must advance in order to support patients that largely do not fit into the "young, healthy" category and to support patients throughout difficult surgical procedures.

Safe anesthesia no longer means recovering as many patients as we anesthetize. Instead, we must focus on what happens to the patient during the anesthetic period—which starts when the patient is admitted for anesthesia and ends when the patient is fully conscious and free of pain.

Necessary advances in anesthesia include better preparation of the patient for anesthesia (including the use of preanesthetic tranquilizers [see Chapter 5] and analgesic agents [see Chapters 5, 6, 9, and 10]), improved support of the patient during the anesthetic period (including advanced monitoring [see Chapter 2], and use of supportive drugs like colloids and positive inotropic agents [see Chapters 11 and 12]), and increased attention to events in the recovery period (including emergence delirium and bouts of pain [see Chapters 4 and 13]).

Anesthetic drug concerns, patient support, and monitoring are similar for a large number of the compromised or critical patients. An overview of both topics are presented. More specific information is presented with each disease or condition, and an in-depth discussion of sedative, anesthetic, and

analgesic drugs (see Chapters 5 through 10) is available; in-depth monitoring (see Chapter 2) and support (see Chapter 11) are also reviewed elsewhere.

Dosages (Table 13.1) and the use of sedative and anesthetic drugs in compromised, very young, and aged patients differ from those in normal, healthy young adult patients (i.e., are lower). Reducing dosages in compromised patients is critical, often even more critical than the actual anesthetic drugs that are selected.

PHARMACOLOGY OVERVIEW FOR THE AGED OR CRITICAL PATIENT

All tranquilizers, induction agents, and inhalation agents cause some degree of dose-dependent central nervous system (CNS) depression, and most cause both respiratory and cardiovascular depression. In healthy patients, many of the physiologic effects of anesthetic drugs are well tolerated or may be counteracted by routine procedures such as administration of oxygen or intravenous (IV) fluids. In compromised patients, these physiologic effects may be exacerbated, further contributing to the morbidity of the patient.

Premedicants: Anticholinergics

Atropine and glycopyrrolate are important for treating vagally mediated bradycardia but should not be used indiscriminately, especially in patients with questionable cardiac function. Increased heart rate (HR) generally contributes to an increased cardiac output, but tachycardia also causes increased cardiac work and oxygen demand, and may actually cause cardiac output to decrease because of decreased

Table 13.1. Drugs, drug dosages, and drug concerns in critical, neonatal, and geriatric patients.

Drug	Dosage (mg/kg; unless noted)	Effects	Cautions
Opioids			
Morphine	0.2–0.5 D; 0.1–0.2 C; IM, SQ	Profound analgesia	Minimal CV and respiratory depression; histamine release IV
Oxymorphone	0.025–0.1 D; 0.025–0.05 C; IM, IV, SQ	Profound analgesia	Same as morphine; no histamine release
Hydromorphone	0.05–0.2 IM, IV, SQ; D and C	Profound analgesia	Same as morphine; no histamine release
Butorphanol	0.1–0.4 IM, IV, SQ; D and C	Moderate analgesia and sedation of short duration	Must supplement with longer lasting analgesic agent
Buprenorphine	0.01–0.03 IM, IV, SQ: D and C; TM in C	Moderate analgesia of long duration, no or minimal sedation	May need to combine with a sedative
Fentanyl	CRI: 1–10 µg/kg/hr IV; D and C	Profound analgesia, short duration of action so generally administered as CRI or TD	Minimal CV and respiratory depression at low doses
Sedatives			
Opioids	See above	See above	See above
Diazepam/midazolam	0.1–0.2 IV, IM; D and C Midazolam also SQ	May provide mild sedation; mild to no CV or respiratory depression	Generally does not provide adequate sedation in healthy patients; may cause excitement
Acepromazine	0.01–0.03 IM, IV, SQ; D and C	Mild to moderate sedation	No analgesia, not reversible, causes vasodilation and hypotension; may have extended duration
Induction			
Propofol	2–4 IV; D and C	Rapid effects; rapidly cleared from body through a variety of routes	Produces CV and respiratory depression of similar magnitude (but shorter duration) to that caused by thiobarbiturates
Ketamine (K)/diazepam (V)	K: 2–8 with V: 0.2–0.5 GIVE TO EFFECT; IV; D and C	Sympathetic nervous system stimulation with CV changes that include increased HR and contractility	Worsening of cardiac function in some patients; may cause tachycardia and hypertension; may contribute to seizures
Etomidate	0.5–1.5 IV	Minimal to no CV changes	Adrenocortical suppression, clinical significance is unknown
Inhalant agents	Dosages are extremely high for induction	Anesthesia in calm patients; excitement in healthy patients; contraindicated in vomiting patient	Excessive hypotension because of large dosages needed for induction
Maintenance			
Isoflurane	0.5–2%	Anesthesia to effect; pungent	All inhalant gases contribute to hypotension, hypoventilation, and hypothermia
Sevoflurane	1–4%	Anesthesia to effect	See Chapter 7
			See Chapter 7

D, dog; C, cat; IV, intravenous; IM, intramuscular; SQ, subcutaneous; TD, transdermal; TM, transmucosal; CRI, constant rate infusion; CV, cardiovascular; HR, heart rate.

ventricular filling time. Myocardial perfusion and oxygen delivery occur during diastole, and tachycardia minimizes the time spent in diastole. If oxygen demand is not met by oxygen delivery, myocardial ischemia and exacerbation of cardiac dysfunction may occur.

Premedicants: Sedatives and Tranquilizers

Sedation may not be necessary in quiet or debilitated patients. However, sedatives alleviate stress in anxious patients and decrease the dosage of drugs needed for induction and maintenance of anesthesia. The side effects of sedatives should be weighed against the side effects of a large dose of induction or maintenance drugs. Drugs that provide both sedation and analgesia (e.g., opioids) are almost always appropriate.

Opioids should be considered for any patient experiencing pain. In general, opioids cause only minimal cardiovascular depression, mild to moderate respiratory depression, and anticholinergic-responsive bradycardia. Opioids provide moderate to profound analgesia (depending on the opioid) that allows reduction of the dosage of induction and maintenance agents, which generally outweighs any direct cardiovascular or respiratory depression caused by the opioids.

Morphine, hydromorphone, oxymorphone, and fentanyl (among others) are pure μ-agonist opioids and provide profound analgesia and moderate sedation in dogs (excitement often occurs in cats). Butorphanol, an agonist-antagonist opioid, provides short-duration moderate-intensity analgesia with mild sedation, whereas buprenorphine, a partial agonist opioid, provides long-duration moderate-intensity analgesia with virtually no sedation and minimal to no cardiovascular and respiratory depression. Because butorphanol and buprenorphine are not as potent as the pure μ-agonists, they are appropriate used alone for mild to moderate pain and are appropriate for severe pain when used as part of a multimodal protocol (e.g., with local anesthetic agents or nonsteroidal anti-inflammatory drugs [NSAIDs]). The effects of opioids may be reversed with pure opioid antagonists such as naloxone and naltrexone. There are no absolute contraindications for opioids.

The benzodiazepines (e.g., midazolam and diazepam) are commonly used as mild tranquilizers and muscle relaxants in compromised patients because they produce minimal or no cardiovascular and respiratory depression and the effects of benzodiazepines are reversible. Benzodiazepines may not provide adequate sedation when used alone in all patients (although they are commonly used alone in compromised patients) but are generally more than adequate when combined with opioids. Most compromised and aged patients do not require sedation beyond that provided by opioids and/or benzodiazepines. If more sedation is necessary, acepromazine and the α_2-agonists (e.g., medetomidine) might be suitable in some healthy patients. However, because of the cardiovascular effects of each of these drugs, they are generally not recommended in compromised patients. Acepromazine causes vasodilation, which may cause hypotension. Acepromazine is not reversible, nor does it provide analgesia. α_2-Agonists cause both increased systemic vascular resistance and bradycardia and are reserved for generally healthy patients. α_2-Agonists are reversible and do provide analgesia.

Induction Drugs

Propofol is generally a good choice for anesthetic induction of compromised patients and of very young or very old patients. Propofol causes myocardial depression and hypotension comparable to that caused by thiobarbiturates; however, this effect is extremely short-lived and normally well tolerated in patients without profound cardiovascular disease. Propofol also causes a brief period of respiratory depression and potential apnea, especially when the drug is administered rapidly. However, propofol is easily titrated "to effect," thus attenuating the likelihood of overdosage. Also, propofol is rapidly cleared form the body via multiple routes and does not depend solely on hepatic metabolism or renal elimination. Recoveries are rapid and complete, thereby minimizing the duration of anesthesia-induced physiologic depression.

Ketamine may be a good choice in some compromised patients because ketamine-induced stimulation of the CNS leads to increased sympathetic outflow. This results in increased HR, myocardial contractility, cardiac output, and arterial blood pressure. However, cardiac work and myocardial oxygen requirements are also increased. Furthermore, the cardiac support is an *indirect* effect modulated through the sympathetic nervous system (SNS).

The direct effect of ketamine is myocardial depression, and this may be manifest in patients that do not have a fully functioning SNS. In critical patients, endogenous catecholamine stores are commonly depleted and SNS mechanisms are exhausted. In aged and extremely young patients, the SNS may be unable to mount an appropriate response to stimulation. Thus, in these patients, ketamine may actually cause a moderate to profound decrease in blood pressure. Also, ketamine may contribute to seizure activity in some patients. The dissociative drug tiletamine, a component of Telazol, has similar effects and side effects as ketamine and has a longer half-life.

Etomidate, which causes minimal or no change in HR, cardiac output, mean arterial blood pressure, and baroreceptor-mediated responses, is a viable option for patients with significant cardiovascular dysfunction. Etomidate is rapidly hydrolyzed by the liver, so patients with normal hepatic function recover from anesthesia quickly. Etomidate may cause some excitement at induction and should be preceded by a tranquilizer. Interestingly, etomidate causes adrenocortical suppression. It may be an excellent choice for suppressing the stress associated with anesthesia and surgery, but possibly a poor choice for patients that need to mount an adrenocortical response for survival (e.g., trauma patients, patients with sepsis). However, the clinical implication of the adrenocortical suppression is unknown and there are no absolute guidelines of when to use or not use etomidate.

Ultrashort-acting thiobarbiturates (e.g., thiopental, methohexital) cause moderate to profound respiratory and cardiovascular depression and should be used with caution in compromised patients.

Mask induction with inhalant anesthetic agents is not recommended for most patients and is completely contraindicated in compromised patients that resist induction and go through an excitement phase with struggling. Struggling during mask induction may cause tachycardia, hypertension, increased cardiac oxygen demand, catecholamine release, increased incidence of arrhythmias, and tachypnea. Furthermore, a very high concentration of inhalant anesthetic is necessary to induce the patient to anesthesia when the inhalant is used alone. This may cause a precipitous decrease in arterial blood pressure and ventilatory function. Therefore, this method of induction is not appropriate for patients with cardiac disease, compromised cardiac function secondary to other disease (e.g., endotoxemia, hypocalcemia), or hypovolemia. Although the technique *may* be appropriate for moribund or heavily sedated patients since struggling is not expected, the high concentration of anesthetic gas needed for induction is still extremely dangerous.

Maintenance Drugs

The inhalant anesthetic agents produce dose-dependent cardiovascular and respiratory depression in all patients and should always be delivered at the lowest possible dose needed to maintain appropriate anesthetic depth. Fortunately, the gases are fairly easily titrated "to effect" and the necessary dose may be drastically reduced by the use of tranquilizers (when appropriate) and analgesic agents (almost always appropriate). The best inhalant agents are those with minimal hepatic metabolism and low solubility, which allows a rapid induction to and recovery from anesthesia, and a rapid change of anesthetic depth during the operative period. The most appropriate inhalants are isoflurane, sevoflurane, and desflurane. Desflurane is rarely used in veterinary medicine and is not covered in this chapter.

Analgesia

Analgesia is often wrongly withheld from critical and traumatized patients for a variety of reasons, including fear of "masking" underlying disease processes and lack of understanding of the effects and side effects of the drugs themselves. Pain causes a myriad of side effects (Table 13.2), including SNS stimulation and catecholamine release, which may lead to tachycardia, vasoconstriction, and arrhythmias. Pain causes tachypnea, impaired pulmonary function, decreased gastrointestinal (GI) motility, and increased incidence of GI ulceration. Pain impairs healing through a variety of mechanisms, including cortisol release and immunosuppression. Adequate analgesia allows patients to recover from surgery more quickly, and with fewer side effects, than patients that have not had their pain treated appropriately. Pain has the potential to contribute to the demise of the patient and may mask other signs (e.g., a trauma patient that presents with tachycardia, pale mucous membranes, and a prolonged CRT could be in hemodynamic crisis or in pain). Analgesic agents may be used not only to relieve the

Table 13.2. Sequelae of pain.*

GI compromise	*Renal dysfunction*
Gastric ulceration	Renal hypertension
Ileus	Decreased renal blood flow
Anorexia	Renal ischemia
Nausea/vomiting	
Fluid imbalance	*Pulmonary compromise*
Electrolyte imbalance	Tachypnea
Acid-base imbalance	Respiratory acid-base imbalance
	Pulmonary hypertension
Cardiovascular compromise	$\dot{V}/\dot{Q}$ mismatch
Tachycardia	Pulmonary edema
Hypertension	
Arrhythmias	
Increased cardiac work	*Other effects*
Increased oxygen demand	Impaired wound healing
	Immune system dysfunction
Increased metabolic rate	Hemostasis disorders
Increased oxygen demand	
Negative nitrogen balance	
Cachexia	

*"One of the psychological curiosities of therapeutic decision making is the withholding of analgesic drugs because the clinician is not absolutely certain that the animal is experiencing pain. Yet the same individual will administer antibiotics without documenting the presence of a bacterial infection. Pain and suffering constitute the only situation in which I believe that, if in doubt, one should go ahead and treat." LE Davis, clinical pharmacologist, University of Illinois.

patient's suffering but also to make the patient more tractable for an exam, and as part of the initial diagnostic process. If the symptoms described above are relieved with analgesia, pain was probably the cause. If they are not relieved, further diagnostics must proceed rapidly.

> Analgesia may be used diagnostically. As the effects of pain are alleviated and the signs of pain are eliminated from the overall clinical presentation, the signs of other complications generally become more apparent.

The use of preemptive analgesia will decrease the necessary dosage of induction and inhalant drugs. Because these drugs cause dose-dependent cardiovascular and respiratory depression, use of the lowest possible dosage improves anesthetic safety. Opioids and local anesthetic agents are appropriate in almost all compromised patients and nonsteroidal antiinflammatory drugs (NSAIDs) are appropriate in some compromised patients. Other analgesic agents (e.g., ketamine) may be appropriate as detailed previously (see Chapters 5, 6, and 9).

Opioid administration (see Chapters 5 and 9) should be considered in every painful patient. There are few patients in which opioids would be inappropriate. Routes of administration of opioids are numerous and include IV (as a single bolus or as a constant rate infusion [CRI]), intramuscularly, subcutaneously, orally, epidurally or spinally, transmucosally, and transdermally. Maintenance of anesthesia with a fentanyl CRI (1 to 10μg/kg/hr) supplemented with very low dosages of an inhalant anesthetic agent is a safe and effective protocol for extremely compromised patients.

Local anesthetic agents are an excellent addition to anesthetic/analgesic protocols because local blockade of a nerve decreases transmission of painful impulses from injured or incised tissue to the central nervous system. Thus, pain is alleviated for the duration of action of the local anesthetic drug and beyond; hypersensitivity or "windup" (see Chapters 8 and 9) is less likely to occur. Local anesthetic techniques include field (i.e., block of surgery field), intercostal, intrapleural, oral, and intra-articular blocks. Local anesthetic agents are often used in conjunction with the opioids for spinal and epidural anesthesia/analgesia. Epidural opioids provide long-duration analgesia with little to no systemic effects. Epidural local anesthetic agents will cause sympathetic blockade with vasodilation, which may exacerbate hypotension. Patients should have adequate circulating volume prior to administration of local anesthetics in the epidural space.

Lidocaine (but NOT bupivacaine) may also be administered as a CRI in dogs to provide systemic analgesia in surgical and trauma patients. Ketamine and numerous opioids (e.g., morphine, fentanyl) may also be used in CRIs. CRIs provide the patient with a steady plane of analgesia without the peaks and troughs of pain/pain relief associated with intermittent injections.

NSAIDs provide analgesia and decrease inflammation. This class of drugs is appropriate for most healthy patients and may be appropriate for compromised patients with inflammatory pain. However, NSAIDs should be used only after rehydration and serum chemistry assessment in compromised patients. NSAIDs are inappropriate in patients with acute hepatic or renal dysfunction.

PATIENT PREPARATION AND MONITORING OVERVIEW

Appropriate preparation for anesthesia, monitoring, and support during anesthesia and in recovery reduces the anesthetic risk in ALL patients and is absolutely critical in compromised, pediatric, and geriatric patients. A thorough physical exam is required, and the components of a good basic exam are listed in Table 13.3. A complete blood count

Table 13.3. Preanesthesia examination and testing for compromised, very young, and aged patients.

Minimum database for all patients:
  Thorough physical exam
    General exam
    Heart rate and rhythm
    Pulse strength and quality
    Mucous membrane color and capillary refill time
    Respiratory rate, depth and pattern
    Thoracic ausculation
      Heart sounds
      Lung sounds
    Abdominal palpation
  Chemistry
    Complete blood count (CBC)
    Complete serum chemistry including
      Total protein, albumin, BUN, Creatinine, ALP, ALT, ALT, glucose, electrolytes (K^+, Na^+, Ca^{2+}, Cl^-)
    Complete urinalysis
  Other monitoring
    ECG
    Blood pressure (recommended)
Other tests for specific patients
  Thoracic radiographs (cardiac or respiratory disease; trauma)
  Abdominal fluid collection (trauma or abdominal disease)
  Echocardiogram (cardiac disease or cardiac complications from other diseases [e.g., hyperthyroidism]
    or trauma)
  Other tests as needed

(CBC) and full serum chemistry blood panel (including measurement of electrolytes) are required, and a urinalysis is recommended for most patients. An electrocardiogram (ECG) should be recorded and evaluated in all patients. Arterial blood pressure (ABP) should also be measured in all compromised, very young, and aged patients. Other tests (e.g., thoracic radiographs, echocardiograms, bile acid assay) should be performed as needed.

In all compromised patients, intraoperative patient monitoring should include basic monitoring (HR and rhythm; respiratory rate [RR], depth, and pattern; mucous membrane [MM] color, capillary refill time [CRT], and body temperature) and more advanced monitoring (e.g., ECG, arterial blood pressure [ABP], end-tidal CO_2 [ETCO$_2$] and/or pulse oximetry). Blood pressure monitoring is critical and invasive monitoring should be considered. However, if placement of catheters takes excessive time, invasive monitoring should be abandoned so that anesthesia time is not prolonged. Prolonged anesthesia may be extremely detrimental, especially in compromised patients. Monitoring should begin at induction and some monitors (e.g., the ECG) should be placed on the patient prior to anesthesia and maintained throughout recovery. Central venous pressure (CVP) and urinary output are recommended for some patients. Monitoring tools and techniques are listed in Table 13.4 and described in more detail (see Chapter 2).

Despite all of the electronic monitors available to us, the best "monitor" is still an actual staff member who is dedicated to anesthesia. The presence of a person dedicated to anesthetic monitoring has been shown to decrease the anesthetic complication and mortality rates (Dyson et al. 1998). A technician should be totally dedicated to support and monitoring of the anesthetized patient, especially in critical patients.

PATIENT SUPPORT OVERVIEW

Support for all patients should include the administration of IV fluids and analgesia. Oxygen administration and active warming are necessary in most compromised patients. Other support drugs, including antiarrhythmic drugs and inotropic drugs may be necessary in some patients. Because fluid therapy (see Chapter 11) is critical in compromised patients, a brief review will be provided here.

Table 13.4. Intraoperative monitoring and support for compromised, very young, and aged patients.

Basic monitoring for all patients
Heart rate and rhythm
Pulse strength and quality
Mucous membrane color and capillary refill time
Respiratory rate, depth, and pattern
Electronic monitoring for all patients
ECG
Blood pressure
Pulse oximetry
End-tidal CO_2 (recommended)
Monitoring for specific patients
Urine output
Central venous pressure
Invasive monitoring of blood pressure
Arterial blood gases
Serial glucose and/or electrolyte concentration
Basic support for all patients
Intravenous fluids (crystalloids, colloids, or blood products)
Active support of thermoregulatory system
Oxygen and ventilatory support
Support for specific patients
Positive-pressure ventilation
Electrolyte supplementation
Positive inotropic agents
Antiarrhythmic agents
Antibiotics
Other support as needed

In compromised or traumatized patients, rapid initiation of IV fluids is often necessary and appropriate fluid therapy (both type of fluids and rate of administration) is frequently critical for a successful outcome. Two IV catheters are generally necessary in critical patients, especially those going to surgery. One catheter may be dedicated to fluid therapy, while the other may be dedicated to collection of blood for analysis and delivery of supportive and/or emergency drugs. CVP is the most ideal measure of fluid balance. Normal CVP is −3 to +5 cm H_2O and fluid administration should be slowed or stopped if CVP is greater than 10 cm H_2O. If CVP is not available, packed cell volume (PCV) and total protein (TP) values may be combined with diligent and thorough thoracic auscultation to guide fluid therapy.

Fluid choices include crystalloids, hypertonic saline, synthetic colloids, and blood products. Isotonic crystalloids (e.g., lactated Ringer's solution [LRS], Normosol-R, 0.9% saline) are generally the first line of fluid therapy in most patients. During anesthesia, crystalloids are usually administered at 10 to 15 ml/kg/hr IV. However, rapid fluid resuscitation is often necessary, especially during patient stabilization prior to anesthesia and in time of profound hypovolemia. In these instances, a "shock" dose of crystalloids should be administered. A typical shock dose of crystalloids is defined as administration of 1 blood volume (90 ml/kg in dogs and 60 ml/kg in cats) in 1 hour. Hypertonic saline produces rapid expansion of the circulating volume and may be administered (4 ml/kg over 15 minutes) in acute hypovolemic episodes. Crystalloid administration must follow hypertonic saline administration. Contraindications for hypertonic saline include uncontrolled hemorrhage, cardiogenic shock, and renal failure. Thus, hypertonic saline may be used in many, but not all, critical patients. Hypotonic solutions (e.g., 0.45% saline, 5% dextrose) may be used in special circumstances, like advanced cardiac disease.

Traumatized and critically ill patients often present with hypoproteinemia and hypoalbuminemia. If plasma protein is less than 4.0 g/dl or serum albumin concentration is less than 1.5 g/dl, synthetic colloids or plasma should be used to increase plasma oncotic pressure and to maintain plasma volume. Dextran 70 and hydroxyethyl starch (hetastarch) are commonly used synthetic colloids. The total daily dose of both colloids in dogs is 20 ml/kg/day IV, and all of this or a portion (5 to 10 ml/kg IV) may be administered during surgery. Smaller boluses (4 to 5 ml/kg) may be administered semirapidly over 15 to 30 minutes if rapid volume expansion is necessary. The dosage of colloids in cats is slightly less (10 to 15 ml/kg/day IV), and a small bolus (1 to 3 ml/kg IV) may be administered semirapidly over 15 to 30 minutes if rapid volume expansion is necessary. When colloids are administered during surgery, acute hypotensive crises should still be treated with a rapid infusion of crystalloids. Although more often attributed to dextran containing solutions, both dextrans and hetastarch may dilute existing clotting factors and alter hemostasis.

If impaired clotting is already present or the patient needs clotting factors, plasma should be administered. Ideally, the patient should be cross-matched prior to administration of any blood product. Plasma should be administered through a filter and the patient should be monitored for anaphylactoid reactions. Whole blood is indicated in patients that are hypoalbuminemic and have a low PCV (less than 18% to 20%). When whole blood is administered, the recipient's PCV should increase by 1% for every 2.2 ml of blood/kg of body weight that is administered (Carroll 2003). Oxyglobin is a hemoglobin-based oxygen carrying fluid that may be used to increase plasma and total hemoglobin concentration and arterial oxygen content. Oxyglobin is approved in dogs but not in cats. The recommended total dose (15 ml/kg IV) is lower than the label dose (30 ml/kg) and the recommended administration rate (5 ml/kg/hr) is also lower than the label rate (10 ml/kg/hr) (Carroll 2003).

Patients that have been traumatized or that are critically ill often have difficulty ventilating, whether from effects of injury (e.g., flail chest, diaphragmatic hernia, head trauma) or the effects of disease (e.g., weakness of the ventilatory muscles or pulmonary edema). Any patient that is weak or debilitated is highly likely to have respiratory impairment and must be supported. Clearly, if the patient is not ventilating at all or is unconscious, it should be intubated and supported with intermittent positive-pressure ventilation (IPPV) and supplemental oxygen. Even patients that are ventilating are likely to be hypoxic due to a variety of factors, including decreased ventilation due to muscle weakness or impaired thoracic movements (e.g., limited diaphragmatic movement secondary to pressure on the diaphragm by ascites), decreased hemoglobin concentration due to acute hemorrhage or anemia of chronic disease, impaired responsiveness to hypercarbia (e.g., head trauma), ventilation/perfusion ($\dot{V}/\dot{Q}$) mismatch, and hypermetabolic diseases or conditions (e.g., hyperthyroidism or shock). Stress or excitement from any cause (e.g., pain, hospitalization) may exacerbate hypoxia. Oxygen therapy is required in almost all critical and seriously traumatized patients. If the patient is ventilating and is conscious, supplemental oxygen should be administered through a mask, nasal cannula, hood, or even "blow-by," which is the simple placement of an oxygen-filled hose (e.g., the rebreathing hose on an anesthesia machine) near the patient's nose. This technique increases the inspired oxygen to approximately 40% and, in the words of a prominent criticalist, "'blow-by' oxygen delivery may be one of the best initial treatments in critically ill or injured patients" (Crowe 2003). If the patient is going on to anesthesia, the hypoventilation from induction drugs may cause further oxygen desaturation, and this may reach a critical point if there is any delay of intubation and oxygen delivery. Thus, critical patients should be preoxygenated for 2 to 5 minutes prior to induction.

Compromised patients are often hypothermic. Hypothermia causes a variety of complications, including clotting dysfunction (impaired platelet function and decreased activation of the coagulation cascade), increased risk of infection, slowed drug metabolism, tissue hypoxia (secondary to vasoconstriction), acidosis, abnormal electrical conduction in the heart, and myocardial ischemia. Hypothermia also causes cerebral effects that decrease the patient's anesthetic needs. Unfortunately, the decreased anesthetic need is not always recognized and the delivery of anesthesia is not changed, resulting in an overdosage of anesthetic agents. Although shivering in recovery may increase the body temperature, the intensive muscle movements associated with shivering cause discomfort and increase oxygen consumption by as much as 200% (Sessler 2002). In fact, in human medicine, an active area of research centers on prevention of shivering in the postoperative period. Finally, hypothermia is the main cause of prolonged recoveries from anesthesia in small animal patients. In almost all patients, active warming should begin as soon as the patient is anesthetized and should continue well into the recovery period (until body temperature ≥36.7°C or ≥98°F).

Other drugs are necessary for many critical patients (see Chapters 11 and 12). This category includes positive inotropic agents (e.g., dopamine, dobutamine) and antiarrhythmic drugs (e.g., lidocaine, esmolol). Electrolytes and acid-base regulators (e.g., sodium bicarbonate) are also often required.

RECOVERY FROM ANESTHESIA

Monitoring and support must continue throughout the recovery period until the patient is fully conscious. Compromised patients may recover slowly from anesthesia and prolonged support may be necessary. Unfortunately, most unexpected anesthetic deaths occur in recovery, and most of these are attributed to the known side effects of anesthetic drugs (e.g., cardiovascular and respiratory depression) and the lack of monitoring and support. In anesthetized humans, a 26% overall complication rate occurred when intraoperative and postoperative complications were combined. Of the 26%, only 3% occurred intraoperatively and 23% occurred in recovery (Tarrac 2006). Complications that occur most commonly in anesthetized humans (Mayson, et al. 2005) include respiratory compromise (15.2%), cardiovascular abnormalities (12.3%), and excessive pain (7.2%). There are few risk studies in veterinary medicine that look directly at the percentage of complications that occur in recovery. However, because all mammals are affected similarly by most anesthetic drugs, we would expect postanesthetic complications that occur in veterinary patients to be similar to those that occur in humans.

ANESTHESIA FOR PATIENTS WITH CARDIOVASCULAR DISEASE

Cardiovascular Physiology/Pharmacology

In every tissue of the body, oxygen is required for normal cellular function, and it is delivery of this oxygen that drives the cardiovascular system. Autoregulation of cardiac output, changes in vascular tone, production of red blood cells, and hemoglobin loading and unloading all occur in response to tissue oxygen needs. The cardiovascular system is comprised of the heart, the vasculature, and the blood. Dysfunction of any or all of these components may occur in patients with cardiovascular disease, disease that secondarily affects the cardiovascular system (e.g., hyperthyroidism), and in patients with healthy hearts that have suffered trauma or are in shock. Unfortunately, anesthesia may exacerbate this dysfunction and contribute to the demise of the patient.

Most physiologic (e.g., autoregulation) or pathologic (e.g., cardiac disease) changes ultimately affect cardiac output. Cardiac output (Fig. 13.1) is the amount of blood pumped by the left ventricle into the aorta each minute, and it is a product of HR and stroke volume (SV). SV is a product of preload, afterload, and myocardial contractility (inotropy). Most of the drugs associated with sedation or tranquilization and anesthesia cause some degree of

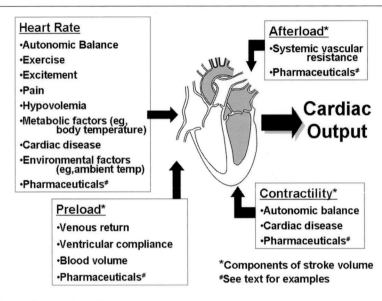

Heart Rate
- **Autonomic Balance**
- **Exercise**
- **Excitement**
- **Pain**
- **Hypovolemia**
- **Metabolic factors (eg, body temperature)**
- **Cardiac disease**
- **Environmental factors (eg, ambient temp)**
- **Pharmaceuticals#**

Preload*
- **Venous return**
- **Ventricular compliance**
- **Blood volume**
- **Pharmaceuticals#**

Afterload*
- **Systemic vascular resistance**
- **Pharmaceuticals#**

Cardiac Output

Contractility*
- **Autonomic balance**
- **Cardiac disease**
- **Pharmaceuticals#**

*Components of stroke volume
#See text for examples

Figure 13.1. Determinants of cardiac output.

dose-dependent cardiovascular depression, which may be manifest as changes in HR, SV, or both.

Profound bradycardia may cause a significant decrease in cardiac output if SV does not increase to compensate for the lower rate. Conversely, tachycardia (e.g., following anticholinergic administration) may be as hazardous as bradycardia, especially if the patient is suffering from cardiac dysfunction.

> Tachycardia causes increased cardiac work and decreases the time that the heart spends in diastole. Because ventricular filling and myocardial perfusion occur during diastole, tachycardia may result in a decrease of both cardiac output and oxygen delivery to the myocardium.

Preload, or cardiac filling (or venous return), is dictated by blood flow, blood volume, and venous capacitance. An ideal preload volume will fill the ventricle just enough to cause slight stretch of the myocardium, which will improve contractility and increase SV (because of Starling's law[1]). The volume of venous return is extremely important because (1) the heart can only eject the amount of blood that is returned to it, making cardiac output

highly dependent on preload, and (2) the heart must eject the amount of blood returned to it or congestion will occur. Excessive or even moderate vasodilation causes hypotension and may lead to "pooling" of the blood in the vasculature with minimal cardiac return and inadequate preload. Afterload, or resistance to ejection or systemic vascular resistance, is dictated primarily by vascular tone. The arterial tree must maintain some degree of tone in order to support flow of blood all the way from the aorta to the capillaries out in the tissues. However, excessive tone will increase the amount of cardiac work because the heart must work harder to eject blood into the constricted vessels than it works ejecting blood into dilated vessels. Excessive tone will cause a decrease in cardiac output. Slight vasodilation generally results in decreased afterload with subsequent increased cardiac output and decreased cardiac work. Drugs that affect preload and afterload include those drugs that cause vasodilation (e.g., acepromazine, inhalant anesthetic agents) and vasoconstriction (e.g., α_2-agonists). Myocardial contractility is impaired by most anesthetic drugs including propofol, thiopental, and the inhalant anesthetic agents. Clearly, a decrease in myocardial contractility will cause a decrease in cardiac output. Effects of anesthetic drugs on cardiovascular function are listed in Table 13.5.

Table 13.5. Cardiovascular effects of some commonly used anesthetic drugs.

Drug	Heart rate	Heart rhythm	Preload	Afterload	Inotropy	Cardiac output
Acepromazine	↑	—	↓	↓	— or ↓	↓ or ↑
Medetomidine	↓↓	+ or —	↑	↑	— or ↓	↓
Diazepam and midazolam	—	—	—	—	—	—
Opioids	— or ↓	—	— or ↓	—	— or ↓	— or ↓
Thiopental	↑	+ or —	↓	↓	↓	↓
Propofol	— or ↓	+ or —	↓	↓	↓	↓
Ketamine and tiletamine	↑	+ or —	↑	↑	↑	↑ or — or ↓
Etomidate	—	—	—	—	—	—
Isoflurane	↓	—	↓	↓	↓	↓
Sevoflurane	↓	—	↓	↓	↓	↓

↑, increased; ↓, decreased; —, no change; +, potentially arrhythmogenic.
Adapted from Muir (1998).

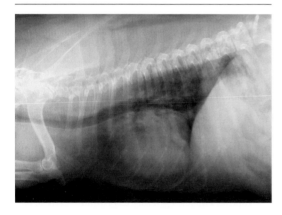

Figure 13.2. Thoracic radiograph of patient with mitral valve insufficiency and an enlarged heart. This patient is at increased anesthetic risk.

Patient Assessment

Patients with cardiac disease are at increased risk for morbidity and mortality. Thus, all elective procedures should be delayed until appropriate diagnostics and therapy are completed. In addition to the basic preoperative exam and laboratory analysis described in Table 13.3, patients with cardiac disease require thoracic radiographs (Fig. 13.2) and blood pressure measurement. The thorax should be carefully auscultated and evaluated for both cardiac (e.g., murmurs) and pulmonary (e.g., edema) abnormalities. Assessment of pulse quality and strength and thorough evaluation of the ECG tracing are required. Thoracic ultrasound or echocardiography is recommended in patients with moderate to advanced disease.

Patient Preparation for Anesthesia

Clearly, decreased circulating volume will lead to decreased tissue perfusion, especially in patients with inadequate pump function. Hydration should be critically assessed and preoperative fluids administered if necessary. Oxygen should be delivered through a face mask for 5 minutes prior to induction of anesthesia. However, if the patient does not readily accept the face mask, this technique should be abandoned as struggling and excitement are extremely hazardous for the patient with cardiac disease.

Preoperative treatment may also include the administration of inotropic agents (e.g., dopamine or dobutamine) and/or antiarrhythmic agents (see Chapter 11). Acid-base and electrolyte imbalances may affect cardiac function, and these should be corrected prior to anesthesia.

Because induction drugs may cause tremendous cardiovascular changes, the ECG and blood pressure monitor should be attached to the patient and in use prior to induction of anesthesia.

Monitoring and Support

Patients with cardiovascular disease are at high risk for anesthetic complications, and all of the monitoring techniques and tools described in Table 13.4 should be used. In particular, patients with cardiovascular disease require continuous monitoring of HR and rhythm (ECG) and ABP.

In patients with adequate pump function, anesthetic drug–induced cardiovascular depression may generally be overcome by counteracting the decrease in cardiac output with an increase in circulating volume. Crystalloids are appropriate in most patients, but colloids may be necessary in patients with low protein, and whole blood or packed cells are necessary in anemic patients. Half-strength saline is often recommended for short-term therapy in patients with severe disease. Patients with impaired pump function cannot handle a volume overload and should not be overhydrated. CVP measurement is ideal for monitoring appropriate fluid administration and should be considered in patients with cardiovascular disease. Cardiac output measurement would be ideal for assessment of cardiac function but is generally not practical in veterinary medicine, except in the research setting.

> Patients with impaired pump function cannot handle a volume overload and should not be overhydrated.

Arrhythmias and hypotension should be treated appropriately. The treatment of arrhythmias depends on the source and type of arrhythmia and is reviewed elsewhere (Cote and Ettinger 2005). Hypotension should be treated with judicious boluses of IV fluids and a CRI of a positive inotropic agent like dopamine or dobutamine. Drugs that increase systemic vascular resistance (SVR), like phenylephrine, are not generally the first-choice therapy for hypotension in patients with cardiovascular disease, but exceptions occur. Electrolytes should be assessed, especially if the patient is receiving diuretics.

Anesthesia

PREMEDICANTS

Pain is a tremendous stressor (see Table 13.2) and analgesia should be provided preemptively. Opioids are an excellent choice for patients with cardiovascular disease. Choice of opioid is based on intensity and duration of expected pain. Benzodiazepines may be added to the opioid if necessary. A low dose of acepromazine may cause a decrease in afterload and may be appropriate in some patients. α_2-Agonists cause profound cardiovascular effects and are not recommended. Anticholinergics are rarely used and should not be used indiscriminately. Vagally mediated bradycardia should be treated if the bradycardia is contributing to hypotension.

INDUCTION AGENTS

Ketamine and tiletamine are the exceptions to the rule that sedative-anesthetic agents cause cardiovascular depression. These agents promote increased HR and contractility, both of which contribute to increased cardiac output but also contribute to increased cardiac work. Ketamine causes direct myocardial depression in patients without a fully functional sympathetic nervous system, which often occurs in critically ill patients. Thus, ketamine is generally a good choice for patients with normal cardiovascular function or compensated dilatative cardiac disease, but is not the best choice for diseases with cardiac hypertrophy, tachycardia, or hypertension (e.g., hypertrophic cardiomyopathy or hyperthyroidism). Ketamine is almost always used with a benzodiazepine, which will blunt the response of the SNS.

Propofol causes moderate to profound cardiovascular depression that is equal to that caused by thiobarbiturates. However, the effects of propofol are short-lived and the hypotension may be alleviated by adequate fluid loading.

Etomidate causes virtually no cardiovascular changes (neither suppression nor stimulation) and is the best choice for patients with severe cardiovascular disease or instability. In the absence of etomidate or in patients with mild disease, a balanced technique using low dosages of appropriate premedicants (e.g., opioids and benzodiazepines) with low dosages of appropriate injectable induction agents (e.g., propofol or ketamine/diazepam) is perfectly acceptable.

As previously discussed, the stress and excitement associated with struggling during mask induction and the high dosages of anesthetic gas required for mask induction make this technique unacceptable in most critical patients, especially in those with cardiac disease.

Maintenance Drugs

All of the inhalant anesthetic agents cause mild to moderate cardiovascular depression that is dose dependent; thus, it is imperative to maintain the inhalant anesthetics at the lowest concentration possible. This is best accomplished by inclusion of appropriate analgesic agents in the anesthetic protocol. Boluses or CRIs of opioids, a CRI of lidocaine or ketamine, epidural analgesia, and local anesthetic blockade are all appropriate in most patients with cardiovascular disease. A CRI of fentanyl with minimal use of inhalants is an excellent anesthetic technique for patients with cardiovascular disease.

> Use analgesic agents as part of a balanced anesthetic protocol to decrease the need for high concentrations of injectable and inhalant anesthetic agents.

Anesthesia for Specific Cardiovascular Diseases

The most commonly encountered cardiovascular diseases in dogs and cats include mitral valve insufficiency, dilated cardiomyopathy, and hypertrophic cardiomyopathy. Anesthesia for patients with other conditions, including aortic and pulmonic stenosis and congenital cardiac defects, is reviewed elsewhere (McMurphy 1993).

MITRAL VALVE INSUFFICIENCY

Mitral valve insufficiency (MVI) is the most common cardiac disease in dogs. Small to medium-sized dogs older than 16 years are most commonly affected (Haggstrom et al. 2005). The incidence of disease is low in cats. MVI is usually caused by a progressive degeneration of the atrioventricular valves that allows regurgitant flow of blood into the left atrium during left ventricular systole. Valvular regurgitation causes further pathology including dilation of the left atrium and eccentric hypertrophy of the left ventricle. Depending on progression of the disease, patients may present with a wide variety of signs that range from a soft systolic murmur with no signs of cardiac disease to complications from end-stage heart failure. Stabilization will depend on stage of the disease at presentation and includes diuretics, angiotensin-converting enzyme (ACE) inhibitors, and positive inotropic agents (Haggstrom et al. 2005).

Considerations for Anesthesia

A slightly increased HR (NOT tachycardia) is advantageous in patients with MVI because increased ventricular filling and distention may occur during times of bradycardia. In a normal ventricle, increased distention is generally met with increased force of contraction. In patients with MVI, increased distention may cause additional enlargement of the atrioventricular orifice and further increase of the regurgitant volume. SVR or afterload should be kept to a minimum in order to promote more flow into the systemic vasculature with (hopefully) less flow through the mitral valve. Low-dose acepromazine may be used to decrease afterload but is not indicated if significant cardiovascular disease exists. After anesthesia, when additional cardiovascular depressing drugs will not be given, low-dose acepromazine may be appropriate.

Recommended Regimens

- Anticholinergic only if needed.
- Compromised patient: opioid ± benzodiazepines; etomidate or propofol; isoflurane or sevoflurane. May need to decrease vaporizer settings by using opioid/benzodiazepine CRI. If contractility is significantly decreased, may need to support with positive inotrope.
- In the absense of significant cardiovascular disease: opioid ± low-dose acepromazine; thiopental; isoflurane or sevoflurane.
- In all cases, be mindful of fluid overload: decrease fluids.

DILATED CARDIOMYOPATHY

Dilated cardiomyopathy (DCM) is the most common myocardial disease in the dog, with adult medium-size and large breed dogs most commonly affected. With the discovery and correction of taurine-deficient diets, DCM has become uncommon in cats. DCM is characterized by cardiac enlargement and impaired systolic function of one or both ven-tricles (most commonly, the left ventricle). The clinical presentation is highly variable depending on the stage of the disease. Stabilization includes ACE inhibitors and treatment for congestive heart failure (CHF), like diuretics (Meurs 2005).

A progressive decrease in myocardial contractil-ity with impaired systolic ventricular function occurs in patients with DCM. Measures of pump function such as ejection fraction, fractional short-ening, rate of ejection, and rate of ventricular pressure development are all reduced, whereas end-diastolic ventricular volume is increased (McMurphy 2003). Ventricular relaxation is also impaired. Contractility, SV, and cardiac output continue to decline as the disease progresses and mitral and tricuspid valve insufficiency, ventricular arrhythmias, and/or atrial fibrillation occurs in a significant number of patients.

Considerations for Anesthesia

Clearly, patients with advanced DCM are at high risk for anesthetic complications and stabilization prior to anesthesia is critical. A thorough evaluation of cardiac function, including echocardiography, is recommended. ABP should be measured and the ECG thoroughly evaluated. Arrhythmias and hypo-tension should be corrected prior to anesthesia. IV fluids should be administered, but fluid balance may be difficult to achieve in advanced stages of the disease. Adequate circulation and appropriate preload volume is critical because an adequate preload is necessary to compensate for decreased pump function. Yet, because pump function is poor, the heart cannot eject excess fluid load and overhy-dration should not occur. Also, poor pump function means that increased afterload may severely limit cardiac output.

Recommended Regimens

- Anticholinergic only if needed.
- Compromised patient: opioid ± benzodiazepines; etomidate or propofol; isoflurane or sevoflurane. May need to decrease vaporizer settings by using opioid/benzodiazepine CRI. If significant func-tion is decreased, may need to support with posi-tive inotrope.
- If atrial fibrillation: avoid drugs that speed atrio-ventricular nodal conduction such as dobutamine.

Use drugs that do not speed ventricular response rate (e.g., opioids).
- Be mindful of fluid overload: decrease fluids.

HYPERTROPHIC CARDIOMYOPATHY

Hypertrophic cardiomyopathy (HCM) is the most commonly diagnosed cardiac disease in cats but is uncommon in dogs. Although the frequency of the disease is equal in male and female cats, males tend to develop the disease at a younger age and develop a more severe form of the disease (Kittleson 2005). The exact cause of primary HCM is unknown, but it may be familial in some breeds. Conditions like hyperthyroidism, systemic arterial hypertension, and aortic stenosis may lead to a hypertrophied left ventricle and secondary HCM. Concentric hyper-trophy of the ventricles (primarily the left ventricle) with small ventricular chamber size is characteristic of HCM. Atrial enlargement may also occur. The cardiac chambers become stiff, resulting in increased pressure for any given volume during diastolic filling, and this will eventually lead to CHF with pulmonary edema and pleural effusion. Coronary circulation to the thickened myocardium decreases, predisposing the patient to myocardial ischemia. Thromboembolism may develop. Myocardial relax-ation is impaired but contractility usually is normal. The clinical presentation is highly variable depend-ing on the stage of the disease. Stabilization may include diuretics, ACE inhibitors, diltiazem, and β-adrenergic blockers (Kittleson 2005). The prog-nosis of severe HCM is poor, and sudden death is not uncommon.

Considerations for Anesthesia

In HCM, myocardial contractility or pump function is adequate. Decreased cardiac output and perfusion occur because of inadequate diastolic ventricular volume that occurs due to the small ventricular chamber size. Anesthetic goals include prevention of tachycardia, which will decrease ventricular filling time and increase cardiac work, and minimi-zation of afterload. Thus, drugs that increase rate or force of contraction (e.g., anticholinergics, ket-amine, dobutamine, dopamine) are not generally used. However, vasodilation (e.g., as occurs with acepromazine or propofol) may cause marked hypotension because of a limited ability of the heart to increase SV. Appropriate (but judicious) fluid therapy both before and during anesthetic drug administration is required for adequate preload. Hypotension that is unresponsive to fluid therapy may be treated with a CRI of phenylephrine, which will promote adequate filling but is not ideal in that the drug will also increase afterload. Clearly, treatment of hypotension in HCM patients is difficult.

Recommended Regimens
- Anticholinergic only if needed.
- Compromised patient: opioid ± benzodiazepines; etomidate or propofol; isoflurane or sevoflurane.
- Avoid drugs that speed HR or contractility: anticholinergics, inotropes, ketamine.
- Judicious fluids for adequate preload.
- Avoid hypotension and increased SVR.

ANESTHESIA FOR PATIENTS WITH RENAL DISEASE

Renal Physiology

The kidneys play a major role in the maintenance of homeostasis in the body through filtration of body fluids, reabsorption of filtered solutes, and excretion of the byproducts of cellular metabolism. Hormones secreted by the kidney are involved in regulation of systemic and renal hemodynamics; promotion of red blood cell production; and regulation of calcium, phosphorous, and bone metabolism. Interestingly, the kidneys, which comprise as little as 0.4% of total body mass, receive 20% to 25% of the cardiac output. This constitutes more blood per gram of tissue than any other organ in the body, including exercising muscle. Substantial renal blood flow (RBF) is imperative for normal renal function because the oxygen consumption per gram of tissue is higher in the kidney than in any other organ. This high oxygen requirement makes the kidney particularly susceptible to ischemic insults. If renal oxygen delivery is inadequate, whether due to decreased renal blood flow or decreased arterial oxygen content, the kidneys may experience an ischemic episode, which could cause renal damage or exacerbate existing renal disease. Thus, support of both the respiratory and the circulatory systems is extremely important in the anesthetized patient. Unfortunately, as previously mentioned, most anesthetic agents cause dose-dependent depression of these two systems.

All measures of urinary function, including RBF, glomerular filtration rate (GFR), urinary output, and electrolyte excretion, are temporarily decreased after general anesthesia. These changes are generally completely reversible and RBF and GFR return to normal within several hours of short, uncomplicated procedures. However, if surgery is extensive, or anesthesia is prolonged, the inability to concentrate urine may last for several days. Pain, hypoxia, hemorrhage, and other forms of stress also induce large decreases in both RBF and GFR. These changes are most likely mediated by changes in sympathetic activity and cardiovascular function. SNS stimulation selectively induces renal vascular constriction, which may markedly decrease the RBF, even when mean arterial pressure is within the range associated with renal autoregulation. Even in a patient with healthy kidneys, stress associated with anesthesia, surgery, and pain may be extremely detrimental to renal function.

Patient Assessment

In addition to the basic preoperative exam and laboratory analysis described in Table 13.3, patients with renal disease require preoperative assessment of urine output. Thorough evaluation of the serum chemistry analysis and urinalysis is critical. Blood urea nitrogen (BUN), creatinine, and electrolytes should be carefully evaluated. The PCV and TP should be measured because chronic renal disease may cause anemia and loss of protein in the urine.

The patient should also be evaluated for common side effects of chronic renal disease, including hypertension, vomiting, and muscle wasting.

Patient Preparation for Anesthesia

The anesthesia-induced impairment of renal function is mediated in part by depression of the cardiovascular system and subsequent decreased RBF. These effects may be minimized by adequate fluid loading with isotonic crystalloids prior to the induction of anesthesia. Ideally, the patient should be in a mild state of diuresis prior to anesthesia. Urine output should be measured and maintained between 0.5 and 2.0 ml/kg/hr. IV fluid administration should continue throughout the anesthetic period and into the postoperative period to promote diuresis. Because the kidneys may not be able to handle excess fluids, the patient should not be overhydrated.

> Urine output should be 0.5 to 2.0 ml/kg/hr.

The use of diuretics is somewhat controversial in the treatment of renal failure because the diuretics may not alter the course of the underlying disease. The management of patients with nonoliguric or high-output renal failure is less complicated and carries a better prognosis than patients with oliguric renal failure. Fluid overload (whether an absolute overdose of fluids or a relative overdose due to decreased urinary excretion of fluids) may lead to pulmonary edema, which requires diuretic therapy. It is not unreasonable and may be necessary to use diuretic therapy in patients with renal failure. Diuretic therapy should *always* be accompanied by evaluation of hydration status, serum electrolyte concentration, and acid-base balance.

Dopamine is often used to treat patients with renal dysfunction. Low dosages (1 to 3 μg/kg/min IV) of dopamine stimulate renal dopaminergic receptors and improve renal function by increasing the RBF, GFR, urine output, and sodium excretion and by decreasing renal vascular resistance. Dopamine at moderate dosages (5 to 10 μg/kg/min IV)

may also activate β-adrenergic receptors, which may increase cardiac output and cause dilation of renal arterial beds.

Patients with renal disease are often hypoproteinemic, anemic, hyperkalemic, and acidotic, and all of these derangements must be addressed prior to anesthesia. Hypoproteinemia leads to increased free fractions of highly protein-bound drugs and reduces oncotic pressure, making drug and fluid administration more challenging. Anemia, due to decreased erythropoietin production and bone marrow suppression, will lead to a decreased cardiac reserve and impaired renal oxygen delivery. Anemia is poorly tolerated in patients with renal disease, and a blood transfusion prior to anesthesia should be considered in patients with a hematocrit less than 18% to 20%. The effect of anemia on oxygen delivery to the cells is further described in Table 13.6.

Hyperkalemia leads to unstable cardiac electrical activity, and patients with serum potassium greater than 5.5 to 6.0 mEq/L should not be anesthetized. Calcium gluconate may be added to the fluids or calcium chloride may be administered as a bolus (0.1 mg/kg IV) if hyperkalemia is present. Acidosis

Table 13.6. Effects of decreased hemoglobin concentration and oxygen saturation on tissue oxygen delivery.

Cardiac output (Q) and arterial oxygen content (CaO_2) determine the amount of oxygen that is delivered to the tissues (Do_2). CaO_2 is a product of both the cardiovascular system (through red blood cells and hemoglobin) and the respiratory system (through adequate gas exchange). Both decreased red blood cell mass (or function) and impaired respiratory function can decrease the CaO_2, but the red cells have a greater impact. Normal CaO_2 is a component of the saturation of hemoglobin with oxygen (SaO_2); the amount of hemoglobin (Hb) present in the blood, a constant that dictates the amount of oxygen that can be bound by Hb (approximately 1.36–1.39 in horses); the amount of oxygen dissolved in the blood (PaO_2); and the solubility constant (0.003).

Thus, CaO_2 is determined by:

$$(SaO_2 \ [\%] \times [HB] \ g/dl \times 1.36) + (PaO_2 \times 0.003)$$

And the normal CaO_2 is:

$$(0.98 \times 15 \times 1.36) + (98 \times 0.003) = 20.28 \ ml/dl$$

CaO_2 subsequent to decreased available oxygen might be similar to:

$$(0.85 \times 15 \times 1.36) + (85 \times 0.003) = 17.60 \ ml/dl$$

And CaO_2 subsequent to decreased number of red blood cells might be similar to:

$$(0.98 \times 6 \times 1.36) + (98 \times 0.003) = 8.29 \ ml/dl$$

Thus, adequate oxygenation is important but a critical mass of circulating red cells is imperative for tissue oxygenation.

Table 13.7. Hyperkalemia: ECG changes and treatment.

Serum K$^+$ concentration (mEq/L)	ECG changes	Treatment and treatment effect
Normal (4.0–5.0)	None	None
Mild hyperkalemia (<6.0) 5.5	T waves become large and peaked	Administer 0.9% NaCl to dilute K$^+$, and increase GFR and urinary K$^+$ excretion (LRS will suffice because K$^+$ concentration is low in LRS).
Moderate hyperkalemia (6.0–8.0) 6.5 7.0	Decreased R amplitude; prolonged QRS and PR intervals; ST-segment depression Decreased P wave amplitude	1. Administer 0.9% saline. 2. Administer 1–2 mEq/L sodium bicarbonate slowly over 20 minutes (drives K$^+$ into cell in exchange for H$^+$). 3. Administer 1.5 g/kg dextrose (20%–50%) as an IV bolus (stimulates insulin release, which promotes movement of K$^+$ into cells). 4. Administer insulin (0.1–0.25 U/kg) with 20–50% dextrose (1–2 g/U insulin) IV (promotes movement of K$^+$ into the cell).
Severe hyperkalemia (>8.0) 8.5 10.0	No P waves Wide QRS wave; flutter, fibrillation, and/or asystole may occur	1. Continue treatment described for moderate hyperkalemia. 2. Administer 10% calcium gluconate (0.5–1.0 ml/kg IV) over 10–15 minutes (antagonist of cardiac effects of K$^+$) monitor ECG during calcium therapy.

will exacerbate hyperkalemia and will change the free fraction of many anesthetic drugs. An overview of the effects and treatment of hyperkalemia is presented in Table 13.7.

Patient Monitoring and Support

In addition to the monitoring tools and techniques described in Table 13.3, patients with renal disease require evaluation of urine production. Also, measurement of CVP is ideal but in its absence appropriate fluid therapy may be gauged by assessing urine output, periodically auscultating lungs for fluid build-up, and serially measuring the PCV and TP. Because of the numerous metabolic derangements associated with renal disease, electrolyte and acid-base status should be checked periodically throughout the anesthetic episode and into recovery. These derangements frequently lead to arrhythmias and cardiovascular compromise. The ECG should

be placed on the patient prior to induction and used throughout the induction, maintenance, and recovery periods. Frequent measurement of arterial blood pressure is also required. In fact, because of the high risk of ischemic insult to the kidney, both oxygenation and blood pressure monitoring are absolutely critical. Arterial blood gas monitoring is ideal, but the combination of a pulse oximeter and an ETCO$_2$ monitor will suffice and should be used in all patients. Blood pressure monitoring is vital and mean arterial pressure should be maintained at 70 to 80 mm Hg or higher because this is the presumed lower limit of renal blood flow autoregulation. The exact mechanisms of autoregulation are not known, but what is known is that the kidney is able to regulate its own blood flow by altering resistance in the renal afferent arterioles within a mean arterial pressure range of 70 to 140 mm Hg (some report the range as 80 to 180 mm Hg), thus allowing the kidney to protect the glomerular capillaries during periods of hypertension and preserve renal function during periods of hypotension. Appropriate fluid therapy and a dopamine CRI should be used to treat hypotension.

> Mean arterial pressure should be maintained at or above 70 to 80 mm Hg because this is the lower limit at which renal autoregulation of blood flow may occur.

Patients with chronic renal disease are often debilitated and underweight, and loss of muscle mass makes the patient more prone to pressure injury, peripheral nerve damage, and hypothermia. The patient should be placed carefully on a well-padded operating table and actively warmed.

Anesthesia

Anesthetic agents that preserve cardiovascular function and that are eliminated by routes other than the urine are ideal. Most drugs are weak electrolytes and are lipid soluble in the unionized state and are, therefore, extensively reabsorbed by renal tubules. Fortunately, most drugs are not dependent on renal excretion for termination of their action, depending instead on redistribution and metabolism for this effect. After biotransformation, these drugs are generally inactive and are excreted in the urine as polar, water-soluble forms of the parent compound. The majority of drugs with prominent central and peripheral nervous system activity fall into this category, including most opioids, barbiturates, phenothiazines, benzodiazepines, and local anesthetic agents. Ketamine falls into this category in humans and dogs but is excreted primarily unchanged in the urine of cats.

A reduced dosage of drugs is critical because of several factors: hypoproteinemia leads to increased free fractions of highly protein-bound drugs, muscle wasting leads to decreased tissue for redistribution of drugs, and impaired renal clearance will lead to recirculation and prolonged duration of activity of renally cleared drugs.

PREMEDICATION

Stress and pain should be avoided in all patients and avoidance is even more critical in patients with renal disease, as both stress and pain cause increased sympathetic tone with subsequent vasoconstriction and decreased renal blood flow. Opioid agonists (e.g., oxymorphone, morphine), agonist-antagonists (e.g., butorphanol), and partial agonists (buprenorphine) cause minimal depression of the cardiovascular system when used in low doses. These drugs provide analgesia, are reversible, and are generally highly metabolized by the liver with only a small portion excreted unchanged by the kidneys. Most opioids are only slightly (morphine, 35%) to moderately (fentanyl, 84%) protein bound. Opioid free fraction and activity are only slightly to moderately changed by hypoproteinemia. Pain is a stressor that may cause a decrease in RBF and GFR. Thus, opioid-induced analgesia is an extremely valuable means of alleviating or eliminating pain-induced renal damage.

> Pain is detrimental in *all* patients but may be even more detrimental in those with renal disease. Pain causes catecholamine release with subsequent vasoconstriction and decreased renal blood flow, which may exacerbate renal dysfunction.

Benzodiazepines (e.g., diazepam, midazolam) cause minimal cardiovascular depression and, thus, minimal alteration of renal blood flow. Although benzodiazepines are extensively metabolized in the liver, some benzodiazepines (e.g., diazepam) depend on renal elimination of active metabolites. Prolonged effects could occur if urinary excretion of the active metabolites is impaired. Fortunately, the depressant effects of benzodiazepines are minimal and prolonged activity is generally not detrimental. Also, benzodiazepines and many of their metabolites may be reversed with the drug flumazenil.

Acepromazine causes α-adrenergic blockade with subsequent vasodilation. A low dose of acepromazine might be an appropriate tranquilizer choice in a patient with renal disease that was fluid loaded and the α-blockade may protect the renal cortex from the vasoconstriction that occurs secondary to sympathetic stimulation and endogenous catecholamine release. α_2-Agonists do promote diuresis but also increase SVR and decrease cardiac output and are not recommended.

Approximately 20% to 50% of a dose of atropine is recovered unchanged in the urine or in the form of active metabolites. The same is true for quaternary ammonium compounds like glycopyrrolate. There is a potential for accumulation of these drugs in patients with renal failure. However, a single dose will not generally cause clinical difficulties and bradycardia should be treated with an anticholinergic if the HR is low enough to affect blood pressure. Glycopyrrolate may be a better choice because vomiting is common in these patients and glycopyrrolate decreases gastric fluid volume and acidity.

INDUCTION AGENTS

Because patients with renal disease are often nauseated, vomiting or regurgitation with subsequent aspiration may occur during induction. Therefore, induction and intubation should occur rapidly to prevent aspiration and ensure a patent airway. Because induction of anesthesia using inhalant anesthetic agents delivered by a mask occurs relatively slowly, this technique is not recommended for induction in patients in which rapid intubation is necessary. As previously discussed, the stress and excitement associated with struggling during mask induction and the high dosages of anesthetic gas required for mask induction make this technique unacceptable in most critical patients, especially in those with renal disease.

Propofol, because of its multiple routes of elimination, may be the best choice for induction of patients with renal disease. In humans, less than 0.3% (Stoelting 1999) of propofol is excreted unchanged in the urine and renal dysfunction does not influence the clearance of propofol. Other than phenobarbital, most barbiturates depend almost exclusively on redistribution to tissues and hepatic metabolism for termination of anesthetic action and thus are not affected by renal disease. Barbiturates are moderately protein bound (e.g., 75% to 85% of thiopental is bound to albumin). Thiopental is a weak acid with its pK_a in the physiologic range. Acidosis, which is common in patients with renal disease, will result in more unionized, nonbound, active thiopental. If used in patients with renal disease, barbiturate dosages should be greatly reduced and repeat boluses should be avoided. Barbiturates cause mild to moderate myocardial depression with a subsequent decrease in cardiac output.

Ketamine and tiletamine produce stimulation of the SNS leading to increased cardiac output and arterial blood pressure. Although this should lead to increased renal perfusion, perfusion may actually decrease due to catecholamine-induced increases in renal vascular resistance. Ketamine is eliminated in the urine as the parent compound in cats and as an active metabolite in other species. Ketamine may not be the best choice in patients with renal disease.

MAINTENANCE DRUGS

All inhaled anesthetics are biotransformed to some extent and the nonvolatile products of metabolism are eliminated almost entirely by the kidney. Termination of the CNS effects of inhaled anesthetics is dependent on pulmonary excretion so that impaired kidney function will not alter the response to these agents. Inhalant anesthetics are generally the best choice for maintenance of anesthesia in patients with renal disease. Fluoride concentrations after isoflurane, halothane, and sevoflurane are all well below the nephrotoxic threshold of 50 μmol/L. Although sevoflurane may produce a potentially nephrotoxic compound (Compound A) when combined with carbon dioxide absorbents, this phenomenon does not appear to be a common clinical problem and the inhalant has been used without adverse effects in numerous patients with renal disease.

Renal blood flow is best preserved with light planes of anesthesia, and inhalant anesthetic concentrations should absolutely be maintained as low as possible. This is best accomplished by inclusion of appropriate analgesic agents in the anesthetic protocol. Boluses or CRIs of opioids, epidural analgesia, and local anesthetic blockade are all appropriate in most patients with renal disease.

Stress, including the stress caused by pain, should be avoided in the recovery period. The patient should be allowed to recover quietly (tranquilize if necessary) and should be adequately analgesed.

Anesthesia for Patients With Urethral Obstruction

Urethral obstruction occurs most commonly in male cats, and patients may present in a wide variety of clinical conditions. If owners are astute, the patient may present with acute blockage and severe pain but minimal medical compromise. As the disease progresses, patients become hyperkalemic, azotemic, acidotic, hyponatremic, hypocalcemic, and hyperglycemic. Hypertension and arrhythmias occur early, with hypotension and even shock occurring as the disease progresses. Renal compromise may occur with prolonged block, and a ruptured bladder is not uncommon. Patients who are obstructed generally require emergency anesthesia and only minimal stabilization is possible. Hyperkalemia is generally the main concern and treatment prior to anesthesia is necessary (see Table 13.7). Careful cystocentesis may also be necessary.

Healthy but painful cats may tolerate almost any anesthetic protocol but the protocol should include analgesia. Analgesia may help to relieve urethral spasm, which will make the patient more tolerant of catheter placement and may make the blockage easier to dislodge. Buprenorphine is a good choice in cats. As cats become progressively compromised, anesthesia becomes more dangerous and no anesthetic protocol is ideal. Propofol provides rapid induction and is readily cleared even in patients with renal compromise. Propofol also causes muscle relaxation, which may be beneficial in relief of urethral spasm. However, propofol causes fairly profound cardiovascular depression, which may not be well tolerated in patients that are extremely compromised. Ketamine may provide cardiovascular support in early phases of the disease but contribute to cardiac dysfunction in later phases as the SNS becomes unable to respond. Ketamine is cleared by the urine in cats and clearance may be prolonged in patients with secondary renal compromise. As with propofol, ketamine is appropriate (with diazepam) in early stages of the disease but may not be well tolerated in patients that are extremely compromised. A low dose of either drug, following appropriate dosages of analgesics, is generally acceptable.

ANESTHESIA FOR PATIENTS WITH HEPATIC DISEASE

Hepatic Physiology

The liver has many functions, including synthesis of proteins (e.g., albumin and clotting factors) and detoxification of exogenous (e.g., drugs) and endogenous (e.g., ammonia) substances. Also, the liver plays an important role in regulation of glucose concentrations and is a major site for glycogen storage. The liver is the exclusive site of albumin synthesis, and hepatocytes synthesize all of the coagulation factors (except factor VIII) as well as inhibitors of coagulation and fibrinolysis (antithrombin III, antiplasmin) and fibrinolytic proteins (plasminogen). The liver is also the site of vitamin K–dependent activation of factors II, VII, IX, and X and protein C. Some of the clinical consequences of decreased hepatic protein synthesis that are important to the anesthetist include decreased plasma oncotic pressure due to hypoalbuminemia, bleeding tendencies secondary to coagulation protein deficiencies, and the development of hepatic encephalopathy due to ammonia retention.

The liver has a tremendous reserve, and the appearance of clinical signs of hepatic disease (e.g., icterus, hypoglycemia, bleeding tendencies, hepatic encephalopathy, and/or ascites) generally occur late in the disease process, when hepatic reserves are exhausted. Early clinical signs of hepatic disease (e.g., anorexia, polyuria [pu]/polydypsia [pd], vomiting, and lethargy) are very nonspecific and may not be attributed to hepatic disease. Thus, hepatic disease may not be suspected without adequate preanesthesia testing.

All anesthetic protocols have been shown to have the potential to cause transient abnormalities in liver function tests in humans, even in those without preexisting liver disease, and the function test abnormalities were highest in patients following intra-abdominal surgery (Stoelting 1999). Both patients with healthy and those with compromised livers may be at risk for some degree of liver dysfunction following anesthesia and surgery, especially following intra-abdominal procedures.

Patient Assessment

In addition to the basic preoperative exam and laboratory analysis described in Table 13.3, patients with hepatic disease require preoperative assessment of clotting function. Hypoglycemia and hypoalbuminemia occur fairly commonly in patients with liver disease, and blood glucose and albumin concentrations must be critically evaluated. If liver function is questionable, bile acid assays and liver biopsies should be considered.

Serum enzymes commonly associated with hepatic disease include the leakage enzymes (ALT and SDH) associated with hepatocellular disease and the enzymes associated with cholestatic disease

(ALP and GGT). These enzymes are consistently increased after hepatobiliary injury. However, these enzymes have high sensitivity but low specificity for detection of true hepatic disease. Because the liver has an extensive role in metabolism and has an extremely high blood flow, it is very sensitive to secondary injury. Thus, liver enzymes may be elevated without the presence of significant hepatic disease. Conversely, quite severe hepatopathies may have only minimal enzyme abnormalities because replacement of hepatocytes by fibrosis, prolonged enzyme leakage, or both results in depletion of total liver enzyme content (Webster 2005). Commonly measured liver enzymes may not accurately predict the degree of hepatic dysfunction. None of the enzymes previously mentioned assess liver function. Screening tests of hepatic function (e.g., serum concentrations of albumin, protein, bilirubin, and glucose) are required in order to determine whether liver disease is indeed present. Paired preprandial and postprandial determinations of serum bile acids are the preferred methods for assessment of hepatobiliary function in both dogs and cats. Quantification of bile acids is sensitive and specific for liver function because the synthesis, secretion, extraction from portal blood, and re-excretion of bile acids all depend on adequate liver function. Elevated concentrations of bile acids may be observed with portosystemic shunts, liver failure, and cholestasis. A liver biopsy is generally required to differentiate between these diseases.

Because the liver synthesizes most clotting factors, evaluation of coagulation is indicated. Several tests are available, including prothrombin time (PT; for evaluation of extrinsic and common pathways), activated partial thromboplastin time (aPTT), and activated coagulation time (ACT; for evaluation of intrinsic or common pathways). The clotting cascade and assessment of hemostasis is covered elsewhere (Carr 2005).

Patient Preparation for Anesthesia

Appropriate patient stabilization is critical, as evidenced from data in human patients with portal hypertension in which mortality associated with anesthesia was 50% when preoperative serum albumin concentrations were lower than 3 g/dl, serum bilirubin levels were greater than 3 mg/dl, and ascites and hepatic encephalopathy were present. However, mortality significantly decreased (to 10%) when preoperative serum albumin levels were 3 to 3.5 g/dl, serum bilirubin was 2 to 3 mg/dl, prothrombin time was normal, and hepatic encephalopathy was absent (Roizen 2000).

Blood glucose concentrations should be measured prior to, during, and following anesthesia and dextrose-containing fluids should be administered in hypoglycemic patients. If abnormalities of coagulation are present, vitamin K, plasma (fresh or frozen), or fresh whole blood may be indicated prior to anesthesia and surgery.

In the patient with normal albumin concentration, isotonic fluids should be administered prior to surgery to insure adequate circulating volume and hepatic blood flow. Although lactated Ringer's solution is a balanced electrolyte solution that is appropriate for most patients, patients with hepatic disease may not be able to metabolize lactate, so a lactate-free solution is recommended (e.g., normal saline, Normosol-R). Dextrose containing solutions are necessary in hypoglycemic patients.

Ascites is common in patients with moderate to severe liver disease. Causes of ascites include hypoalbuminemia, portal hypertension, inflammation, or hepatic neoplasia. Fluid in the abdomen exerts pressure on the diaphragm in the recumbent or anesthetized patient, and this pressure may inhibit diaphragmatic movement and impair ventilation. A portion of the ascitic fluid may need to be removed prior to anesthesia. Rapid removal of large volumes of abdominal fluid is extremely dangerous, as hemodynamic instability may occur when fluid shifts from the vascular space to the abdominal cavity to replace the abdominal fluid that has been removed. The fluid should be removed slowly and IV fluids should be administered as the fluid is removed to prevent cardiovascular collapse.

> A large volume of ascitic fluid may impair diaphragmatic movement and ventilation, requiring partial removal of the fluid prior to anesthesia. In order to prevent circulatory collapse, the fluid must be withdrawn slowly and with concurrent administration of IV fluids.

Finally, seizures may occur in patients with hepatic encephalopathy, and these seizures should be controlled prior to anesthesia. Diazepam may be an acceptable choice for seizure control.[2]

Patient Monitoring and Support

In addition to the monitoring tools and techniques described in Table 13.4, patients with hepatic disease generally require serial measurement of blood glucose and albumin and may require serial evaluation of clotting function. To avoid hepatic ischemia, blood pressure and arterial oxygenation must be critically evaluated and supported.

IV fluids should be continued throughout the intraoperative and postoperative periods. Isotonic crystalloids are generally a good choice, but colloids or plasma may be used in hypoalbuminemic patients. Because synthetic colloids may affect hemostasis, plasma may be a better choice in some patients. A brief review of the administration of fluids is included at the beginning of this chapter, and a more in-depth review is available in Chapter 11.

Because hypothermia causes impaired coagulation and slowed drug metabolism, the effects of hepatic disease may be compounded in hypothermic patients. Active warming should begin during the anesthetic period and continue well in to recovery.

Anesthesia

Almost all drugs used to provide sedation, anesthesia, and analgesia are metabolized to some extent by the liver. Drugs with minimal hepatic metabolism and reversible drugs should be used when possible.

> Almost all anesthetic and sedative drugs are metabolized, to some extent, by the liver.

PREMEDICANTS

Surgical stimulation and pain cause decreases in hepatic blood flow independent of the anesthetic drug administered. The greatest decreases in hepatic blood flow occur during intraabdominal procedures, presumably due to mechanical interference of blood flow produced by retraction in the operative area, as well as to the release of vasoconstricting substances such as catecholamines (Stoelting 1999). Because pain and stress also cause the release of catecholamines, it is likely that they compound the decrease in hepatic blood flow. Low-dose opioids

are appropriate for patients with hepatic disease, but there are some cautions associated with opioid use. Opioids are generally highly metabolized by the liver, and the effects of a standard dose may be exaggerated or prolonged. The effects of opioids may be reversed with opioid antagonists like naloxone, if necessary. Opioids may cause an increase in intrabiliary pressure by increasing biliary sphincter tone, but this appears to be of much greater significance in humans than it is in dogs. Endogenous opioids (endorphins, enkaphalins) have been associated with hepatic encephalopathy (HE) and opioids should perhaps be avoided in patients with HE.

Benzodiazepines are also appropriate sedatives in patients with hepatic disease; however, benzodiazepines require hepatic metabolism for termination of activity and the duration of action may be prolonged. Benzodiazepines are highly (96% to 98%) protein bound and may have exaggerated effects in hypoproteinemic patients. There is some evidence that patients with hepatic disease may also have increased CNS sensitivity to the benzodiazepines due to the presence of endogenous benzodiazepine receptor ligands (EBRLs), which are compounds derived from the diet that interact with the same CNS receptors as diazepam and midazolam (Dodam 2003). The liver normally removes EBRLs from the portal blood, but increased concentrations of EBRLs have been found in the blood of dogs with portosystemic shunt. Increased concentrations of EBRLs may contribute to HE. In cats, diazepam has been associated with severe, fatal hepatocellular necrosis (Center et al. 1996; Hughes et al. 1996). However, this condition is extremely rare and occurred after multiple doses of oral diazepam. A single dose of zolazepam (in Telazol) has also been associated with hepatocellular necrosis (Hughes et al. 1996). Despite the precautions in both species, benzodiazepines are appropriate for most patients with hepatic disease but they should be used at low dosages and prolonged and exaggerated effects should be expected. Benzodiazepines may need to be avoided in patients with HE.

Acepromazine is extensively metabolized by the liver, may induce hypotension, and may potentiate seizures. Thus, acepromazine is not recommended in patients with hepatic disease. α_2-Agonists are attractive because the drug effects are reversible. However, α_2-agonists may cause decreased hepatic blood flow secondary to vasoconstriction and are probably best avoided.

INDUCTION DRUGS

Thiopental (in dogs and cats) and ketamine (in dogs) are highly hepatically metabolized and may have a prolonged duration of action in patients with hepatic disease. Ketamine and tiletamine are associated with seizure activity and should not be used in patients with HE. Although propofol is cleared in part by hepatic metabolism, clearance also occurs through a variety of other processes and organs, including the kidneys and the lung. The duration of action of propofol is not prolonged in patients with hepatic disease. Furthermore, propofol has also been used to control refractory status epilepticus in cats and dogs and may be used in patients with HE. Etomidate undergoes extensive redistribution to the tissues for initial termination of activity, followed by rapid and complete hydrolysis in the liver. Hepatic dysfunction does not appear to affect the clearance of etomidate, making it a reasonable choice for induction in patients with hepatic disease.

MAINTENANCE AGENTS

The liver is highly perfused, receiving approximately 30% of the total cardiac output through two sources (hepatic artery and portal vein). The liver may contain up to 10% of the total blood volume at any given time and is an important source of additional blood during acute hemorrhage. Oxygenated blood is delivered through the hepatic artery (roughly 25% of the flow with 45% to 50% of the total oxygen) and slightly deoxygenated blood is delivered through the portal vein (roughly 75% of the flow but only 50% to 55% of the total oxygen). All inhalant anesthetic agents cause a decrease of blood flow through the portal vein. With isoflurane, sevoflurane, and desflurane, hepatic artery flow increases and overall flow is stable. With halothane, hepatic artery flow does not increase and total flow decreases, thus decreasing hepatic oxygen delivery. Hypoxia of the hepatocytes is considered to be a major contributor to the multifactorial etiology of postoperative hepatic dysfunction; thus, decreased oxygen delivery may be extremely detrimental. Furthermore, fulminant hepatic necrosis following halothane administration has been reported in humans, and it appears that decreased hepatic

oxygen delivery may play a role in its genesis (although the exact mechanism is unknown). This condition has not been described in small animal veterinary patients. Isoflurane or sevoflurane should be used to maintain anesthesia because recovery from these drugs depends on exhalation of active drug and not on hepatic metabolism. Halothane is more extensively metabolized than the other inhalant anesthetic agents and is not ideal.

OTHER ANESTHESIA-RELATED DRUGS

Local anesthetic agents that are of the ester class (procaine, tetracaine) are metabolized by plasma cholinesterases produced by the liver, whereas those from the amide class (lidocaine, mepivacaine, bupivacaine) are directly metabolized by the liver. Duration of action of local anesthetics may be prolonged, but this is unlikely to be recognized clinically. Recommended protocol: low dose opioids; propofol or etomidate; isoflurane or sevoflurane.

Anesthesia for Patients With Portosystemic Shunt

All of the assessment, preparation, monitoring, support, and anesthetic information just presented is appropriate for the patient with portosystemic shunt. Patients are usually young and small, so hypoglycemia and hypothermia are common. Preoxygenation is recommended, and active warming is required. Recommended protocol: opioids (e.g., butorphanol, buprenorphine); propofol; isoflurane or sevoflurane. Maximize circulating volume; check clotting.

Anesthesia for Patients With Hepatic Lipidosis

All of the assessment, preparation, monitoring, support, and anesthetic information just presented is appropriate for the patient with hepatic lipidosis. Hepatic lipidosis occurs in cats that are systemically ill, so overall health status and the effects of concurrent disease (e.g., diabetes) (Fig. 13.3) must be evaluated. Cats commonly become hypothermic during anesthesia. Preoxygenation is recommended and active warming is required. Recommended protocol: opioids (e.g., buprenorphine); propofol; isoflurane or sevoflurane.

ANESTHESIA FOR PATIENTS WITH ENDOCRINE DISEASE

In all patients, including those without preexisting disease, the stress of anesthesia and surgery

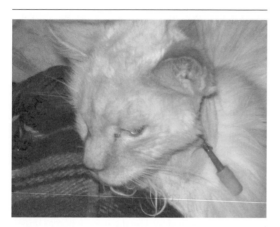

Figure 13.3. Cat with diabetes mellitus and hepatic lipidosis who was anesthetized for placement of a feeding tube. Concurrent illnesses are common in compromised patients and can complicate the physiologic effects of anesthesia. Furthermore, almost all anesthetic agents are metabolized to some extent by the liver and hepatic dysfunction may cause exaggerated or prolonged effects of anesthetic drugs. This patient recovered extremely slowly from anesthesia.

produces changes in the endocrine system that is characterized by increased secretion of pituitary hormones and activation of the SNS. Cortisol, vasopressin, and glucagon are among the hormones secreted during stress, and increased catabolism is the overall metabolic effect. These stress-related changes may further exacerbate the pathology of endocrine disease, and it is important to understand the pathophysiology of the various diseases in order to formulate a logical and safe anesthetic plan. Often, appropriate patient management is more critical than actual anesthetic drug selection. Endocrine disorders encountered in veterinary patients include disorders of the pancreas (diabetes mellitus and insulinoma), disorders of the thyroid gland (hyperthyroidism and hypothyroidism), and disorders of the adrenal gland (hyperadrenocorticism, hypoadrenocorticism, and pheochromocytoma).

> Stress and pain should be minimized in patients with endocrine disease. Even in healthy patients, anesthesia, surgery, and pain may cause a profound endocrine and metabolic response.

Diabetes Mellitus

PATHOPHYSIOLOGY

Insulin, excreted by the beta cells in the islets of Langerhans in the pancreas, is essential for normal cell and tissue function. Insulin deficiency, as occurs with diabetes mellitus, results in a variety of disorders that must be considered in the patient presented for anesthesia. Diabetes mellitus is one of the most common endocrine disorders in dogs and cats and the most common endocrine disorder in humans. In human medicine, diabetes mellitus is generally classified as "type 1" (failure of endogenous insulin production) or "type 2" (insulin resistance), but in veterinary medicine, most clinicians agree that classification of diabetes as insulin-dependent diabetes mellitus (IDDM) or non–insulin-dependent diabetes mellitus (NIDDM) is more useful. The most common type of diabetes in dogs and cats is IDDM. NIDDM occurs in cats but is rare in dogs (Nelson 2005). The overall rate of diabetes appears to occur with similar frequency in dogs and cats, with the reported rate varying from 1 : 100 to 1 : 500 (Nelson 2005).

With insulin deficiency, transportation of glucose across cell membranes is decreased, resulting in hyperglycemia and osmotic diuresis; protein from skeletal muscle is used to make glucose, resulting in muscle wasting; fatty acids are used by the insulin-deficient liver to produce ketones for energy, resulting in ketoacidosis; and intracellular potassium ions are exchanged for extracellular hydrogen ions to compensate for the acidosis, resulting in serum hyperkalemia (but whole body hypokalemia may occur). Prolonged hyperglycemia and ketonemia may lead to metabolic acidosis, dehydration, circulatory collapse, renal failure, and even to coma and/or death (Nelson 2005). Interestingly, hepatic lipolysis is blocked with even low concentrations of insulin; thus, ketone bodies are not always produced in the insulin-deficient patient.

PATIENT ASSESSMENT

All of the components of the basic preoperative exam and laboratory analysis described in Table 13.3 should be used. Careful assessment of serum chemistry (including blood glucose, acid-base status, electrolytes) and the urinalysis (including urine specific gravity, glycosuria, proteinuria, and ketonuria) is required. Serum fructosamine may be measured, and high concentrations occur with sustained hyperglycemia.

Serial blood glucose monitoring is required in diabetic patients but, unfortunately, portable blood glucose monitors, point-of-care analyzers, and reagent test strips that are commonly used in veterinary medicine are not always accurate (Cohn et al. 2000). In a study comparing monitors (Cohn et al. 2000), one portable blood glucose monitor was off by as much as 15% and the point-of-care unit was the most accurate.

PATIENT PREPARATION FOR ANESTHESIA

Diabetic patients scheduled for elective procedures should be stabilized and regulated prior to anesthesia with appropriate insulin therapy and blood glucose monitoring. Stabilization of diabetic patients presented for emergency surgery may include administration of insulin as a bolus or a CRI. Dosages and techniques for emergency treatment are reviewed elsewhere (Robertson 2003).

Management goals include minimal disruption of food intake with return to eating as soon as possible postoperatively. The surgical procedure should be scheduled early in the morning, allowing a full day of hospitalization for monitoring the patient. One-half of the patient's normal dose of insulin should be administered on the morning of surgery with a few bites of easily digested food. The patient may be treated as a "full stomach" patient for intubation (see Chapter 16).

Stress hormones have an "anti-insulin" effect that leads to alterations in glucose homeostasis and hyperglycemia; thus, the stress response to surgery should be minimized. Appropriate preoperative sedatives and perioperative analgesic agents should be used. Also, all incisions, wounds, and catheter sites should be scrubbed and kept extremely clean because diabetic patients are at increased risk for infections and impaired wound healing. The mechanism of the increased risk is not completely understood, but elevated blood glucose levels may be associated with decreased white blood cell function and chemotaxis.

SUPPORT AND MONITORING

In addition to the monitoring tools and techniques described in Table 13.4, patients with diabetes mellitus require serial monitoring of blood glucose, which should be measured preoperatively, post induction, and at least once per hour intraoperatively and postoperatively. Ideally, the blood glucose should be maintained between 150 and 250 mg/dl.

> To avoid erroneous glucose values, use two catheters in a diabetic patient: one catheter for administration of dextrose containing fluids and the other catheter for blood collection for glucose monitoring.

Fluid therapy will depend on the serum concentrations of glucose, but 5% dextrose in a balanced electrolyte solution is often administered intraoperatively to prevent hypoglycemia. Serial blood glucose measurements with appropriate fluid therapy should be continued until the patient is completely recovered from anesthesia. Acute hypoglycemia is more critical than acute hyperglycemia. Unfortunately, the common signs of hypoglycemia (e.g., salivation, vomiting, tremors, weakness, seizures, and collapse) may be masked under anesthesia and the patient must be carefully monitored for other changes associated with hypoglycemic stress (e.g., tachycardia and hypertension).

> The signs of hypoglycemia may be masked in the anesthetized patient. Acute tachycardia and hypertension with no concurrent change in surgical stimulus provide a clue that the patient may be hypoglycemic and blood glucose concentrations should be analyzed immediately.

ANESTHESIA

Even in well-regulated patients, some decompensation will occur; thus, the goal of anesthesia is to recover the patient quickly and as stress free as possible and to allow the patient to resume a normal feeding schedule. With anesthesia of diabetic patients, the actual choice of anesthetic drugs is not as critical as patient support. However, drugs that are reversible (e.g., opioids) and drugs that are rapidly cleared from the body (e.g., propofol) should be considered. Because a stress-free recovery is optimal, analgesia should be addressed both intraoperatively and throughout the anesthetic period. Opioids should be included in the protocol, and buprenorphine, because of its long duration of action and minimal sedative properties is often a good choice for mild to moderate pain, especially in cats. Local anesthetic agents are ideal additions to the anesthetic protocol and should be used whenever possible (e.g., use oral blocks for dental extractions). NSAIDs may be used in patients that do not have concurrent renal compromise.

Acepromazine generally provides prolonged sedation that is not optimal. α_2-Agonists cause transient hyperglycemia, and although they are reversible and reversal provides a rapid recovery, this class of drugs should probably be avoided in diabetic patients.

Propofol is cleared quickly and does not cause residual sedation or "hangover" and is a good choice for diabetic patients. Ketamine/valium, thiopental, and etomidate are all acceptable, and choice should be based on concurrent disease processes and personal preference. Recovery from isoflurane and sevoflurane is rapid and either inhalant may be used in diabetic patients.

Support throughout recovery is critical and should include continued measurement of blood glucose concentrations, evaluation and treatment of pain, and active rewarming of the patient.

> The goal of anesthetic management for diabetic patients is to achieve a rapid, but stress free, recovery and to resume a normal feeding schedule as soon as possible.

Insulinoma

Insulin-secreting tumors (or beta cell tumors) are rare but have occurred in middle-aged and older dogs. Profound hypoglycemia should be considered an emergency and treatment should be instituted quickly in order to prevent brain damage. Acute hypoglycemia is treated with an IV bolus (1 ml/kg) of 50% dextrose. However, stabilization of patients with insulinoma may be difficult because necessary therapy (IV administration of dextrose) may cause stimulation of the tumor, which leads to further insulin release and worsening of the hypoglycemia. The goal of stabilization is to alleviate clinical signs but not to establish normal blood glucose concen-

trations. A more detailed description of stabilization is found elsewhere (Robertson 2003).

Patient Assessment, Preparation, Monitoring, and Support and Anesthesia

In addition to the basic preoperative exam and laboratory analysis described in Table 13.3, patients with insulinoma require serial blood glucose monitoring every 15 to 30 minutes. Hypoglycemia must be avoided or treated quickly. Generally, preoperative fasting is not recommended, but a small meal of easily digested food should be fed 2 to 3 hours preoperatively (Robertson 2003). Dextrose-containing fluids should be administered throughout the procedure and well into recovery. Full stabilization following tumor removal may take several days of medical therapy.

Anesthetic protocols should be chosen based on the fact that tumor removal requires major abdominal surgery. Opioids should be administered preoperatively, and acepromazine or benzodiazepines may be added, if necessary. Propofol, thiopental, and etomidate all provide cerebral protection during times of hypoglycemia and would all be appropriate for induction. Low dosages of isoflurane or sevoflurane should be used for maintenance. Readdress analgesia in recovery and continue analgesia for at least 3 to 5 days following all major surgeries.

THYROID DISEASE

Hypothyroidism

Pathophysiology, Patient Assessment, and Preparation for Anesthesia

Hypothyroidism, or decreased thyroid production of thyroxine (T_4) and triiodothyronine (T_3), is common in dogs but rare in cats. Clinical signs of hypothyroidism occur secondary to a decrease in metabolic rate. Clinical signs that affect anesthesia include mild to moderate obesity (which may affect ventilation due to abdominal fat weighing against the diaphragm), anemia, arrhythmias (primarily bradycardia), and hypothermia. L-Thyroxine therapy is used to treat hypothyroidism and, when possible, the patient should be normalized prior to surgery. However, hypothyroidism is generally not life threatening and anesthesia may proceed without stabilization, if necessary.

PATIENT SUPPORT AND MONITORING AND ANESTHESIA

All of the monitoring tools and techniques described in Table 13.4 should be used with emphasis on ventilation and body temperature. Both of these should be supported as necessary. Blood transfusions (see Chapters 11 and 16) should be considered in anemic patients.

Anesthetic drug choice is not as important as drug dosage because hypothyroid patients generally have exaggerated responses to tranquilizers and anesthetic agents. Use low dosages of all drugs. Opioids provide analgesia and allow a reduction of induction and maintenance drugs, so opioids are often used as premedicants. Anticholinergics may be used, if necessary, but hypothyroidism affects atropine pharmacokinetics, causing a significant increase in peak serum concentration and drug bioavailability with decreased clearance (Smallridge et al. 1989). Thus, lower doses and/or a longer dosing interval of atropine is warranted. Ketamine works indirectly through the SNS to support cardiovascular function by increased contractility and rate. Ketamine with diazepam is a good choice for induction. Propofol and thiopental are also acceptable. The inhalant anesthetic agents isoflurane and sevoflurane are a good choice for maintenance. Although inhalant anesthetic agents may cause marked cardiovascular depression in hypothyroid humans, they may not cause a profound effect in dogs (Robertson 2003). Support and monitoring must continue well into recovery, and active rewarming is almost always required. Emergence from anesthesia may be prolonged in these patients.

Hyperthyroidism

PATHOPHYSIOLOGY

Hyperthyroidism is the most common endocrine disease in cats but is not as common in dogs. It is a disease of older cats (12 to 13 years) and dogs (10 years). The etiology of the disease is unclear. Hyperthyroidism is a multisystemic disease with varied and wide-ranging effects. Organ systems affected include the cardiovascular, respiratory, urinary, and hepatic systems, although almost any organ system may be involved. Thyroid hormones are involved in regulation of heat production and metabolism of carbohydrates, proteins, and lipids.

They also interact with the nervous system, increasing overall sympathetic drive. Clinical signs are numerous and varied and usually include weight loss (despite an increased appetite), pu/pd, and hyperactivity. Cardiac function is often normal in the early stages of the disease, but sinus tachycardia, arrhythmias, and hypertrophic changes occur as the disease progresses and some hyperthyroid patients will present in CHF. Death in untreated patients is most often related to a cardiac event. "Thyroid storms" are life-threatening events that occur secondary to stress-induced exacerbation of hyperthyroidism and present as acute tachycardia, tachypnea, hyperthermia, and alterations in consciousness. Thyroid storms are rare in people and may not occur in animals.

Medical therapy for hyperthyroidism includes the use of antithyroid drugs and radioactive iodine (Mooney 2005). Surgical removal of the thyroid gland is a viable option in many patients.

PATIENT ASSESSMENT

The diagnosis of hyperthyroidism is confirmed by thyroid testing, which is reviewed elsewhere (Mooney 2005). Hyperthyroidism increases minute oxygen consumption (up to 100% above normal) in all tissues except the brain. Thus, any organ may be affected by the disease and complete patient evaluation is required. In addition to thyroid testing and the basic preoperative exam and laboratory analysis described in Table 13.3, patients with hyperthyroidism may require thoracic radiographs and an echocardiography. Common cardiovascular concerns include tachycardia, arrhythmias, hypertension, and possible HCM; thus, a full cardiac exam is necessary. The serum chemistry profile should be thoroughly assessed as elevations in hepatic enzymes, BUN, and creatinine are common. In fact, in one study, 97% of hyperthyroid cats had elevations in one or more hepatic enzymes (ALP, LDH, ALT; Peterson et al. 1983), and in another study, 42% were azotemic. Electrolytes, especially potassium and calcium, should be evaluated. Ventilatory function should be evaluated.

PREPARATION FOR ANESTHESIA

Intraoperative or immediate postoperative deaths in hyperthyroid cats have been reported to be 10% (Peterson et al. 1984) to 14%. Thus, elective procedures should be postponed until the patient may be made euthyroid with appropriate medical therapy. Although the therapy is reviewed elsewhere, it is worth mentioning that methimazole, carbimazole, and ipodate are the most commonly used antithyroid drugs, and cats receiving methimazole before surgery may present with anorexia, vomiting, thrombocytopenia, hepatopathy, and elevated serum creatinine values (Robertson 2003).

MONITORING AND SUPPORT

Diligent monitoring of hyperthyroid patients is essential, and all of the monitoring techniques and tools described in Table 13.4 should be used. Because tachycardia, arrhythmias, and changes in blood pressure are fairly common, the HR and rhythm (ECG) and arterial blood pressure should be assessed frequently. Severe tachycardia (HR greater than 200 beats/min) and ventricular arrhythmias should be treated. Recommendations for treatment include a bolus of propranolol (0.01 to 0.05 mg/kg IV) or a CRI of the short-acting β-blocker esmolol (Robertson 2003). Changes in body temperature are also common, and core body temperature should be monitored throughout the procedure with active cooling (or warming) of the patient as needed. Hyperthyroid patients are hypermetabolic and have an elevated oxygen consumption, yet the metabolic derangements and the catabolic state associated with severe hyperthyroidism often cause weakness of the muscles associated with ventilation, leading to a reduction in vital capacity and lung compliance. However, the hypermetabolic state leads to increased carbon dioxide production, which, in conjunction with a decrease in tidal volume, may cause hypercarbia. Thus, ventilatory function must be assessed (i.e., pulse oximeter, ETCO$_2$ monitor, possibly arterial blood gases) and supported. Although the phenomenon seems to be uncommon in animals, the previously described thyroid storm could occur with manipulation of the thyroid gland. Attentive monitoring during thyroid manipulation is critical.

ANESTHESIA

Stress and excitement exacerbate thyrotoxicosis and appropriate sedation and analgesia should be used perioperatively. An opioid (e.g., buprenorphine or hydromorphone) plus acepromazine produces good sedation and analgesia, and the acepromazine may provide some protection against arrhythmias. Anticholinergics are rarely, if ever, necessary and are not recommended because tachycardia is extremely detrimental in patients with hypertrophic disease (see more under Hypertrophic Cardiomyopathy). Recommended induction agents include propofol, thiopental, and etomidate. Thiopental may have an advantage in hyperthyroid patients because the thiourea structures have some antithyroid activity; however, a single induction bolus probably does not have any significant effect. Drugs like ketamine and tiletamine that increase sympathetic tone are not the best choice, but combining ketamine with valium decreases the degree of sympathetic stimulation and a ketamine/valium combination is generally acceptable in the early stages of the disease. These patients should absolutely not be mask induced unless they are extremely sedate or moribund.

Isoflurane and sevoflurane are suitable for maintenance but halothane, because of the myocardial sensitization to the arrhythmic effects of catecholamines, is not a good choice. *All* of the inhalant anesthetic agents cause mild to moderate cardiovascular depression that is dose dependent; thus, it is imperative to maintain the inhalant anesthetics at the lowest concentration possible. This is best accomplished by inclusion of appropriate analgesic agents in the anesthetic protocol. Boluses or CRIs of opioids are most appropriate for patients with hyperthyroidism. Local anesthetic agents are also appropriate and should be used whenever possible. NSAIDs may be used in patients with normal renal function.

In recovery, supplemental oxygen should be administered, an ECG should remain attached to the patient, and any emergent pain or excitement should be treated. Postoperative complications following thyroid surgery commonly involve the airway. Extubation should be followed by a period of observation as airway obstruction from laryngeal nerve paralysis, hypocalcemia-induced vocal cord tetanus, or hematoma formation at the surgical site may occur. If the patient cannot ventilate, a reinduction to anesthesia and reintubation may be necessary. The airway obstruction may then be addressed while the patient is stable, rather than in crisis. Supplemental oxygen should be administered while the patient is reanesthetized. Severe cases may require a tracheostomy tube.[3] Electrolytes should be monitored because acute muscle weakness secondary to hypokalemia and hypocalcemic tetany may occur in recovery. If a hyperthyroid patient has cardiovascular (CV) disease, use CV regimen. Most dog's thyroid tumors are not active.

Hyperadrenocorticism (Cushing's Disease)

Hyperadrenocorticism, or Cushing's disease, is one of the most common endocrinopathies in dogs but it is rare in cats. The disease most commonly occurs in middle-aged to older dogs (9 to 11 years). Naturally occurring hyperadrenocorticism occurs in two forms, the most common of which is pituitary-dependent hyperadrenocorticism (PDH), characterized by overproduction of adrenocorticotropic hormone (ACTH). The second most common type occurs secondary to a functional adrenocortical tumor, characterized by cortisol secretion that is independent of pituitary control. Iatrogenic hyperadrenocorticism following chronic glucocorticoid therapy may be the most common form of the disease in veterinary medicine (Reusch 2005).

Clinical signs and laboratory abnormalities are generally caused by chronic glucocorticoid excess and, to a small extent, excess adrenal androgens. Clinical signs that affect anesthesia include fluid and sodium retention, hypokalemia, hypertension, impaired respiratory function (from muscle weakness), tachypnea, hepatomegaly, and excessive fat depositions.

PATIENT ASSESSMENT

Initial diagnosis and stabilization may be complicated and is reviewed elsewhere (Reusch 2005). Hyperadrenocortical patients may present for anesthesia in different stages of disease, with a variety of concurrent illnesses (e.g., diabetes mellitus, pancreatitis, urinary tract infections) and with varying side effects from treatment. Thus, each patient must be assessed individually. In addition to the basic preoperative exam and laboratory analysis described in Table 13.3, patients with hyperadrenocorticism require serial measurement of blood glucose concentrations and blood pressure monitoring.

PREPARATION FOR ANESTHESIA

Hyperglycemia with or without overt diabetes mellitus is common, and blood glucose should be measured and abnormalities corrected. Electrolyte imbalances should also be corrected. Hypertension is common in these patients, and blood pressure should be measured prior to anesthesia. Up to 86% of dogs with untreated hyperadrenocorticism may be hypertensive (systolic BP greater than 100 mm Hg) and the blood pressure may not decrease in response to standard therapy (Ortega, et al. 1996).

Life-threatening pulmonary thromboemboli may occur in patients with hyperadrenocorticism, and the risk of thromboemboli is increased during surgery and anesthesia. Although thromboemboli may occur in any organ system, pulmonary emboli are the most common. Hypertension and obesity play a role in the development of the emboli, but the primary cause appears to be hypercoaguability associated with hyperadrenocorticism. The incidence of this complication is unknown and may be hard to diagnosis because the emboli often lead to nonspecific signs of respiratory distress, and ancillary diagnostic tools, like thoracic radiology, may not show any evidence of the emboli. Thus, an acute episode of respiratory distress (tachypnea, dyspnea, cyanosis, hypoxemia, and hypocapnia) in hyperadrenocortical patients is generally attributed to pulmonary emboli. Treatment is only moderately successful, but there is some indication that *pretreatment* with antithrombolic agents may be beneficial (Reusch 2005).

Patients with glucocorticoid excess are prone to infection and bruising; thus wounds, surgical incisions, and IV catheter sites must be thoroughly scrubbed and the tissue handled carefully.

Because patients with hyperadrenocorticism are at risk of hypoventilation, oxygenation with 100% oxygen by facemask is recommended for roughly 5 minutes prior to induction, but only if the patient will accept the mask without struggling.

SUPPORT AND MONITORING

Vigilant monitoring is essential in these patients. All of the monitoring techniques and tools described in Table 13.4 should be used. Frequent blood pressure monitoring is crucial. Some patients may be hypertensive at the beginning of the procedure and suddenly hypotensive following removal of the adrenal gland. Furthermore, some adrenal tumors are invasive and require resection from surrounding structures, including the vena cava. Unstable blood pressure is common because of physical interference with venous return to the heart and severe hemorrhage may occur. Direct blood pressure has the advantage of providing continuous information and should be considered when possible. Ventilatory function may be assessed using arterial blood gases if possible, or pulse oximetry and ETCO$_2$ if blood gases are not available. If the PaCO$_2$ is greater than 60 mm Hg, manual or mechanical ventilation is required. If pulmonary emboli occur, the emboli effectively block circulation to a portion of the alveoli, preventing them from participating in gas exchange. This shunting of blood away from alveoli will make ETCO$_2$ gas monitors inaccurate (see Chapters 2 and 3).

Fluid therapy initiated preoperatively should continue throughout the anesthesia period and well in to the recovery period.

SURGERY

The surgical treatment of the disease deserves a brief comment here because the anesthesiologist will need to provide treatment during the anesthetic episode. Surgical removal of adrenal tumors (adrenalectomy) is a viable option, especially in cats. However, the surgery is technically challenging and severe postoperative complications are common. When the tumor is located, the anesthesiologist will need to administer dexamethasone (0.1 mg/kg IV over 6 hours). Repeat dosages are necessary and both dosages and dosing intervals have been described (Reusch 2005). Hypophysectomy is even more challenging and the success rate is low.

ANESTHESIA

Preoperative sedation may be achieved with a low dose of either acepromazine or a benzodiazepine combined with an opioid, or with an opioid used alone. Opioid analgesia will allow a decrease in the dose of induction and maintenance drugs. Because tumor removal requires highly invasive surgery with associated pain, potent opioids (e.g., morphine, hydromorphone) are recommended but opioids of lesser potency (e.g., butorphanol, buprenorphine) may be acceptable if used as part of multimodal therapy. Thiopental and propofol are appropriate for induction. Ketamine and tiletamine may be acceptable but are not ideal choices for hypertensive patients. Etomidate may be a good choice because it causes adrenocortical suppression, but the clinical significance of the suppression is unknown. Both isoflurane and sevoflurane are appropriate for maintenance.

Hypoadrenocorticism (Addison's Disease)

Hypoadrenocorticism, or Addison's disease, is uncommon in the dog and rare in the cat. It is a disease of young to middle-aged patients (4 to 6 years). Idiopathic adrenocortical atrophy is the most common cause of hypoadrenocorticism in the dog and is thought to be the end result of immune-mediated destruction of the adrenal cortices. The disease may also be caused by other immune-mediated diseases or drug-induced adrenocortical necrosis (e.g., following mitotane or trilostane therapy).

PATHOPHYSIOLOGY AND PATIENT ASSESSMENT

Primary hypoadrenocorticism, in which adrenal gland production of both glucocorticoids and mineralocorticoids is deficient, is the most common form of the disease. In the secondary and some atypical forms of the disease, only glucocorticoids are deficient. Deficiency of aldosterone, the primary mineralocorticoid, causes an impaired ability to conserve sodium and water and a failure to excrete potassium, which leads to hyponatremia and hyperkalemia. Lethargy, nausea, hypovolemia, hypotension, reduced cardiac output, and decreased renal perfusion are common sequelae of hyponatremia. Hyperkalemia causes muscle weakness, hyporeflexia, and impaired cardiac conduction. Glucocorticoid deficiency causes decreased tolerance of stress, loss of appetite, vomiting, diarrhea, abdominal pain, and lethargy (Herrtage 2005).

All of the components of the basic preoperative exam and laboratory analysis described in Table 13.3 should be used. Patients with hypoadrenocorticism require careful assessment of hydration status, serum electrolytes, and glucose concentration. In addition, an ECG should be recorded and carefully evaluated because these patients are commonly bradycardic and have ECG abnormalities, including sinoatrial standstill and first-degree atrioventricular block as a result of hyperkalemia.

An Addisonian crisis is life threatening and occurs when there is a significant stress to which the patient cannot mount an appropriate response. The patient is usually found totally collapsed with weak pulses, profound bradycardia, abdominal pain, vomiting, diarrhea, dehydration, and hypothermia. Profound bradycardia is unusual in a patient who has collapsed, and this is often the clue that the patient is experiencing an Addisonian crisis. Patients must be stabilized before anesthesia and surgery may be considered. Both long-term stabilization and treatment of patients in an Addisonian crisis are reviewed elsewhere (Herrtage 2005). Unfortunately, any stressor may precipitate an adrenal crisis in patients with adrenal suppression, including surgery, trauma, and sepsis. Thus, a stabilized patient may still respond adversely in the perioperative period.

PREPARATION FOR ANESTHESIA

Hypovolemia, electrolyte imbalance, and glucose abnormalities should be corrected in all patients. Volume replacement with normal saline (0.9% sodium chloride) should start immediately on admission of the patient to the hospital. Normal saline provides sodium and chloride but contains no potassium. "Shock" rates (60 to 90 ml/kg/hr IV) may be required initially. Fluid therapy may correct acidosis and hyperkalemia, but if these still exist or if ECG abnormalities are present during initial therapy, treatment for hyperkalemia should be initiated (see Table 13.7). Glucocorticoids may be administered once normovolemia has been restored. Stabilization and glucocorticoid treatment is covered elsewhere (Herrtage 2005; Roberson 2003).

PATIENT MONITORING AND SUPPORT

In addition to the monitoring techniques and tools described in Table 13.4, patients with hypoadrenocorticism require arterial blood pressure and ECG monitoring. Serum electrolyte and glucose concentrations should be analyzed every 1 to 4 hours, depending on the severity of the disease. Hypovolemia, hypotension, electrolyte abnormalities, and hypoglycemia should be anticipated and prevented (if possible) or treated. Fluid therapy initiated preoperatively should continue throughout the anesthesia period and through the recovery period. Choice of fluid should be based on lab results, but fluid rate may need to be higher in these patients (15 to 20 ml/kg/hr IV) than in many other surgical patients. If hypotension occurs despite adequate crystalloid therapy, colloids (e.g., hetastarch or dextran) should be administered and an infusion of a positive inotrope (e.g., dopamine or dobutamine) should be considered.

ANESTHESIA

The choice of anesthetic drugs is not as critical as stabilization of the patient. The stress level should be kept at a minimum; thus, preoperative tranquilizers and perioperative analgesic agents should be used. Opioids and local anesthetics should be used for analgesia. Propofol and thiopental are appropriate for induction. Etomidate is questionable because the drug causes adrenocortical suppression. Isoflurane and sevoflurane are both acceptable for maintenance. Dexamethasone (2 to 4 mg/kg SQ/IV) should be administered at premedication. During surgery, a rapid-acting glucocorticoid (e.g., prednisolone sodium succinate) should be administered every 2 to 4 hours (Robertson 2003). Recovery should also be stress free and tranquilizers and analgesic agents should be used as needed.

Pheochromocytoma

PATHOPHYSIOLOGY, PATIENT ASSESSMENT, AND PREPARATION FOR ANESTHESIA

Pheochromocytomas, which are catecholamine secreting tumors of the chromaffin cells of the adrenal medulla, are rare in dogs and cats. When they occur, it is generally in aged dogs and cats (average age at diagnosis, 10 to 11 years). Clinical signs may be absent (some tumors are diagnosed as an incidental finding on necropsy or at surgery) or complicated by concurrent disease (e.g., hyperadrenocorticism, diabetes mellitus, renal failure, and hepatic disease; McNiel and Husbands 2005). Patients with uncomplicated pheochromocytoma may present with a variety of problems, including weakness, collapse, GI disorders (weight loss, vomiting), CNS disorders (nervousness, seizures), pu/pd, proteinuria, and hypertension. Surgical excision is the treatment of choice, but medical therapy is acceptable and is described elsewhere (McNiel and Husbands 2005). Due to the complexity of the surgery, these cases are rarely anesthetized in private practice and are only covered briefly here. However, an excellent review of stabilization and anesthesia for patients with pheochromocytoma is available (Robertson 2003).

PATIENT SUPPORT AND MONITORING AND ANESTHESIA

Anesthetic complications are common but may be minimized with appropriate preoperative stabilization and treatment, including control of hypertension and arrhythmias. Blood pressure and rhythm disturbances should be stabilized for 1 to 2 weeks prior to anesthesia.

For anesthesia, all of the monitoring tools and techniques described in Table 13.4 should be used, with vigilant monitoring of blood pressure, cardiac rhythm, and circulating volume, especially during manipulation of the tumor when catecholamine release may cause or exacerbate hypertension and arrhythmias. Nitroprusside may be needed for α-blockade prior to the tumor removal. Following resection of a pheochromocytoma, hypovolemia and hypotension may occur as the circulating catecholamine concentrations decrease and loss of vascular tone occurs. Hypotension is generally managed by administration of large volumes of IV crystalloids, but colloids or whole blood may be needed and unresponsive hypotension may be treated with dopamine or dobutamine. Arrhythmias should be treated according to the location and type (e.g., lidocaine for ventricular tachycardia).

When making anesthetic choices, drugs that stimulate the release of catecholamines or are known to cause arrhythmias (e.g., ketamine) should be avoided. Anesthetic agents used in humans include opioids, propofol, isoflurane, and sevoflurane. Etomidate may be a good choice. Appropriate analgesia is critical, and the opioids, local anesthetics, and NSAIDs are all good choices. Postoperative care includes maintenance of fluid balance and provision of analgesia. Monitoring of ABP, HR, and rhythm should continue in recovery; in fact, monitoring and medical therapy may continue for several days, or even several weeks, before the patient is ready to be discharged.

ANESTHESIA FOR NEONATAL, PEDIATRIC, AND GERIATRIC PATIENTS

Improved medical knowledge about preventative care and support of aging patients has led to longer life spans and a subsequent increase in the number of geriatric patients admitted for veterinary care. On the other end of the age spectrum, the desire to neuter pets at an extremely young age and the surgical skill to repair congenital defects, such as patent ductus arteriosus (PDA) and cleft palate, have led to an increase in the number of neonatal and pediatric patients requiring anesthesia. However, most of the knowledge regarding the physiologic and pharmacokinetic-pharmacodynamic responses to anesthesia and anesthetic drugs is based on data collected in young to middle-aged pets or extrapolated from data collected in anesthetized humans. Although our knowledge base is incomplete, we do know that because of limited organ reserve and altered responses to anesthesia and anesthetic drugs, neonatal, pediatric, and geriatric patients may be at a greater anesthetic risk than young to middle-aged adult patients. To provide safe and effective anesthesia, it is imperative that the differences in these groups of patients be understood.

The rate of aging is dependent on both the species and breed of the patient, and there may be little correlation between chronologic age and physiologic age. However, the neonatal, pediatric, and geriatric life stages may be roughly defined. Puppies and kittens are generally considered "neonates" for the first 6 weeks of life and "pediatrics" for the first 12 weeks of life (Robinson 1983). The "geriatric" life stage of dogs and cats is more difficult to define because of the tremendous individual, species, and breed variation but is generally considered to be the last 20% to 25% of the animal's normal expected life span (Dodman et al. 1984).

Physiologic and Pharmacokinetic-Pharmacodynamic Considerations

Compared to young and middle-aged adult patients, pediatric and geriatric patients have limited organ reserve, decreased ability to respond to a physiologic challenge or change, and increased "sensitivity" to anesthetic drugs that is manifest as exaggerated or prolonged effects after the administration of drug dosages appropriate for young adults. The differences between young adult patients and pediatric, neonatal, and geriatric patients are numerous and generally culminate in increased anesthetic risk in the very young and the very old. A brief review of pertinent changes and their effects on anesthesia is presented here and summarized in Tables 13.8 and 13.9.

PEDIATRIC AND NEONATAL PATIENTS

In the neonatal small animal, organ function and physiologic responses gradually mature during the first 4 weeks of life, becoming similar to those found in adults by 6 to 8 weeks of life (Breazile 1978; Dodman et al. 1984) (Table 13.8). Neonates are considered to be more "sensitive" to the effects

Table 13.8. Unique physiologic characteristics of neonatal and pediatric patients that may affect anesthesia.

Physiologic characteristic	Effect on anesthesia

General characteristics
  Hypoalbuminemia
  Increased permeability of blood-brain barrier
  Low percentage of body fat
  Circulating fluid volume is centralized
  Immature thermoregulatory system
	Exaggerated effect from standard drug dosage for young adult patients, decreased dosage required; decreased tolerance to fluid load, do not overhydrate; Hypothermia contributes to delayed recovery, keep warm.

Renal/urinary system Immature renal function	Prolonged duration of action of renally cleared drugs, may prolong recovery time; decreased tolerance to fluid load, do not overhydrate.
Hepatic system Immature hepatic function	Prolonged duration of hepatically cleared drugs, may prolong recovery time.

Respiratory system
  High metabolic rate with high oxygen
    consumption
  High minute volume
  Limited pulmonary reserve
  Pliable rib cage
	Decreased respiratory reserve, both oxygen and ventilatory support are required for most patients. Mask induction occurs extremely quickly, induction must be closely supervised.

Cardiovascular system
  Limited myocardial contractile tissue
  Low ventricular compliance
  Limited cardiac reserve
  Cardiac output heart rate dependent
  Poor vasomotor control
	Decreased cardiac reserve, cardiovascular system must be supported with IV fluids, and some patients may need chronotropic support.

of sedative and anesthetic drugs (Fig. 13.4). Reasons for this "sensitivity" include (1) a lower percentage of drug bound to plasma proteins (due to neonatal hypoalbuminemia) with a subsequent increase in the free, active portion of highly protein bound drugs (such as barbiturates, ketamine, and etomidate); (2) an increased permeability of the blood-brain barrier; and (3) a low percentage of body fat resulting in an insignificant adipose tissue compartment for redistribution (Baggot 1992). In dogs and cats, renal function, including both glomerular filtration and tubular function, is not fully developed at birth and does not reach full function for 1 to 2 months after birth. Thus, the effects of drugs dependent on renal excretion for termination of activity are prolonged. Hepatic metabolism is immature for the first 3 to 4 weeks (and perhaps up to 12 weeks of life) (Baggot 1992) and metabolism of many

drugs may be slowed, thereby extending the duration of drugs or active metabolites of drugs that require hepatic metabolism for termination of activity. Most of the currently used injectable sedative and anesthetic drugs fall into this category. Finally, circulating fluid volume in the very young is fixed and relatively centralized, allowing greater delivery of anesthetic agents to the highly perfused tissues, including the brain. This contributes to the exaggerated effects of sedative and anesthetic drugs.

Pediatric and neonatal patients have a high metabolic rate with subsequent high oxygen consumption, necessitating alveolar ventilation that is much greater than that of adults. Because of the increased alveolar ventilation, anesthetic induction with inhalant anesthetic agents may occur very quickly in neonates, and mask inductions should be closely supervised. Pulmonary reserve is minimal in this

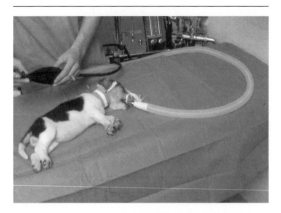

Figure 13.4. Neonatal dog anesthetized for emergency laparotomy. Neonatal and geriatric patients are at increased anesthetic risk over young adult patients because of a variety of physiologic characteristics that result in an exaggerated and/or prolonged response to anesthetic drugs. Because of its small body size, this patient is also highly likely to become hypothermic, which will also cause an altered response to anesthetic drugs.

age group, increasing the possibility of hypoxia during apnea or airway obstruction. The neonatal rib cage is pliable, resulting in less efficient ventilation and greater work of breathing and predisposing young patients to hypoxia and ventilatory fatigue during airway obstruction (e.g., endotracheal tube plugged with mucus) or respiratory disease. All of these factors contribute to the need for ventilatory support in the very young patient.

> Mask inductions in neonatal patients occur *very* quickly and must be monitored closely to avoid overdose of the inhalant anesthetic agent.

The neonatal heart has less contractile tissue per gram of myocardial tissue than the adult heart and ventricular compliance is limited. Thus, SV and cardiac reserve are limited in pediatric patients, and cardiac output is dependent on the HR. Adding to the limited cardiac reserve is the fact that neonates have a resting cardiac index (CI; which is cardiac output divided by body weight or body surface area) that is greater than in the CI in adults and is very close to maximal cardiac output. Also, the

SNS is not fully developed in neonates, leading to (1) minimal increases in HR and contractility in response to sympathetic stimulation, (2) limited vasomotor control, and (3) limited baroreceptor reflexes in response to hypotension.

Circulating fluid volume in the very young is fixed and relatively centralized, making the pediatric patient more susceptible to hypovolemia. However, for the first 1 to 2 weeks of life, the neonatal kidney may be less efficient than the adult kidney at eliminating fluid loads and regulating electrolytes. Thus, balancing fluid need with fluid load may be somewhat complicated and the judicious use of appropriate IV fluids is important.

GERIATRIC PATIENTS

Although advanced age is not a disease in itself, aging results in decreased physiologic adaptation to change or stress and reduced functional organ reserve and may be accompanied by age-related diseases. Furthermore, advanced age has been linked to increased anesthetic risk in dogs (Gaynor et al. 1999), although cats may be at higher risk from other factors (Dyson et al. 1998).

Geriatric patients are also considered to be more "sensitive" to the effects of sedative and anesthetic drugs (Table 13.9). Reasons for this "sensitivity" include (1) a lower percentage of drug bound to plasma proteins (due to lower concentrations of plasma albumin) with a subsequent increase in the free, active portion of highly bound protein drugs; (2) age-related CNS effects that include neuronal degeneration, decreased rate of synthesis and increased rate of destruction of neurotransmitters, and decreased number of receptors and affinity of the receptors for neurotransmitters; (3) a decrease in skeletal muscle (resulting in less tissue for initial redistribution of drugs, which delays initial termination of drug activity); and (4) an increase in body fat (resulting in greater sequestration of fat-soluble drugs, which slows their elimination and prolongs recovery). Renal blood flow, kidney mass, GFR, and tubular function all decline. Decreased filtration rate and excretory capacity of the kidney prolong half-life and duration of effect of drugs that are primarily eliminated by the kidney. With age, hepatic mass and total hepatic blood flow decrease, resulting in a reduction of hepatic clearance of drugs and prolonged duration of effect of many drugs, including many

Table 13.9. Unique physiologic characteristics of geriatric patients that may affect anesthesia.

Physiologic characteristic	Effect on anesthesia
General characteristics 　Hypoalbuminemia 　Neuronal degeneration 　Decrease in neurons and neurotransmitters 　Decrease in skeletal muscle 　Increase in body fat 　Impaired thermoregulatory system	Exaggerated effect from standard drug dosage for young adult patients, decreased dosage required; decreased tolerance to fluid load, do not overhydrate. Fat may act as drug reservoir and contribute to delayed recovery. Hypothermia contributes to delayed recovery, keep warm.
Renal/urinary system 　Decreased RBF, GFR and tubular function 　Decreased filtration rate and excretory capacity	Prolonged duration of action of renally cleared drugs, may prolong recovery time; decreased tolerance to fluid load, do not overhydrate.
Hepatic system 　Decreased hepatic mass and hepatic blood flow	Prolonged duration of action of hepatically cleared drugs, may prolong recovery time.
Respiratory system 　Loss of strength of muscles of ventilation 　Thorax becomes rigid, lungs lose elasticity 　Increased closing volume 　Reduction in arterial oxygen	Decreased respiratory reserve, both oxygen and ventilatory support are required for most patients.
Cardiovascular system 　Myocardial atrophy 　Fibrosis of the endocardium 　Decreased myocardial contractility 　Loss of vascular distensibility 　Maximum heart rate decreases, cardiac output is SV dependent SNS less responsive to stress 　Decreased vasoconstrictor and baroreceptor responses	Decreased cardiac reserve, cardiovascular system must be supported with IV fluids, and some patients may need chronotropic or inotropic support.

RBF, renal blood flow; GFR, glomerular filtration rate; SV, stroke volume; SNS, sympathetic nervous system.
NOTE: The changes listed here are general changes associated with aging but may not be present in all aged patients.

anesthetic agents. Finally, the blood volume decreases by 20% to 30% (because of loss of total body water), allowing a greater percentage of the drug to be delivered to the highly perfused tissues, including the brain.

With age, the muscles of ventilation lose strength and the thorax becomes rigid, decreasing the efficiency of breathing. Functional alveoli are lost and elasticity declines, resulting in an increased closing volume and trapping of air in the lung that leads to or worsens $\dot{V}/\dot{Q}$ mismatch. These changes cause a reduction in arterial oxygen concentration, thereby decreasing oxygen reserve and predisposing the geriatric patient to hypoxia during times of reduced ventilation. Also, PaO_2 decreases with age.

Myocardial atrophy and fibrosis of the endocardium occur with age, resulting in decreased myocardial contractility and compliance. The vasculature loses elasticity and becomes less distensible, resulting in increased afterload and hypertension. These factors combine to decrease the cardiac reserve.

With age, the maximum HR that may be generated decreases and the cardiac output in the geriatric patient becomes dependent on SV and the end-diastolic blood volume (or preload). The conduction system of the heart is also affected by aging, and this may make the geriatric patient more prone to anesthetic-induced cardiac arrhythmias. Furthermore, the ability of the autonomic nervous system, especially the SNS, loses some of its ability respond to stress. Geriatric patients have decreased baroreceptor activity and a decreased vasoconstrictor response to hypotension.

Because of the decreased blood volume, decreased renal blood flow, and dependence on preload for cardiac output, the geriatric patient is fairly intolerant of hypovolemia. However, the geriatric kidney is not efficient at excreting a fluid load and excessive fluid therapy is not well tolerated. Thus, balancing fluid need with fluid load may be somewhat complicated and the judicious use of appropriate IV fluids is important.

Preparation for Anesthesia (Neonatal, Pediatric, and Geriatric Patients)

All of the components of the preoperative exam and laboratory analysis described in Table 13.3 should be used. A thorough physical examination, CBC and serum chemistry evaluation are critical for all patients. An ECG and UA are highly recommended, especially in geriatric patients who may have concurrent disease. Other tests should be performed based on the patient's overall health status (e.g., thoracic radiographs for cardiac disease).

Hydration status should be critically evaluated. Because both groups of patients adapt poorly to hypovolemia, preoperative fluid therapy may be necessary. However, because protein is low and renal clearance may be compromised, overhydration may occur if fluid needs are not carefully calculated. Geriatric and pediatric patients are generally fasted before surgery. However, neonates are highly susceptible to hypoglycemia and should not be fasted. Blood glucose concentrations must be evaluated in neonates, diabetics, and any patient with prolonged recovery. Because of low oxygen reserve, both groups of patients may need to be preoxygenated for 2 to 5 minutes before induction and receive oxygen for as long as possible after the surgical procedure.

Monitoring and Support (Neonatal, Pediatric, and Geriatric Patients)

The limited physiologic reserves in neonatal, pediatric, and geriatric patients increase the possibility of anesthetic complications, and these must be prevented if at all possible or recognized early if they do occur. All of the monitoring techniques and tools described in Table 13.4 should be used. A staff member should be dedicated to careful monitoring of the patient throughout the entire procedure. Because of their large body surface area compared with body mass, neonates and pediatric patients may lose heat rapidly. Neonates may not be able to shiver and warm themselves. In those patients that may shiver, shivering greatly increases oxygen consumption and may contribute to hypoxia. Thus, every attempt should be made to avoid hypothermia. Oxygen and fluid therapy should proceed as described in the previous section.

Analgesia is imperative and absolutely should not be withheld from these patients because of misconceptions about pain perception in the very young or very old or because of fear of the side effects of analgesic agents. Pain itself may cause tachycardia, hypertension, decreased renal blood flow, and myriad other effects (see Table 13.2) that may not be well tolerated in very young and very old patients with minimal physiologic reserve. Local anesthetic agents and opioids may be used in any age group; however, dosage must be calculated carefully and, in neonates and other extremely small patients, the drug may need to be diluted with sterile water or sterile saline in order to provide a volume large enough for injection.

> Do not withhold analgesia from neonatal, pediatric, or geriatric patients. As with middle-aged patients, very young and very old patients feel pain.

Anesthesia (Neonatal, Pediatric, and Geriatric Patients)

Because of the decreased physiologic reserves and increased sensitivity to the effects of many drugs, anesthetic agents for neonates, pediatric patients, and geriatric patients are chosen carefully and dosed conservatively. For healthy patients, most of the currently used sedative and anesthetic drugs are appropriate, but drug dosages are lower than those used for young and middle-aged adults. In compromised patients, drug selection may be more critical and the guidelines for concurrent disease conditions outlined in this chapter are recommended.

PREMEDICANTS

Opioids alone are often suitable for preoperative analgesia and tranquilization. Full μ-agonists like morphine and hydromorphone should be considered for healthy patients scheduled for painful procedures. Dosages may need to be decreased and ventilation supported. Partial-agonist opioids like buprenorphine may not provide adequate sedation when used alone but contribution to cardiovascular or respiratory depression is minimal. Buprenorphine is an excellent choice in patients that require minimal sedation (e.g., most neonates, compromised geriatric patients) and is especially good in cats. Butorphanol provides moderate sedation but must be supplemented with other drugs because the duration of action is very short. Benzodiazepines (e.g., diazepam, midazolam), which cause minimal respiratory and cardiovascular depression, may be added to the opioids if more sedation is needed. Acepromazine might be used in some cases, but the duration of action may be extremely prolonged and acepromazine-mediated vasodilation is likely to result in hypotension in patients with minimal vascular and baroreceptor control. Thus, acepromazine is generally not used in the very young or very old patients. The α_2-agonists (e.g., medetomidine) may be suitable for healthy geriatric patients that need moderate to profound sedation (Muir et al. 1999), but the α_2-agonist–induced cardiovascular changes preclude its use in compromised patients.

INDUCTION AGENTS

When used at reduced dosages, any of the currently available injectable induction agents (e.g., propofol, ketamine/valium, thiopental) are appropriate in healthy patients. Because of the multiple routes of elimination, propofol is often the best choice because compromised or immature metabolic and clearance mechanisms will not affect elimination of the drug. Appropriate ventilatory and circulatory support is required to compensate for the depression caused by propofol. Cautious mask induction may be appropriate in sedate or lethargic patients, but excitement and struggling will greatly increase oxygen demand and, as already stated, these patients have only minimal ventilatory reserve. As has been discussed, mask inductions are appropriate only in patients that will accept induction calmly.

MAINTENANCE DRUGS

Isoflurane and sevoflurane are appropriate choices for maintenance of anesthesia. As with other patients, inhalant anesthetic concentrations during maintenance of anesthesia should be kept to a minimum because inhalant anesthetics are major contributors to hypotension, hypoventilation, and hypothermia. Adequate analgesia may allow a significant decrease in the dose of inhalant anesthetic agents necessary for anesthesia. Intraoperative analgesia may include supplemental dosages of opioids and blockade with local anesthetic agents. CRIs of fentanyl, ketamine, lidocaine, or other drugs are also appropriate in some patients.

Patient monitoring and support must continue throughout the recovery period. Active warming is generally necessary. Blood glucose concentrations should be rechecked, especially in neonatal and diabetic patients, in patients with severe liver compromise, and in any patient that is having a prolonged recovery.

ANESTHESIA FOR CRITICALLY ILL AND TRAUMATIZED PATIENTS AND PATIENTS IN SHOCK

When critically ill or traumatized patients or patients in shock are presented to the hospital, their physiologic status must be thoroughly evaluated prior to the administration of tranquilizers or anesthetic agents. Judicious dosages of analgesic agents, however, are often appropriate in the early assessment phase and may aid in the determination of prognosis as the side effects of pain are alleviated. Whether the crisis is medical or surgical in nature, stabilization of all patients should begin immediately.

Patient Assessment

In addition to the components of the preoperative exam and laboratory analysis described in Table 13.3, patients with trauma or severe systemic disease require a thorough but rapid exam of organ systems thought to be affected by the disease or trauma. In a triage type of approach using a team of caregivers, organ systems that could result in imminent death should be examined first (e.g.,

CNS, cardiovascular, respiratory), while systems that might be affected but that will not cause immediate death (e.g., hepatic, renal, gastrointestinal, musculoskeletal) should be evaluated second. The exception to this rule is active hemorrhage from any organ or tissue. Clearly, hemorrhage must be stopped as soon as possible. The first-line exam should include a rapid assessment of breathing (movement of air in and out of respiratory tract, respiratory rate and depth) and of cardiovascular function (brief cardiac auscultation, palpation of pulses, and assessment of CRT). The second-line exam should include a brief neurologic exam to assess consciousness and mentation, an ECG to evaluate cardiac rhythm, and an evaluation of the abdomen, including abdominocentesis to assess bowel, bladder, and spleen integrity. As these evaluations are occurring, another member of the team should draw blood for a complete CBC and serum chemistry. An IV catheter should be prepared and placed as soon as possible. Once these tasks have been completed, other tests (e.g., thoracic radiographs, abdominal ultrasound) may proceed as needed.

Patient Stabilization and Preparation for Anesthesia

Life-threatening abnormalities should be addressed immediately. For example, hemorrhage should be controlled, nonventilatory patients should be intubated and ventilated with supplemental oxygen, and patients with cardiac compromise should receive appropriate treatment (e.g., CPR for cardiac arrest, antiarrhythmic therapy for arrhythmias). Once these crises have been controlled, the stabilization and preparation for anesthesia may begin. Obviously, patients with active hemorrhage that cannot be controlled should be anesthetized immediately. All other patients should be stabilized prior to anesthesia. Anesthetizing patients prior to stabilization is totally counterproductive as the increased anesthetic risk will increase the likelihood of anesthesia-related morbidity and mortality. Stabilization includes appropriate fluid therapy with necessary electrolytes and acid-base components, assessment of pain, administration of support drugs like dobutamine or lidocaine, administration of oxygen, and attention to the overall well-being of the patient.

Aggressive fluid therapy should be instituted as soon as possible. Crystalloids, synthetic colloids, hypertonic saline, and blood products are all appropriate choices depending on the circumstances. Fluid administration should be guided by serial monitoring of arterial blood pressure, CVP, PCV, and total protein/serum albumin concentrations and by the presenting patient complaint. Patients with active hemorrhage should not receive hypertonic saline, and glucose-containing solutions are not recommended for patients with head trauma.

Critical patients are extremely likely to be hypoxemic. Causes of hypoxemia are numerous and include (1) decreased ventilation due to inability to move the thorax or muscles of ventilation (e.g., thoracic trauma, diaphragmatic hernia, muscle weakness); (2) decreased ventilation due to the inability to mount a ventilatory response (e.g., head trauma); (3) $\dot{V}/\dot{Q}$ mismatch; (4) poor perfusion of tissues secondary to hypovolemia, hypotension, or sludging of blood; and (5) increased metabolic demand. In most patients, a combination of these issues will be present. Thus, supplemental oxygen should be supplied to all critical and traumatized patients, and the ability to ventilate absolutely must be assessed (Fig. 13.5).

Severe pain may cause a myriad of problems (see Table 13.2) that may contribute to the demise of the

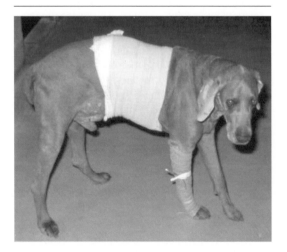

Figure 13.5. Patient with obvious signs of pain following thoracic trauma. Ventilation was impaired (as evidenced by low PaO_2 and high $PaCO_2$ on arterial blood gas analysis) prior to analgesia but all ventilatory parameters returned to normal within 20 minutes of the administration of 0.3 mg/kg, IM morphine.

patient. Patients with limited physiologic reserve, such as traumatized or critically ill patients, are limited in their ability to respond to the physiologic changes produced by pain and, thus, have the greatest need for analgesic therapy. A low dose of an opioid is appropriate in almost every patient and may aid in diagnostic evaluation of the patient. As the clinical signs associated with pain are relieved, the clinical signs associated with other problems become apparent. Figure 13.5 shows a patient following thoracic trauma with obvious signs of pain. Pain in this patient caused impaired ventilation, but alleviation of the pain (0.3 mg/kg morphine IM) allowed the patient to ventilate and improved the arterial blood gas profile. Local anesthetic blockade is also appropriate in almost every patient, and this class of drugs should be used whenever possible. Some examples of the use of local anesthetic blockade in traumatized patients include intercostal blocks for chest tube placement and oral blocks for facial trauma; CRIs are appropriate in most patients, and choices for CRI include opioids (e.g., fentanyl or morphine), ketamine, and lidocaine. NSAIDs are generally not used until the patient is stable and the serum chemistry has been evaluated.

Ancillary support drugs are often necessary in critical and traumatized patients. Tissue perfusion must be supported and patients that are still hypotensive (mean arterial pressure less than 80 mm Hg) following fluid resuscitation should receive a positive inotropic agent (e.g., dopamine or dobutamine). Antiarrhythmic agents, antibiotics, and other drugs should be administered as needed.

Some complications may not appear at admission but may manifest after stabilization begins (e.g., hemorrhage may increase as perfusion pressure is improved) and some may not manifest for several days (e.g., sepsis). Thus, traumatized and critically ill patients may require vigilant monitoring and support for days to weeks.

Patient Monitoring and Support

Continuous monitoring of this group of patients is absolutely critical. In addition to the monitoring techniques and tools described in Table 13.4, patients with trauma or shock may require further monitoring specific to the organ systems affected. For example, continual evaluation and support of breathing are critical in patients with head trauma or thoracic trauma; serial glucose and acid-base measurements may be required in patients with shock; and all patients require a continuous ECG, blood pressure, and oxygen saturation monitor. An $ETCO_2$ is highly recommended in all intubated patients and required for patients with ventilatory dysfunction.

Anesthesia

No drugs are absolutely contraindicated in trauma or shock patients, but drug dosage should be reduced in most patients and drug choice should be based on underlying abnormalities.

PREMEDICANTS

Patients that are extremely debilitated generally do not require premedicants for sedation; however, a low dose of an opioid is almost always recommended to alleviate pain and to allow a decreased dosage of induction and maintenance drugs. Opioid agonists (e.g., oxymorphone, morphine, fentanyl), agonist-antagonists (e.g., butorphanol), and partial agonists (buprenorphine) cause minimal depression of the cardiovascular system when used in low doses. Benzodiazepines (e.g., diazepam, midazolam) cause minimal cardiovascular depression and may be added to the opioids to increase the degree of sedation. The hypotension produced by acepromazine and the profound cardiovascular changes caused by α_2-agonists are not well tolerated in critical patients and these drugs are not recommended. Anticholinergics are rarely needed and should not be used indiscriminately.

INDUCTION AGENTS

In critical patients, vomiting is fairly common and hypoventilation is very common, so induction to anesthesia should occur rapidly and efficiently and intubation should be performed immediately to prevent aspiration and ensure a patent airway. Because induction of anesthesia using inhalant anesthetic agents delivered by a mask occurs relatively slowly, this technique is not recommended for induction in patients in which rapid intubation is necessary. Also, the stress and excitement associated with struggling during mask induction should absolutely be avoided.

Propofol is a good choice for induction in traumatized patients, but preoperative fluid therapy may be required to offset the propofol-induced cardiovascular depression. Ketamine mediates improvement in cardiovascular function through stimulation of the SNS. In patients with mild to moderate disease or trauma, the SNS is probably not impaired and ketamine is a good choice. In patients with severe disease or trauma, the SNS is likely to be impaired and the cardiac depressant effects of ketamine may be pronounced. Ketamine may cause an increase in cerebral blood flow and accentuate seizure activity; thus, it is not the best choice for patients with head trauma or seizures. Etomidate is a good choice for most patients, although the etomidate-mediated adrenocortical suppression may be detrimental in severely compromised patients. The significance of this suppression is unknown.

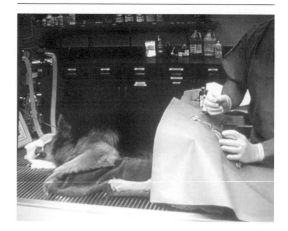

Figure 13.6. Epidural analgesia in a dog following a cesarean section. Although epidurals are generally administered prior to surgery, administration following delivery of the fetuses and skin closure is acceptable. Epidural analgesia provides prolonged pain relief with minimal to no systemic uptake of drugs and no uptake of drug by the nursing puppies.

MAINTENANCE DRUGS

Low-dose isoflurane and sevoflurane are appropriate for maintenance of anesthesia in critical patients. Patients often have little to no physiologic reserve, especially if emergency surgery is necessary and patients must be anesthetized before they are fully stabilized. Concentration of the inhalant anesthetic agents is especially critical, and analgesia should be used to reduce the dosage of inhalant anesthetic agents. A fentanyl CRI with minimal supplemental inhalant gas is a safe and effective technique in these patients. Local anesthetic agents should be used whenever possible. An epidural is also appropriate if the patient is not septic; the patient should be stabilized and fluid loaded prior to the epidural (Fig. 13.6).

Fluids and support drugs should be continued throughout anesthesia and the recovery period. In fact, because of ongoing complications, support and monitoring may need to continue for several days.

Patients in Shock

Patients who have suffered profound trauma or who are critically ill are at risk for developing shock. Types of shock include hemorrhagic, nonhemorrhagic, neurogenic, anaphylactic, and septic. Obviously, hemorrhagic shock occurs with blood loss. Nonhemorrhagic shock occurs with loss of plasma, as with severe burns or intestinal obstruction with loss of plasma into the gastrointestinal tract. No fluid loss occurs in neurogenic shock, but the vasculature loses all tone and the vascular capacity expands to the point that a normal blood volume

cannot maintain adequate venous return and cardiac output. This may occur with acute transection of the spinal cord or with blockade of the peripheral SNS following epidural or spinal administration of a local anesthetic agent in a volume-depleted patient. Anaphylactic shock also causes a loss of vascular tone and abnormalities in blood distribution. Septic shock occurs secondary to overwhelming endotoxemia (i.e., from release of endotoxins from ischemic bowel) or bacteremia (e.g., from extensive infections). Hemorrhagic and neurogenic shock are the most commonly encountered types of shock in trauma patients, whereas septic and nonhemorrhagic shock are more common in critically ill patients.

Ultimately, all types of shock result in inadequate tissue perfusion with subsequent tissue oxygen debt, and the probability of recovery is related to the magnitude of the oxygen debt (Carroll 2003). In order to compensate for the oxygen debt, a hypermetabolic state generally develops as the patient is resuscitated. Interestingly, in humans suffering from shock, return of hemodynamic variables to normal may still be associated with death. Instead, in one study of patients that survived, restoration of blood volume to 16% to 18% in excess of normal values and cardiac index that increased 50% were required to meet the increased metabolic demand of fever and tissue repair in post-trauma and post-operative patients (Shoemaker 1986).

Inadequate resuscitation, another major insult (anesthesia and surgery), or several small insults during the period of shock or even during the hyper-metabolic period may result in death (Carroll 2003).

Aggressive fluid therapy should start as soon as the patient is admitted to the hospital. As with other patients, choice of fluid will depend on the underlying reason for shock and overall patient condition. Crystalloids, colloids, and blood products are all appropriate choices. Support of cardiovascular function will almost always include administration of positive inotropic agents like dopamine and dobutamine. Vasoactive drugs, like phenylephrine or vasopressin, may be needed in forms of shock characterized by excessive vasodilation. Hypoglycemia and hypokalemia are common sequelae of shock. Dextrose (2.5% or 5% IV) in saline or lactated Ringer's saline may be used as maintenance fluids in hypoglycemic patients, and a bolus of dextrose (2 to 4 ml/kg of 50% dextrose or 20 ml/kg of 10% dextrose IV) may be administered in an emergency (Carroll 2003). The need for potassium replacement therapy prior to anesthesia is controversial (Carroll 2003). There are two excellent reviews of support and stabilization of patients in shock (Carroll 2003; Martin 1996).

Patients in shock should not be anesthetized.

ANESTHESIA FOR CESAREAN SECTION

Anesthesia of pregnant patients, whether for cesarean section or for surgeries unrelated to the pregnancy, may be complicated by the physiologic effects of pregnancy and by the fact that fetal health will be affected by anesthesia and the physiologic changes that occur during anesthesia. Pregnancy causes a variety of physiologic changes that are discussed below and summarized in Table 13.10. Three thorough reviews of the changes during pregnancy and anesthesia of the pregnant patient are available (Lumb and Jones 1996; Moon 2003; Ryan and Wagner 2006a, 2006b).

Most of the information that we have regarding the effects of pregnancy is extrapolated from data obtained in pregnant humans and sheep. However, because of the similarity of the mammalian organ systems across species, the same changes that occur in women and ewes are expected to occur in bitches and queens.

Physiology of Pregnancy

As with neonatal and geriatric patients, pregnant patients are deemed to be more "sensitive" to the effects of anesthetic drugs. This "sensitivity" may be due to increased concentrations of progesterone and endorphins, which appear to cause a decreased need for inhalant and local anesthetic agents. In pregnant ewes and humans, the concentration of inhalant gas required for maintenance of anesthesia is drastically reduced (e.g., isoflurane reduction in pregnant ewes is 40%; Palahniuk et al. 1974). The decreased need for local anesthetic agents is apparent in both local and regional (i.e., epidural or spinal) blocks and may decrease the total required dose by as much as one third of that necessary for block in nonpregnant patients (Lumb and Jones 1996).

Pregnant patients have a high metabolic rate with subsequent high oxygen consumption (due to the needs of the developing fetus and the increased uptake in the placenta, uterine muscle, and mammary tissue), necessitating alveolar ventilation that is much greater than that in nonpregnant patients. Because of the increased alveolar ventilation, anesthetic induction with inhalant anesthetic agents may occur very quickly; mask inductions are not recommended. The pressure of the gravid uterus causes a decrease in the FRC, which decreases ventilatory reserve and makes the patient more susceptible to hypoxemia and hypercapnia with even minimal decreases in ventilation. Also, the blood volume increases by approximately 40% in the pregnant patient but plasma volume increases more than red cell mass, resulting in a decreased hemoglobin concentration. These factors combine to make the pregnant patient susceptible to hypoxemia and, because the maternal blood supplies all of the fetal oxygen during pregnancy, these factors increase the likelihood of fetal hypoxemia as well. Any increase in oxygen consumption (e.g., labor or struggling and excitement) or decrease in oxygen delivery (e.g., during the administration of anesthetic drugs) may cause an oxygen debt and desaturation in the pregnant patient. Thus, pregnant patients require pre-oxygenation prior to anesthesia and rapid intubation *without struggling*, followed by ventilatory support during the anesthetic period.

Table 13.10. Unique physiologic characteristics of pregnant patients that may affect anesthesia.

Physiologic characteristic	Effect on anesthesia
General characteristics 　Increased concentration of progesterone and endorphins	Decreased need for inhalant anesthetic agents, decrease vaporizer settings and monitor carefully.
Respiratory system 　Increased alveolar ventilation 　Decreased FRC 　Increased oxygen consumption	Decreased respiratory reserve, both oxygen and ventilatory support are required for most patients. Mask induction occurs extremely quickly, induction must be closely supervised.
Cardiovascular system 　Increased heart rate 　Increased stroke volume 　Increased cardiac output 　Increased cardiac work 　Decreased cardiac reserve 　Increased blood volume (more plasma than cells)	Decreased cardiac reserve, cardiovascular system must be supported with IV fluids. Decreased RBCs = lower hemoglobin concentration and this may contribute to hypoxemia, support with oxygen.
Other characteristics 　Delayed gastric emptying 　Increased gastric acid	Regurgitation is common and aspiration can occur, must intubate as quickly as possible following induction to anesthesia
Fetal concerns 　Drugs that cross the BBB to anesthetize the dam or queen also cross the placenta 　The fetus is extremely sensitive to hypovolemia and hypoxia	Drug dosages should be minimal and very short acting or reversible drugs are preferred. Support of the maternal CV and respiratory systems are crucial for fetal health; delivery of the fetus should occur as rapidly as possible to minimize fetal exposure to anesthetic agents

FRC, functional residual capacity; RBC, red blood cell; BBB, blood-brain barrier; CV, cardiovascular.

HR, SV, cardiac output, and cardiac work all increase and cardiac reserve decreases during pregnancy. Pain and stress, like the stress of labor, put a further burden on the cardiovascular system. Also, hypotension generally evokes only a minimal vasomotor and baroreceptor response in pregnant patients.

In the pregnant patient, gastric emptying is delayed (due to physical displacement of the stomach by the gravid uterus, decreased gastric motility, and increased serum progesterone), intragastric pressure is increased and lower esophageal sphincter tone is decreased. Thus, regurgitation is common and may be complicated by aspiration. Unfortunately, gastric acid secretion is high in the pregnant patient, making aspiration extremely dangerous. Rapid induction to anesthesia, rapid intubation, and maintenance of a protected airway

throughout the anesthetic period and into recovery are critical in these patients.

Fetal Considerations

Uterine blood is not autoregulated; thus, uterine and fetal blood supply, with subsequent fetal oxygen delivery, is directly dependent on arterial perfusion pressure and is indirectly related to uterine vascular resistance. Because almost all anesthetic drugs contribute to hypotension and hypoventilation, anesthesia may cause fetal hypoxia if the bitch/queen is not aggressively supported with fluids and oxygen. Furthermore, any stress (e.g., pain, fear, excitement) may cause catecholamine release, resulting in vasoconstriction and a subsequent decrease in uterine blood flow. Thus, in order to maximize fetal viability, maternal needs, including circulating blood volume, ventilatory capacity, and stress, must be addressed.

Patient Assessment

Because cesarean sections often present as emergencies, thorough patient assessment may not be possible. However, all of the components of patient assessment listed in Table 13.3 should be considered and a rapid physical exam with a focus on hydration and cardiovascular and respiratory function is required. The overall state of the bitch/queen should be determined and the owner should be queried as to the duration of labor. The longer the patient has been in labor, the more compromised both the mother and the puppies/kittens will be. If the cesarean section is an elective procedure, all of the components of Table 13.3, including ECG analysis and blood pressure measurement, should be used.

Patient Preparation for Anesthesia

Whether the patient is presented for an elective or an emergency cesarean section, IV fluids should be started and the patient should be preoxygenated. The choice of fluids depends on the underlying health status of the patient but crystalloids are generally appropriate. All patient preparation (e.g., clipping and scrubbing of the surgical site) should occur prior to anesthesia (and while on oxygen) if at all possible, but struggling should be avoided. An ECG and blood pressure monitor should be connected to the patient prior to or immediately after induction to anesthesia.

Patient Monitoring and Support

All of the monitoring techniques and tools described in Table 13.4 should be used with an emphasis on cardiovascular and respiratory monitoring and support. IV fluids are required to combat the hypotensive effects of anesthetic drugs and to ensure adequate blood flow to the fetus. Interestingly, however, only 53% of dogs presented for cesarean in the United States and Canada receive IV fluids (Moon 2000). Blood pressure should be monitored in all patients.

Because hypoxemia is common and the weight of the gravid uterus against the diaphragm makes breathing difficult, ventilation should be supported with limited IPPV or intermittent (every 5 to 15 minutes) "sighs." Hyperventilation is no better than hypoventilation as hyperventilation may cause alkalosis, which may cause uterine vascular resis-

tance to increase with a subsequent decrease in fetal blood flow. Also, IPPV must be applied carefully because aggressive application of positive pressure in the thorax may cause collapse of the vena cava and decreased blood return to the heart and, subsequently, decreased cardiac output (and decreased fetal blood flow). Both the pulse oximeter and the ETCO$_2$ monitor should be used, although the pressure on the diaphragm and lungs from the gravid uterus may create a $\dot{V}/\dot{Q}$ mismatch that may limit the accuracy of the ETCO$_2$ monitor.

> The fetus is extremely sensitive to hypovolemia, and hypoxemia and aggressive support of maternal ventilation and circulation is necessary for fetal survival.

Anesthesia and Analgesia

There are two goals for successful anesthesia for cesarean section: (1) speed (e.g., rapid induction, rapid intubation, and rapid removal of the fetuses) and (2) low dosages of all anesthetic drugs. The second goal is best met by using balanced or multimodal anesthesia and analgesia. However, it is important to remember that all drugs administered to the bitch/queen will not only indirectly affect the fetus (through maternal hypotension and hypoventilation) but also directly affect the fetus because the fetus will receive the same drugs that the mother receives.

> All drugs that cross the blood-brain barrier to cause anesthesia in the bitch or queen will also cross the placental barrier and affect the fetus.

Local/regional anesthetic techniques work in women and in some large animal species (e.g., ruminants) but are not generally recommended as a sole anesthetic technique in small animals unless the patient is extremely calm or moribund. Otherwise, the patient may resist restraint and, as previously stated, the ensuing fear or excitement will cause catecholamine release with subsequent uterine vasoconstriction and a decreased delivery of oxygenated blood to the fetus.

A judicious dose of a premedicant is often recommended in order to (1) decrease the struggling, excitement, and pain that may accompany anesthesia and surgery and (2) decrease the amount of induction and inhalant anesthetic drugs required to obtain and maintain anesthesia. Opioids are recommended because the opioid effect may be reversed in the fetus, if necessary. A low-dose of pure μ-agonists may be administered (e.g., 0.3 mg/kg morphine or 0.1 mg/kg hydromorphone) and the effects of these drugs may be easily reversed with a drop of naloxone applied under the tongue of the fetus. Alternatively, buprenorphine (0.01 to 0.02 mg/kg IM) may be administered. Buprenorphine is tightly bound to the opioid receptors and is difficult to reverse, but little to no sedation occurs with this drug and reversal is rarely necessary. The use of opioids preoperatively is not associated with decreased fetal survival (Moon 2000). Finally, if bradycardia-mediated hypotension occurs secondary to opioid administration (or any other cause), atropine should be administered because this drug crosses the placental barrier and reaches the fetus, whereas glycopyrrolate does not. If drug-induced bradycardia is present in the mother, it is likely also present in the fetus.

> The use of opioids preoperatively is not associated with decreased fetal survival.

Because it is cleared quickly and by many routes, propofol is generally the best choice for induction to anesthesia. However, propofol does cause cardiovascular depression and is not ideal for seriously compromised bitches/queens. Ketamine/valium has been used successfully but, due to the relatively long duration of the combination, some fetal depression may occur. Both sevoflurane and isoflurane are excellent choices for maintenance of anesthesia.

Maternal analgesia absolutely must be addressed in some fashion. If opioids were not administered preoperatively, a dose of opioids should be administered as soon as the puppies or kittens are delivered. A line block of local anesthetic at the surgery site is extremely quick, easy, and inexpensive and is highly recommended for all patients. Epidural analgesia is highly effective and will provide prolonged analgesia for the mother. Preemptive epidural administration is recommended, but the epidural may be administered after skin closure and this will still provide the mother with extended duration analgesia postoperatively.

Fetal Survival and Care

Unfortunately, puppies delivered by cesarean section have an initial mortality rate much higher than that of puppies delivered by natural birth (8% versus 2.2%, respectively; Moon 2003). Clearly, maternal issues (including maternal health and time in labor) and medical issues (including time under anesthesia and support during anesthesia) factor strongly into the high mortality rate. However, neonatal support and resuscitation following birth also play a role. The neonate must be dried and warmed immediately after birth, and the respiratory and cardiovascular systems must be immediately assessed and supported. See Table 13.11 for an overview of neonatal support and resuscitation.

Table 13.11. Steps for neonatal resuscitation following cesarean section.

General actions	1. Make sure neonate is warm and dry.
	2. Remove fetal membranes from nose and swab or suction any fluid in nostrils.
	3. Gently stimulate and rub the neonate until it appears awake and strong.
Respiratory	1. Gentle stimulation and rubbing often stimulates breathing.
	2. If neonate is not breathing or breathing is weak, administer oxygen. A dose doxapram may also be administered.
	3. If still not breathing or breathing is weak, utilize a tight fitting face mask and force oxygen into lungs by squeezing Ambu or rebreathing bag.
	4. If still not breathing or breathing is weak, intubate and ventilate.
Cardiovascular	1. Gentle stimulation and rubbing often stimulates circulation.
	2. If heart is not beating or beating weakly or slowly, initiate cardiac massage by gently compressing the thorax directly over the heart.
	3. If heart is still not beating or beating weakly or slowly, administer epinephrine.

SUMMARY FOR ANESTHESIA FOR PATIENTS WITH SPECIAL CONCERNS

Patients who are extremely compromised or who are very young or very old continue to be an ever-increasing part of the veterinarian's anesthetic caseload. These patients do not have the physiologic reserves that young, healthy adult patients have, and they generally require more intense monitoring and support before, during, and after anesthesia. In fact, monitoring and support are often more critical than the choice of anesthetic drugs, although a thorough knowledge of the physiologic effects of the drugs is important. It is no longer appropriate to think that safe anesthesia means recovering as many patients as we anesthetize. Hopefully, with information presented in this text, we may focus on what happens to the patient during the anesthetic period—which starts when the patient is admitted for anesthesia and does not end until the patient has returned to full consciousness and is free of pain.

ENDNOTES

1 Starling's law: the myocardial muscle will contract with greater force when it has been slightly stretched, as occurs during adequate cardiac filling (a simplified definition).
2 Some anesthesiologists argue that benzodiazepines contribute to hepatic encephalopathy because flumazenil may reverse hepatic coma from PSS.
3 Cats do not typically do well with tracheotomies/tracheostomies, so other options should be pursued.

REFERENCES

Baggot, J.D. 1992. Drug therapy in the neonatal animal. In *Principles of Drug Disposition in Domestic Animals: The Basis of Veterinary Clinical Pharmacology*, edited by J.D. Baggot, pp. 219–224. Philadelphia: W.B. Saunders.

Breazile, J.E. 1978. Neurologic and behavioral development in the puppy. *Vet Clin N Am Small Anim Pract* 8:31–45.

Carr, A.P. 2005. Inherited coagulopathies. In *Textbook of Veterinary Internal Medicine*, edited by S.J. Ettinger and E.C. Feldman, pp. 1929–1932. St. Louis: Elsevier.

Carroll, G.L. 2003. Anesthesia and analgesia for the trauma or shock patient. In *Textbook of Small Animal Surgery*, edited by D. Slatter, pp. 2538–2544. Philadelphia: W.B. Saunders.

Cohn, L.A., McCaw, D.L., Tate, D.J. et al. 2000. Assessment of five portable blood glucose meters, a point-of-care analyzer, and color test strips for measuring blood glucose concentration in dogs. *J Am Vet Med Assoc* 216(2):198–202.

Cote, E., and Ettinger, S.J. 2005. Electrocardiography and cardiac arrhythmias. In *Textbook of Veterinary Internal Medicine*, edited by S.J. Ettinger and E.C. Feldman, pp. 1040–1076. St. Louis: Elsevier.

Crowe, D.T. 2003. Supplemental oxygen therapy in critically ill or injured patients. *Vet Med* 98(11):935–953.

Dodam, J.R. 2003. Hepatic and gastrointestinal surgery. In *Textbook of Small Animal Surgery*, edited by D. Slatter, pp. 2579–2585. Philadelphia: W.B. Saunders.

Dodman, N.H., Seeler, D.C., and Court, M.H. 1984. Aging changes in the geriatric dog and their impact on anesthesia. *Compend Contin Ed Pract Vet* 6:1106–1112.

Dyson, D.H., Maxie, G.M., and Schnurr, D. 1998. Morbidity and mortality associated with anesthetic management in small animal veterinary practice in Ontario. *J Am Anim Hosp Assoc* 34:325–335.

Gaynor, J.S., Dunlop, C.I., Wagner, A.E., et al. 1999. Complications and mortality associated with anesthesia in dogs and cats. *J Am Anim Hosp Assoc* 35:13–17.

Haggstrom, J., Kvart, C., and Pedersen, H.D. 2005. Acquired valvular disease. In *Textbook of Veterinary Internal Medicine*, edited by S.J. Ettinger and E.C. Feldman, pp. 1022–1039. St. Louis: Elsevier.

Herrtage, M.E. 2005. Hypoadrenocorticism. In *Textbook of Veterinary Internal Medicine*, edited by S.J. Ettinger and E.C. Feldman, pp. 1612–1621. St. Louis: Elsevier.

Kittleson, M.D. 2005. Feline myocardial disease. In *Textbook of Veterinary Internal Medicine*, edited by S.J. Ettinger and E.C. Feldman, pp. 1082–1103. St. Louis: Elsevier.

Konhilas, J.P., Irving, T.C., and de Tombe, P.P. 2002. Frank-Starling law of the heart and the cellular mechanisms of length-dependent activation. *Pflugers Arch Eur J Physiol* 446:305–310.

Mayson, K.V., Beestra, J.E., and Choi, P.T. 2005. The incidence of postoperative complications in the PACU. *Can J Anesth* 52(S1):A62.

McMurphy, R. 2003. Cardiovascular system. In *Textbook of Small Animal Surgery*, edited by D. Slatter, pp. 2572–2578. Philadelphia: W.B. Saunders.

McNiel, E., and Husbands, B.D. 2005. Pheochromocytoma. In *Textbook of Veterinary Internal Medicine*, edited by S.J. Ettinger and E.C. Feldman, pp. 1632–1645. St. Louis: Elsevier.

Meurs, K.M. 2005. Primary myocardial disease in the dog. In *Textbook of Veterinary Internal Medicine*, edited by S.J. Ettinger and E.C. Feldman, pp. 1077–1081. St. Louis: Elsevier.

Moon, P.F., Erb, H.N., Ludders, J.W., et al. 2000. Perioperative risk factors for puppies delivered by cesarean section in the United States and Canada. *J Am Anim Hosp Assoc* 36:359–368.

Mooney, C.T. 2005. Hyperthyroidism. In *Textbook of Veterinary Internal Medicine*, edited by S.J. Ettinger and E.C. Feldman, pp. 1544–1559. St. Louis: Elsevier.

Moon-Massatt, P.F. 2003. Cesarean section. In *Textbook of Small Animal Surgery*, edited by D. Slatter, pp. 2597–2602. Philadelphia: W.B. Saunders.

Muir, W.W. 1998. Anesthesia for dogs and cats with cardiovascular disease. *Compend Cont Educ Pract Vet* 20(4):473–484.

Muir, W.W., Ford, J.L., Karpa, G.E., et al. 1999. Effects of intramuscular administration of low doses of medetomidine and medetomidine-butorphanol in middle-aged and old dogs. *J Am Vet Med Assoc* 215(8):1116–1120.

Nelson, R.W. 2005. Diabetes mellitus. In *Textbook of Veterinary Internal Medicine*, edited by S.J. Ettinger and E.C. Feldman, pp. 1563–1591. St. Louis: Elsevier.

Ortega, T.M., Feldman, E.C., Nelson, R.W., et al. 1996. Systemic arterial blood pressure and urine protein/creatinine ratio in dogs with hyperadrenocorticism. *J Am Vet Med Assoc* 209:1724–1729.

Palahniuk, R.J., Shnider, S.M., and Eger, E.I. 1974. Pregnancy decreases the requirement for inhaled anesthetic agents. *Anesthesiology* 41(1):82–83.

Patterson, S.W., and Starling, E.H. 1914. On the mechanical factors which determine the output of the ventricles. *J Physiol* 48(5):357–379.

Peterson, M.E., Kintzer, P.P., Cavanagh, P.G., et al.

1983. Feline hyperthyroidism: Pretreatment clinical and laboratory evaluation of 131 cases. *J Am Vet Med Assoc* 183(1):103–110.

Reusch, C.E. 2005. Hyperadrenocorticism. In *Textbook of Veterinary Internal Medicine*, edited by S.J. Ettinger and E.C. Feldman, pp. 1592–1611. St. Louis: Elsevier.

Robertson, S.A. 2003. Endocrine system. In *Textbook of Small Animal Surgery*, edited by D. Slatter, pp. 2586–2592. Philadelphia: W.B. Saunders.

Robinson, E.P. 1983. Anesthesia of pediatric patients. *Comp Cont Educ Pract Vet* 5:1004–1011.

Roizen, M.F. 2000. Anesthetic implications of concurrent diseases. In *Anesthesia*, edited by R.D. Miller, 5th ed., pp. 903–1016. New York: Churchill Livingstone.

Sessler, D.I. 2002. Temperature disturbances. In *Pediatric Anesthesia*, edited by G.A. Gregory, 4th ed., pp. 53–69. Philadelphia: Churchill Livingstone.

Shoemaker, W.C., and Fleming, A.W. 1986. Resuscitation of the trauma patient: Restoration of hemodynamic functions using clinical algorithms. *Ann Emerg Med* 15:1437–1444.

Stoelting, R.K. 1999. In *Pharmacology and Physiology in Anesthetic Practice*. Philadelphia: Lippincott Williams and Wilkins.

Tarrac, S.E. 2006. A description of intraoperative and postanesthesia complication rates. *J Perianesth Nursing* 21(2):88–96.

Thurmon, J.C., Tranquilli, W.J., and Benson, G.J. 1996. Cesarean section patients. In *Veterinary Anesthesia*, edited by Lumb and Jones, 3rd ed., pp. 818–828. Baltimore: Williams and Wilkins.

Webster, C.R.L. 2005. History, clinical signs, and physical findings in hepatobiliary disease. In *Textbook of Veterinary Internal Medicine*, edited by S.J. Ettinger and E.C. Feldman, pp. 1422–1434. St. Louis: Elsevier.

Chapter 14
Physical Medicine and Its Role in Recovery

M.A. Crist

Physical medicine (PM) encompasses acupuncture, chiropractic care, massage, physical rehabilitation (e.g., stretching, exercise, heat, and cryotherapy), nutraceuticals, and herbology. PM, especially during recovery, is increasingly used. Many practitioners of PM are grounded in Western medicine, so these modalities are adjunctive treatments to the pharmacologic and surgical methods currently available. As with Western medicine, there are no guarantees of treatment success.

This introduction to complementary and alternative medicine is restricted to acupuncture, physical rehabilitation, nutraceuticals, and herbology. These modalities may enhance perioperative pain management and improve outcome in surgical patients by boosting return to function. There are additional resources for treatment alternatives for the management of chronic pain (Schoen 2001). The importance of nutrition in health and well-being is well documented (Schoen and Wynn 1998), but is also outside the scope of this work.

> Check AVMA guidelines and local regulations before practicing any PM modality.

A committee of the American Veterinary Medical Association (AVMA) determines guidelines for veterinarians practicing acupuncture and other forms of alternative and complementary veterinary medicine included in PM. These guidelines are posted on the AVMA Website, www.avma.com. The interpretation and enforcement of any guidelines regarding PM are generally left to the state.[1] These guidelines and regulations are designed to protect the public from charlatanry and the veterinarian from doing harm (potential litigation).

Veterinarians are encouraged to check their state regulations regarding the practice of PM. Most PM modalities will require additional training. Certification is offered in many areas (e.g., rehabilitation, acupuncture, massage, herbology).

> Additional training is recommended before undertaking a PM modality.

Before beginning PM, you should have an accurate diagnosis, a compliant patient, and owners committed to follow-up care. The owners should be involved in setting realist goals for therapy. There should be continual periodic evaluation for the level of discomfort and the appropriateness of the therapy. Good nursing care will always be paramount.

ACUPUNCTURE

In traditional Chinese veterinary medicine (TCVM), the term acupoint or acupuncture point refers to a depression in the skin where an acupuncture needle is inserted to influence an internal organ or process. The acupuncture point communicates with one or more internal organs by way of a meridian. In morphologic studies, investigators have observed either high densities of nerve trunks, neural terminals, or vascular networks in the subcutaneous (SQ) tissue at or near the acupuncture site. Pain management and analgesia provided by acupuncture are believed to result from activation of these acupuncture points by needles inserted into cutaneous areas with high concentrations of nerve endings, capillaries, venules, and mast cells, which have a lower electrical resistance than the surrounding areas (Jaggar 2000; Skarda 2002).

Acupuncture points are found along the pathways of major peripheral nerves. In traditional Chinese medicine (TCM), the pathways (meridians) are a complex network of major channels that connect all parts of the body. The channels include 12 major meridians (e.g., liver, heart, spleen, lung, kidney, pericardium, gallbladder, small intestine, stomach, large intestine, bladder, triple heater), eight extra channels, and the unpaired conception vessel (CV) and governing vessel (GV) channels. *Qi* (pronounced *ché*) is the vital energy that flows through these meridians and nourishes their respective organs.

When the structures located beneath the acupuncture point are stimulated by an acupuncture needle,[2] pathophysiologic changes are communicated through the point and the meridian to the respective organs. This traditional view of interaction between the related acupuncture points resembles the Western medical concept of viscerosomatic and somatovisceral reflexes, as well as trigger point reaction associated with myofascial and visceral pain.

The effects of acupuncture vary from patient to patient. Beneficial effects from acupuncture include the initial vascular effects, which are seconds of local vasoconstriction followed by a prolonged vasodilatory phase that can last for up to 2 weeks. Other benefits from acupuncture are decreased pain, increased perfusion to the area, enhanced humoral immunity, increased white blood cell (WBC) counts, increased phagocytic activity, and increased antibody levels, and analgesia. Acupuncture treatments are usually given weekly or biweekly for approximately six sessions to determine efficacy. During dry needle acupuncture therapy, the needles should remain in the patient for about 10 to 20 minutes, but treatment time varies from patient to patient. Several other types of acupuncture therapy (e.g., aquapuncture, moxibustion, electrostimulation acupuncture, laser therapy, gold bead implantation) are available. The acupuncture sessions may be combined with other treatments, both conventional and complementary, to speed healing, improve function and quality of life, alleviate pain, and improve the human–animal bond.

Aquapuncture

Aquapuncture is the injection of a solution, such as vitamin B-12, into an acupuncture point. Advantages include minimal restraint and owner acceptance of aquapuncture because they are accustomed to seeing their pets receive injections. Other solutions used for aquapuncture are distilled water, electrolyte solutions antibiotics, herbal extracts, vaccines, steroidal, and nonsteroidal drugs (Altman 2001).

Acupressure

Acupressure is the technique of finger pressure applied to the patient's body at designated points or acupuncture points. Acupressure is not routinely used by veterinarians in practice; however, owners may be taught to use specific pressure points in the home setting to help during acupuncture therapy (Altman 2001). There are references (Snow and Zidonis 2000; Zidonis and Snow 1999) that may be available for owners to examine.

Electroacupuncture

The electrical stimulation of acupuncture points provides a stronger signal. It may induce analgesia and benefit recovery for high-risk neurologic and orthopedic surgical patients. Electrostimulation acupuncture is believed to be a good adjunct to traditional analgesics such as opioids, α_2-agonists and local anesthetics, and nonsteroidal antiinflammatory drugs. The role of electrostimulation in pain management is providing comfort to the patient, reducing the amounts of pain medications, and shortening the patient's recovery and hospitalization time (Skarda 2002).

The mechanisms of acupuncture and electrostimulation acupuncture analgesia are not thoroughly understood. Gate, humoral pain mechanisms, neurogenic pain mechanisms, specificity, and summation are several theories that have been hypothesized for acupuncture analgesia. Analgesic effects produced may result from different sites of the peripheral, spinal (the pain inhibition gates) and central (midbrain and hypothalamus) levels of activation of descending brain-based pain inhibition mechanisms (Skarda 2002).

PRECAUTIONS FOR ELECTROACUPUNCTURE

When performing electroacupuncture (Fig. 14.1), the animal should not be wet or placed on a metal table. The clips of the electrodes should be firmly attached to the needles, avoiding any entrapment of hair. The pair of electrodes should not cross the

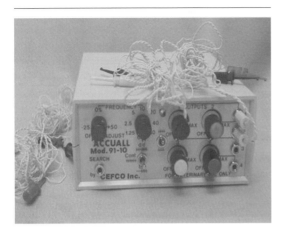

Figure 14.1. Electrostimulation unit.

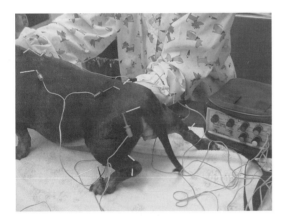

Figure 14.2. Animal with electrostimulation acupuncture and electrostimulation unit.

spinal cord but should remain on the same side and should not cross over the spine in the area of the heart to prevent interruption of cardiac function (Fig. 14.2). It is recommended that acupuncture or electrostimulation acupuncture should be performed in a quiet environment to keep the animal calm.

Complications From Acupuncture and Electroacupuncture

The risks of complications are very low with acupuncture and electrostimulation acupuncture if the techniques are followed properly. Complications may include bleeding, bruising, or hematoma at the acupuncture site, contact dermatitis, localized infection, pneumothorax, seizures, or, on rare occur-

rence, nerve damage. Some contraindications for electrostimulation acupuncture are acute (first 24 hours) traumatic intervertebral disc injury, pregnancy, localized dermatitis, neoplasia, severe blood coagulopathies, epilepsy or seizures, and undiagnosed pain conditions.

Supplies for Acupuncture and Electroacupuncture

Acupuncture needles used for treatment depend on the patient's size and acupuncture point location. Good-quality acupuncture needles are recommended such as Seirin (An Chi; M.E.D. Servi-Systems Canada Ltd., Stittsville, Ontario, Canada). If needles are to be reused, they should be sterilized at 120°C for 30 minutes at 15 pounds of pressure. For dry needling, size 3 needles may be used in dogs and size 5 may be used in cats. The needles are inserted at the acupuncture points to the correct depth by tapping or twirling. The needles used for electrostimulation acupuncture should be stainless steel and 34 gauge and 1 inch for a small dog or cat and 34 gauge and 1.5 inch for a medium-size or large dog. These needles are connected in pairs to the electrostimulator by alligator clips. The positive electrode is usually placed over the trigger point or area of pain and the negative electrode placed over the distal acupuncture point. Lower frequency is applied for 10 to 15 minutes for tonification, and the higher frequency is applied for approximately 10 to 15 minutes for sedation. Different types of electrostimulators are available in the market.

Laser Therapy

Laser, an acronym for Light Amplification by Stimulated Emission of Radiation (Fig. 14.3), is a beneficial adjunct to acupuncture therapy especially if needle placement is difficult or if the patient is fractious. The laser is placed on traditional Chinese acupuncture points on the patient in place of needles to stimulate the acupuncture point. The laser is a safe and painless form of acupuncture and requires minimal restraint for the animal. Efficacy of laser therapy is not yet documented.

Moxibustion

Moxibustion is the burning of an herb on a needle or above acupuncture points to warm the acupuncture point. The herb is usually Mugwart, a plant related to the chrysanthemum plant species. Indirect

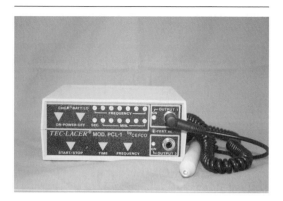

Figure 14.3. Laser unit.

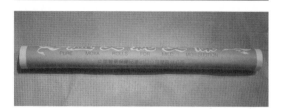

Figure 14.4. Moxa stick.

moxibustion is used in patients with chronic muscular problems or arthritic pain or joint pain caused by cold or dampness. The commercially available moxa stick is the most popular way to apply indirect moxibustion. These moxa sticks (Fig. 14.4) consist of a moxa powder or coarse moxa wool tightly wrapped into cylindrical sticks about 6 to 12 inches long. The end of the roll is ignited and held above the acupuncture point being treated about ½ inch to 1 inch or directly to the needle itself for about 3 to 15 minutes. Moxibustion functions to dispel dampness and cold, help regulate *Qi* and blood, and to help regulate the muscle channels.

PRECAUTIONS FOR MOXIBUSTION

Precautions should be taken with moxibustion. It is contraindicated in patients with febrile conditions, over the caudal back or abdomen of pregnant patients, around the face or mammary areas, or over large blood vessels, large tendons, or major creases in the skin. Be mindful in treating unconscious animals or animals with decreased sensory perception as to prevent burning. Never use moxibustion

with alcohol or in patients on oxygen therapy and care must also be taken with animals with long hair as it can ignite. The newer electroacupuncture machines are equipped with heating devices that can replace the moxa to produce warmth at the acupuncture points (Altman 2001).

Cold therapy has been applied to acupuncture points to provide local analgesia in acutely painful conditions or for trigger point therapy. It is contraindicated in chronically painful conditions.

Bead Implantation

Bead implantation is the technique of implanting sterile beads of gold, silver, or stainless steel into acupuncture points to provide long-term stimulation. The acupuncture points are surgically prepped and the implantation is performed surgically under general anesthesia. This procedure lasts indefinitely (Altman 2001).

> Bead implantation may appear as gunshot on radiographs.

VETERINARY REHABILITATION

Veterinary physical rehabilitation is the noninvasive rehabilitation of injuries in animals. This includes a spectrum of services such as exercise, stretching, electrical stimulation, magnetic field therapy, ultrasonic stimulation, rehabilitative routines, hydrotherapy, and hot and cold compresses. Adequate analgesia must be "on board" prior to rehabilitation. Patients resist treatment and progress slower if allowed to be painful.

> Judicious use of analgesics is required for successful postoperative rehabilitation.

Prior to treatment, the patient needs a complete physical exam by a licensed veterinarian. This should include a complete initial physical rehabilitation assessment and the evaluation recorded and well documented on a detailed physical rehabilitation form. The detailed physical rehabilitation assessment should include a physical exam with good palpation of the limbs and the trunk. A gait and posture analysis, range of motion of the joints, and a neurologic and orthopedic exam should also

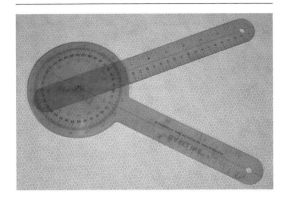

Figure 14.5. Goniometer, an instrument to measure range of motion.

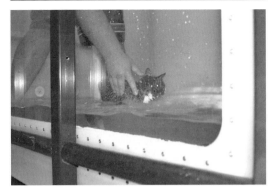

Figure 14.6. Cat on underwater treadmill. Courtesy of David Sessum.

be performed. A treatment plan can then be determined.

Shortly after surgery or trauma, rehabilitation may begin with passive range of motion (PROM). PROM is performed using an external force to move the joint without contraction of muscle within the range of motion. Both stretching and PROM may be utilized with each other to help improve and maintain joint range of motion (ROM) in postoperative patients or patients with chronic issues (Millis et al. 2004). These exercises help prevent adhesions, prevent further injury to ligaments, tendons, muscles and joints, and improve flexibility. The ROM is the full motion through which a joint may be moved and is commonly measured by a goniometer (Fig. 14.5). A goniometer is an instrument that measures angles of extension, flexion, abduction, and adduction of each joint. Muscles also have ROM, which is the distance that a muscle is able to shorten after it has maximally elongated.

The PROM exercises prevent immobilization and nonuse of the joints and muscles. The benefits of continuous passive ROM immediately after joint surgery (barring any contraindication), are decreased pain and improved recovery rate.

Active ROM exercises are active muscle contractions that cross a joint. In addition to the benefits of passive ROM, active ROM maintains elasticity and contractility.

Active assisted ROM is the next phase in rehabilitation and recovery of the progression of the joint motion. Active-assistive exercises are used in patients that need to overcome gravity. Active

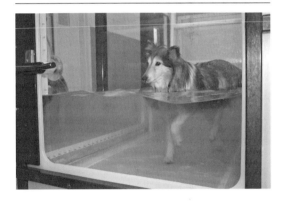

Figure 14.7. Dog on underwater treadmill. Courtesy of Wendy Greathouse.

assisted ROM is performed by placing the animal on an underwater treadmill (Figs. 14.6 and 14.7), ambulatory sling, or Swiss ball (Fig. 14.8) while assisting the animal to place the limb at the appropriate phase of the gait cycle (Millis et al. 2004).

Active resistive ROM exercises are begun when the animal is able to ambulate the affected limb; however, usual joint ROM is restricted during walking and trotting, to prevent the patients' joints from performing a complete ROM. Activities that encourage this active ROM are walking in sand, snow, tall grass, crawling through a tunnel, stair climbing, or walking over cavalettis at various heights (Fig. 14.9). Active resistive exercises restore strength, stamina, and coordination (Millis et al. 2004).

ROM exercises are often combined with various stretching techniques to aid in the role of recovery.

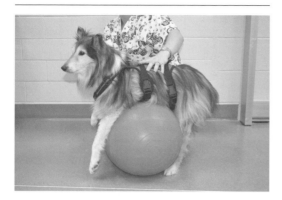

Figure 14.8. Patient using therapeutic ball.

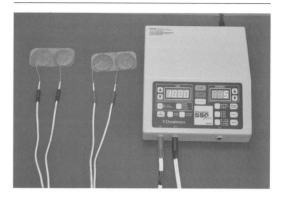

Figure 14.10. Transcutaneous electrical nerve stimulation unit.

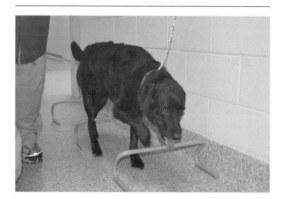

Figure 14.9. Dog going over cavalettis.

These various stretching techniques include static stretching and prolonged mechanical stretching. Heating the tissue before the stretching technique helps improve the effectiveness of the stretching (Millis et al. 2004). Also, therapeutic ultrasound is a good adjunct therapy to enhance the effectiveness of stretching by its ability to warm the tissues. Caution should be used not to force the joints into uncomfortable or painful positions beyond the ROM.

In summary, ROM and stretching exercises aid in the physical rehabilitation recovery program by stretching and realigning connective tissue (Millis et al. 2004).

ELECTRICAL STIMULATION

The application of electrical stimulation (ES) to particular peripheral nerves allows paretic and para-

lyzed muscles to make functional movements. This modality is commonly used in physical rehabilitation to aid in recovery by increasing ROM, increasing muscle strength, muscle reeducation, pain management, and accelerated wound management (Johnson and Levine 2004).

Commonly, the TENS (transcutaneous electrical nerve stimulation) (Fig. 14.10) unit has been used for pain management; EMSs (electrical muscle stimulators) and NMESs (neuromuscular electrical stimulators) are used to reeducate muscles, prevent muscle atrophy, improve joint movement, and decrease pain and muscle spasm associated with intervertebral disc disease. NMESs is a valuable part of postoperative rehabilitation where quick return of muscle mass is beneficial (Johnson and Levine 2004).

Thermal Modalities

Superficial thermal modalities, such as the application of heat or cold, have been used for pain management for decades. This can be accomplished by hot or cold packs, hot or cold whirlpools, infrared, ice massage, or cryokinetics. The application of therapy is most beneficial when applied immediately following trauma (surgical or accidental) to provide analgesia, decrease inflammation, hemostasis control, reduce bruising, and decrease muscle spasm.

Cryotherapy removes heat when applied to the body and results in analgesia by slowed nerve conduction and reduced inflammation by decreased enzyme activity. Various methods are available for cryotherapy application. One economical way to perform icing is by filling a Dixie cup three-fourths full of water and freezing it; the Dixie cup is peeled away as the ice melts. Frozen peas, because they are moldable, and commercial cool packs are also useful cryotherapy applications. Cryokinetics is the combination of motion with cryotherapy to facilitate the patient's rehabilitation exercise pain free.

Superficial heat is applied before initiating flexibility exercises. The benefits of applied heat cause vasodilation in the tissues to help with increased blood circulation, facilitate oxygenation, decrease joint stiffness, increase range of motion, increase enzyme activity, and decrease pain. One recommended method is moist heat. A wash cloth, hand towel, or towel depending on the area and size of the animal is held under warm or hot water. The towel is then placed on the affected area with a dry thick large towel placed over it to hold in the heat. Always be mindful to check the temperature of the skin area being treated to avoid thermal burns, especially in debilitated animals (Heinrichs 2004).

MASSAGE

Massage is incorporated into the recovery process for pain management, to increase mobility, reduce muscle soreness and spasms, and for painful trigger points (Sutton 2004).

Massage can have immediate results but usually requires regular treatment intervals to help with a particular issue. Massage therapy provides pain management and tension relief and helps the body release its natural pain relievers. It has a mechanical effect that relieves muscle tension by decreasing pain, relaxation, and easing decreased mobility. Circulation and lymphatic flow are also improved. It is believed that massage aids in the release of endorphins, activates neuropetides in the central nervous system, and stimulates the immune system, all of which have positive benefits on the patients.

Therapeutic indications for massage therapy can be used for animals suffering from chronic diseases such as osteoarthritis. Massage therapy in these patients increases blood flow to the tissues, relaxes, and decreases muscle tension and discomfort. Surgical candidates also benefit by maintaining muscle tone and condition, flexibility of joints, prevention of adhesion formation, and easing pain and discomfort. Chronic musculoskeletal issues can cause sec-

ondary changes from gait or postural abnormalities that lead to joint dysfunction and painful conditions. Massage can help with pain management in these conditions. Performance animals need their joints to move in all directions and at various impacts. The demands on these competition animals or "weekend warriors" are great. Massage therapy incorporated into a training program is greatly beneficial for the body to perform at peak levels and prevent fatigue, which can lead to injury and pain. Various massage therapies may be applied for relaxation, toning, and precompetition warm-up. During and after competition, massage aids the prevention of musculoskeletal fatigue and soreness.

Massage therapy should not be performed on animals with fever, acute inflammation of the particular area in recovery, infectious diseases, viral disease, or dermatitis and in patients in shock because of the lowered blood pressure that massage therapy produces (Sutton 2004).

DIET AND NUTRACEUTICALS

Therapeutic nutrition for the recovering patient improves healing by providing cells a better environment for regeneration and overcoming the stresses caused by acute or chronic disease or injury. Disease conditions have nutritional components that when managed can aid the healing process through natural means.

Most nutrients may act as therapeutic agents with few side effects. Although nutrients are "slow and gentle," they can potentiate metabolic processes and restore balance and function to the body. Sometimes nutrients may be combined with drug therapy to provide a synergistic effect and improve healing. Although, the risk of drug–nutrient interactions are usually few, the clinical practitioner should be mindful of any adverse interactions (Kendall 1998).

Supplemental nutrients are meant to work collectively with best medicine and practice. No established guidelines for therapeutic nutrition are available. Veterinarians should use high-quality products.

Vitamins and Minerals

Vitamins and minerals may function as therapeutic agents for recovery and pain management. At optimum concentrations vitamins and minerals can aid in the healing processes of the body.

VITAMIN A

Vitamin A is an antioxidant that will protect the body from damage and is beneficial for the immune system. Vitamin A is toxic at high levels so care should be used to prevent overdosing (Kendall 1998).

VITAMIN B

The B complex vitamins are needed for the immune system, energy production and growth. B complex vitamins are also beneficial for acute stress and infections (Kendall 1998).

VITAMIN C

Vitamin C has applications in both preventative and therapeutic health. Vitamin C is required for the production of collagen and can aid in treating degenerative joint disorders, intervertebral disc disease, spondylosis, and hip dysplasia. Vitamin C may also reduce the risk of damage to muscle cells caused by hypoxia and free radicals (Kendall 1998).

VITAMIN E

Vitamin E is an antioxidant that helps prevent inflammatory conditions, myopathies, skin diseases, and cancer. It also enhances muscle strength and endurance in working animals and has been shown to increase disease resistance. Vitamin E is beneficial in treating some occurrences of rhabdomyolysis and nutritional myopathies (Kendall 1998).

Essential and trace minerals improve the health and well-being of cats and dogs by reducing inflammation and enhancing appetite and physical activity in older animals.

Essential amino acids have therapeutic functions in the production of enzymes, hormones, immunoglobulins, neurotransmitters, and proteins found in muscles, tendons, hair, and skin. Supplementation with the branched chain amino acids glutamine, isoleucine, leucine, and valine may help the animal maintain muscle mass during rehabilitation and recovery. Although not essential to protein production, dimethylglycine, glutamine, L-carnitine, and taurine are also beneficial in recovery (Kendall 1998).

DIMETHYLGLYCINE

Dimethylglycine (DMG) has been used in the animal industry to increase performance and enhance the recovery period. It improves the immune response in animals by boosting cell mediated and humoral immunity, enhancing muscle metabolism and oxygen usage, and preventing lactic acid accumulation. Interferon production is enhanced by DMG. When used with other combination therapies, DMG decreased the occurrence of arthritis by reversing some of the inflammatory conditions (Kendall 1998).

GLUTAMINE

Glutamine may be a beneficial supplement to reduce the loss of muscle mass during high endurance events and increased levels of stress or injury (Kendall 1998).

Essential Fatty Acids

Eicosapentaenoic acid (EPA) is an omega-3 fatty acid resulting mainly from marine sources. Gamma-linolenic (GLA) is an omega fatty acid derived from meat and vegetable sources. Other nutritional sources are evening primrose, borage oil, and black currant oils. Fatty acids compete for and prevent the activity of the metabolic enzymes from the arachidonic acid inflammatory cascade, providing potential for the clinical use of EFA in arthritic conditions (Kendall 1998).

Glucosamine

Glucosamine and *N*-acetylglucosamine have therapeutic application by helping protect and regenerate connective tissue and cartilage in affected osteoarthritic joints. They help provide an organized structure for joints with their supporting ligaments, synovial fluid and tendons. Numerous studies have shown glucosamine sulfate is beneficial against degenerative joint disorders and osteoarthritis. Glucosamines are the building blocks of glycaminoglycans (GAG) and proteogylcans that are incorporated into connective tissues and joint tissues.

The GAG, in combination with collagen, forms the molecules responsible for the gelatinous nature of cartilage. The GAG, which includes chondroitin sulfate and hyaluronic acid, allow the cartilage to act as a shock absorber by allowing it to hold water. Both glucosamine sulfate and D-glucosamine are readily absorbed and can be used for GAG synthesis in the chondrocytes of the joints. Both glucosamine HCl (a salt of D-glucosamine) and glucosamine sulfate are beneficial in treating degenerative joint disease by preventing and perhaps reversing cartilage degredation. Glucosamine products are used for many disk degeneration conditions and arthridites to lessen pain and inflammation and provide greater joint mobility (Kendall 1998).

Glycoaminoglycan (GAG) nutritional supplements aid in the treatment of degenerative joint disease in small animals. GAG appears to stabilize the joint by decreasing inflammation, enhancing cartilage synthesis by the chondrocytes and reducing degradation of the surrounding cartilage matrix. GAG is an anti-inflammatory in the connective tissue and aids directly in the structural repair process. They provide chondroitin sulfate and hyaluronic acid precursors to the chondrocytes, which increase the joints' synovial fluid viscosity and aid in the synthesis of the extracellular matrix, thereby slowing down and reversing the destructive process. GAG products provide reduction in pain and inflammation, help normalize synovial fluid viscosity, aid in repair of cartilage, and retard the degenerative process caused by proteolytic enzyme release.

Adequan (Novartis Animal Haealth US, Greensboro, NC 27408) is a partially synthetic polysulfated GAG. Shark and bovine cartilage contain GAG and may be used to help repair damaged joints and treat various types of arthritis. Perna Mussel (*Perna canaliculus*) is a marine mussel produced commercially in New Zealand that contains GAG products to help treat degenerative joint disorders and provide anti-inflammatory effects. GAG products may be used in combination with other modalities to provide regeneration and healing of degenerative joint disease in small animals (Kendall 1998).

Coenzyme Q10

The primary use of coenzyme Q10 is for cardiovascular disorders. Other uses include immune dysfunction and enhancing decreased physical performance. As the animal ages, coenzyme Q10 decreases especially in the heart and liver. Supplementation increases exercise tolerance and energy in older animals and may be beneficial in correcting the age-related decline in the immune system (Kendall 1998).

Digestive Enzymes

Supplemental digestive enzymes help improve digestion and recovery from disease. Enzyme therapy has been beneficial as an analgesic after exercise or soft tissue injury. Geriatric or animals under stress may benefit from the addition of supplemental digestive enzymes (Kendall 1998).

Proanthocyanidin Complex

Proanthocyanidins are a large group of natural plant polyphenolic compounds that have beneficial therapeutic effects. These can be extracted from seeds, fruits, and other plant material. Two commercial products are available from grape seed extract and pine bark extract, one of which is Pycnogenol (Natural Health Science Inc. (NHS), Hoboken, NJ 07030-5722). The antienzyme activity and free radical scavenging action of proanthocyanidins inhibit the activity of proteolytic enzymes that are involved in the destruction of the main building blocks of the extravascular matrix. There may be a therapeutic application for proanthocyanidin com-plex in animals with osteoarthritis or degenerative joint and connective tissue disorders (Kendall 1998).

Free Radical Scavengers

Free radical scavengers such as superoxide dismutase (SOD), dimethylsulfoxide (DMSO), bioflavinoids, and glutathione are beneficial in decreasing inflammation. Oxidative injury causes the destruction of collagen and decreases production of proteoglycans leading to the progression of degenerative joint disease. These free radical scavengers help prevent oxidative destruction, promote improved function, and decrease pain in osteoarthritic dogs (Beale 2004).

Methylsulfonylmethane

Methylsulfonylmethane (MSM) is a tasteless antioxidant beneficial for pain management and inflammation. The possibility of a deficiency of sulfur in the diet is the rational for its use. MSM manufacturers base claims of pain relief, anti-inflammatory effects, and management of osteoarthritis in small animals (Beale 2004).

Creatine

Creatine may boost athletic performance, improve muscle wasting in geriatric animals, and slow the progress of neuromuscular diseases (Lester and Wynn 2004).

Cetyl Myristolate

Cetyl myristolate is an antiarthritic that may improve immune function and act as a tissue lubricant and aids in the treatment of arthritis (Lester and Wynn 2004).

Choline

Phosphatidyl choline or lecithin is a precursor to acetylcholine. It is a structural component of biological membranes, and neurotransmitters and promotes lipid transport. It is beneficial as a performance enhancer (Lester and Wynn 2004).

Phenylalanine

L-Phenylalanine or DL-phenylalanine combination provides analgesic effects and may enhance acupuncture. L-Phenylalanine or DL-phenylalanine combination inhibits decarboxylation of endogenous opioids (Lester and Wynn 2004).

No established guidelines for therapeutic nutrition are available. Veterinarians should use high-quality products.

Herbs

Herbal remedies rarely produce complications when taken alone; however, drug interactions may occur when used in combination with anesthetics, α_2-agonists, and opioids. Herbs should be discontinued 2 weeks prior to surgery to prevent prolonged bleeding times or prolonged anesthetic recovery. Herbal remedies are good for chronic, long-term pain because they are "slow and gentle," but therefore not good for acute injuries.

When herbal remedies are administered in conjunction with anesthetics, α_2-agonists, and opioids, untoward drug reactions may occur.

BOSWELLIA

Boswellia serrato is a beneficial herb for inflammation and arthritis and musculoskeletal pain. A side effect may be gastroenteritis and caution should be used when used in combination with nonsteroidal anti-inflammatory drugs (Lester and Wynn 2004).

CORYDALIS

Corydalis, a Chinese herb, is usually combined in a Chinese herbal formulation for a wide range of pain disorders. A specific mechanism of action is not well described; however, prolonged use may lead to tolerance with opioids (Wynn and Marsden 2003).

DRYNARIA-12

Drynaria-12 is a Chinese herbal formulation used for both the treatment and prevention of degenerative joint disease. It is reported to be highly effective in relieving the pain of osteoarthritis. It is also useful in the role of recovery from injury or surgical treatment of the pelvic limbs (Dharmananda 2000).

LIQUID AMBER-15

Liquid Amber-15 is a Chinese herbal formula designed for the treatment of back pain, disc inflammation, disc extrusion, and spondylitis (Dharmananda 2000).

SAN QI-17

San Qi-17 is a Chinese herbal formula indicated for the treatment of traumatic injury, surgery, or other physical harm. It is usually used for several days to weeks and then other formulas are used for long-term treatment if needed (Dharmananda 2000).

YUNNAN PAIYAO

Yunnan Paiyao (Fig. 14.11) is a classic Chinese formula to stop hemorrhage. The main Chinese herb is a blood mover, and it can be used for pain and bruising due to trauma. Yunnan Paiyao can be administered orally or topically on the traumatized area (Caplan 1998).

DISTRIBUTORS

East Coast Herbs
1-800-283-5191

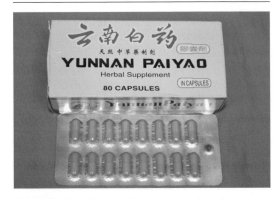

Figure 14.11. Yunnan Paiyao is used orally or topically to decrease or stop hemorrhage.

Mayway USA
1-800-262-9929

Nuherbs
1-800-233-4307

ACUPUNCTURE ORGANIZATIONS

American Academy of Veterinary Acupuncture
  (AAVA)
Suite 320
100 Roscommon Drive
Middletown, CT 06457
Telephone: 860-632-9911
Fax: 860-635-6400
Email: aava@cttel.net
Website: www.aava.org

International Veterinary Acupuncture Society
  (IVAS)
PO Box 271395
Fort Collins, CO 80527
Telephone: 970-266-0666
Fax: 970-266-0777
Email: office@ivas.org
Website: www.ivas.org

Chi Institute Traditional Chinese Veterinary
  Medicine
9700 West Hwy 318
Reddick, FL
Telephone: 800-891-1986
Fax: 866-700-8772
Email: barbara@tcvm.com
Website: www.tcvm.com

ENDNOTES

1 Texas requires that veterinarians have written owner consent forms before practicing any PM modality.
2 Various sensations are described during acupuncture. When an acupuncture point is stimulated by an acupuncture needle, a sensation known as "*Deqi*," a unique needle grasping reaction by the muscle, may be elicited. This particular sensation from an acupuncture needle, believed to be "grasping the *Qi*," is sought during dry needle therapy. However, the therapeutic value and limitations of *Deqi* sensation are not well established.

REFERENCES

Altman, S. 2001. Techniques and instrumentation. In *Veterinary Acupuncture: Ancient Art to Modern Medicine*, edited by A.M. Schoen, et al., 2nd ed., pp. 95–102. St. Louis: Mosby.

Beale, B.S. 2004. Use of nutraceuticals and chondro-protectants in osteoarthritic dogs and cats. *Vet Clin Small Anim* 34:271–289.

Caplan, E. 1998. Integration into surgical practice. In *Complementary and Alternative Veterinary Medicine: Principles and Practice*, edited by A.M. Schoen, S.G. Wynn, et al., p. 668. St. Louis: Mosby.

Dharmananda, S. 2000. *A Bag of Pearls*. Portland, OR, pp. 101, 128, 160.

Heinrichs, K. 2004. Superficial thermal modalities. In *Canine Rehabilitation and Physical Therapy*, edited by D.L. Millis, D. Levine, R.A. Taylor, et al., pp. 277–288. St. Louis: W.B. Saunders.

Jaggar, D.H. 2000. Electro-acupuncture, IVAS certification course, Tampa, Fl.

Johnson, J., and Levine, D. 2004. Electrical stimulation. In *Canine Rehabilitation and Physical Therapy*, edited by D.L. Millis, D. Levine, R.A. Taylor, et al., pp. 289–302, 489. St. Louis: W.B. Saunders.

Kendall, R.V. 1998. Therapeutic nutrition for the cat, dog, and horse. In *Complementary and Alternative Veterinary Medicine: Principles and Practice*, edited by A.M. Schoen, S.G. Wynn, et al., pp. 53–72. St. Louis: Mosby.

Lester, M., and Wynn, S. 2004. Cellular effects of common nutraceuticals and natural food substances. *Vet Clin Small Anim* 34:339–353.

Millis, D.L., Lewelling, A., and Hamilton, S. 2004. Range-of-motion and stretching exercises. In *Canine Rehabilitation and Physical Therapy*, edited by D.L. Millis, D. Levine, R.A. Taylor, et al., pp. 228–243. St. Louis: W.B. Saunders.

Schoen, A.M. (ed.) 2001. *Veterinary Acupuncture: Ancient Art to Modern Medicine*. 2nd ed. St. Louis: Mosby.

Schoen, A.M., and Wynn, S.G. (eds.) 1998. *Complementary and Alternative Veterinary Medicine: Principles and Practice*. St. Louis: Mosby.

Skarda, R.T. 2002. Complementary and alternative (integrative) pain therapy. In *Handbook of Veterinary Pain Management*, edited by J.S. Gaynor, W.W. Muir, et al., pp. 281–326. St. Louis: Mosby.

Snow, A., and Zidonis, N. 1999. *The Well-Connected Dog: A Guide to Canine Acupressure*. Larkspur: Tallgrass.

Sutton, A. 2004. Massage. In *Canine Rehabilitation and Physical Therapy*, edited by D.L. Millis, D.

Levine, R.A. Taylor, et al., pp. 303–323. St. Louis: W.B. Saunders.

Wynn, S.G., and Marsden, S. 2003. Therapies for musculoskeletal disorders. In *Manual of Natural Veterinary Medicine: Science and Tradition*. pp. 341–394. St. Louis: Mosby.

Zidonis, N., and Snow, A. 2000. *Acu-Cat: A Guide to Feline Acupressure.* Larkspur: Tallgrass.

Chapter 15
Clinical Techniques for Anesthesia

Katy W. Waddell and Carin A. Ponder

The techniques described in this chapter are provided for the practitioner who has not used them recently and for the student who is just learning. There are always several ways to accomplish the same task. The best clinical techniques are the ones that reliably work.

PATIENT RESTRAINT

Anesthesia is necessary for most surgical procedures, but physical restraint is needed first. A knowledgeable handler (e.g., veterinary nurse or technician) is paramount to securing venous access (e.g., placement of an intravenous [IV] catheter), anesthetic induction, orotracheal intubation, and anesthetic maintenance without injury to the patient or staff. Most socialized cats and dogs may be easily controlled for examination and preanesthetic preparation. Proper positioning for catheter placement is described below. Fractious cats and small dogs may be wrapped in a bath towel, like a burrito. This is extremely helpful in restraining a cat's limbs to protect the patient and technician from injury. To secure the cat (Fig. 15.1):

- Place the cat on a towel opened lengthwise, perpendicular to the table and perpendicular to the length of the cat. The cat should be placed on the nearest third of the towel to the handler. The cat should be comfortable in sternal recumbency with the forelegs withdrawn.
- Place the nearest free side of the towel over the back of the cat's neck, being sure to secure the perpendicular edge of the towel under the chin of the cat. The forelegs should be trapped in the towel under the chin.
- Pull the side of the towel opposite to the handler over the back of the cat, wrapping that edge of the towel beneath the cat. The two edges of the towel that now cross over the back of the neck should be securely held during the rest of the towel placement.
- Scoop the extra length of towel under the cat. From this position a foreleg may be carefully pulled out for catheter placement. In this position, if the cat is still resisting and the catheter placement appears unlikely, a mask or closed container induction may be accomplished (if there are no contraindications).

Other approaches to restraint include those that are more "hands off." Some patients fight restraint, so the least restraint necessary should be used. These techniques include "baiting" a patient with treats (e.g., processed cheese) or ear twitching in cats (ear twitching is often objectionable, as is "scruffing"). Baiting is rarely used in anesthesia due to fasting requirements. These techniques may produce less stress and resistance from patients. Each patient's temperament should be evaluated before deciding which technique provides the least stress to the patient and maintains a safe working environment for the staff.

Due to temperament and health status, there are some patients that can not be physically handled while they are conscious. For everyone's protection, these patients require chemical restraint. Tranquilizers and sedatives will increase cooperation and decrease the drug requirement for anesthetic induction and maintenance. Common drugs used alone or in combination for chemical restraint include acepromazine, μ-agonists (e.g., hydromorphone, fentanyl), α_2-agonists (e.g., xylazine, medetomidine), dissociative drugs or combinations (e.g., ketamine, tiletamine with zolazepam), and

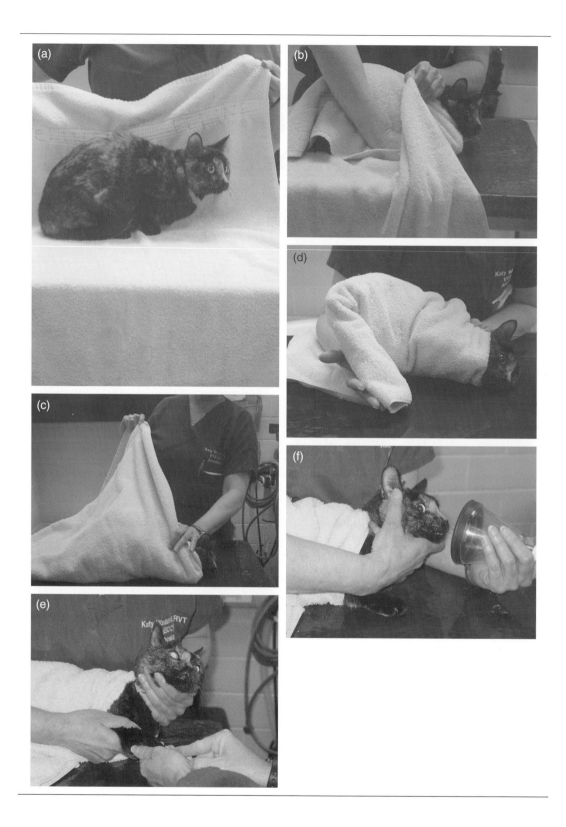

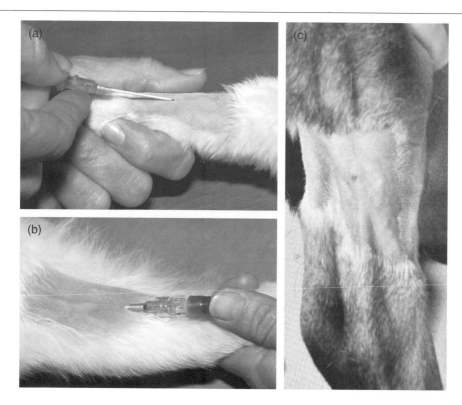

Figure 15.2. (*A*) The cephalic vein may be catheterized in cats and dogs. (*B*) A catheter in the medial saphenous of a cat. (*C*) A shaved lateral saphenous vein in a dog.

rarely alone, benzodiazepines (e.g., diazepam, midazolam) (see Chapter 5).

VENOUS ACCESS

Each patient to be anesthetized should have at least one patent catheter for venous access to administer drugs, fluids, and emergency drugs. Appropriate catheter gauge is determined by patient size; the largest catheter of reasonable size for the patient will provide fastest fluid and drug administration in emergency situations. Smaller catheters are more likely to clot.[1] Generally, the selected vein will be determined by the surgical location (access), patient temperament, and the likelihood of successful catheterization. Common locations for venous access include the cephalic vein in dogs and cats, the medial saphenous in cats, and the lateral saphenous in dogs (Fig. 15.2).

Placing a Peripheral Intravenous Catheter

A surgical blade (No. 40) will provide the smoothest shave; an aseptic preparation should be used to clean the skin.

Figure 15.1. Proper method for restraining a cat using the "burrito" technique: (*A*) the cat is comfortable in sternal recumbency perpendicular to the towel, which is perpendicular to the table. (*B*) The nearest free side of the towel is placed over the back of the cat's neck, securing the perpendicular edge of the towel under the chin of the cat and trapping the forelegs under the chin. (*C*) The side of the towel opposite to the handler is placed over the back of the cat, wrapping that edge of the towel beneath the cat. The two edges of the towel which now cross over the back of the neck should be securely held during the rest of the towel placement. (*D*) Scoop the extra length of towel under the cat. (*E*) From this position, a foreleg may be carefully pulled out for catheter placement. (*F*) If the cat is still resisting and the catheter placement appears unlikely, in the absence of contraindications, a mask induction may be accomplished.

The hair or fur should be shaved over the intended vein. If the entire circumference of the leg is shaved, it will make cleaning the site and securing the catheter easier. However, in show cats and dogs, the amount of hair that is clipped may be an issue. In breeds such as Irish Setters that have "feathers," excessive clipping of hair may be particularly problematic for owners. Discuss the advantages and disadvantages of clipping prior to anesthesia with the owner and document the decision in the record. A surgical blade (No. 40) will provide the cleanest shave. A sterile preparation should be used to clean the skin, alternating surgical scrub and alcohol or water according to the manufacturer's instructions. Percutaneous placement should be easily accomplished.

If a "cutdown" is required to gain venous access (e.g., cardiovascular collapse), a small incision perpendicular to the vessel's course rather than parallel to the vessel will increase visualization.

Choosing a catheter is based on personal preference. If placing a catheter using a tourniquet without assistance with restraint, the Sovereign indwelling canine standard catheter Fig. 15.3*A*) (Tyco Healthcare UK LTD.; e.g., "technician's assistant"[2]) may be the easiest for experienced technicians to place. For beginners, the exposed length of the stylet in the Sovereign indwelling catheter makes it difficult to seat before advancing the catheter. Teflon and polyurethane catheters (Fig. 15.3*B*) are relatively easy for beginners to place. There are also catheters (e.g., Radial Artery Catheterization sets, Arrow International, Inc., Reading, PA 19605) that have a guide wire to facilitate placement. These catheters are typically used for arterial placement (Fig. 15.3*C*).

Placing the Catheter

Securely hold the hub of the catheter and the stylet to keep them from separating, making sure a "flash"[3] will still be visible. If both the stylet and the hub cannot be comfortably held at the same time, hold the stylet when advancing into the vein and the catheter hub when retracting the catheter-stylet. To facilitate placing an intravenous catheter, the catheter should be placed at a 45-degree angle to the skin and vein (Fig. 15.4A). Once the stylet has entered the vein, a "flash" of blood will be seen.

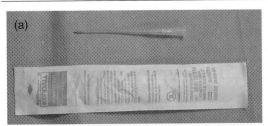
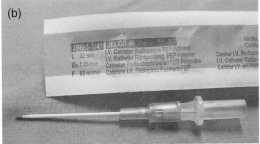
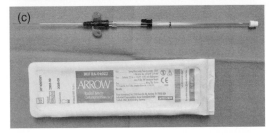

Figure 15.3. (*A*) Kendall Sovereign indwelling canine standard catheter, the "technician's assistant." The stability of the catheter makes it easy for experienced technicians to place without help; the long stylet makes it difficult for inexperienced technicians to seat in the vessel before advancing the catheter. (*B*) Teflon catheters are relatively easy for placement. (*C*) The radial artery catheter set uses a guide wire to feed the catheter in the vessel. Although designed for arteries, they may be useful in catheterizing some difficult peripheral vessels.

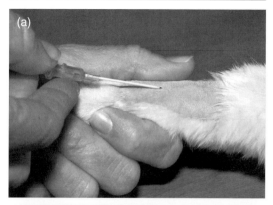

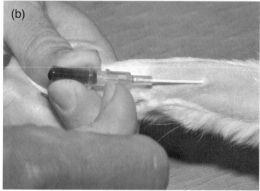

Figure 15.4. (*A*) Hold both the stylet and the hub together or hold the stylet when advancing forward and the hub when backing out. (*B*) Hold the stylet securely when feeding the catheter.

When the flash is seen, position the catheter parallel to the vessel and advance the catheter and stylet together far enough to ensure that the catheter is well seated in the vein. Once well seated, hold the stylet and feed the catheter off the stylet[4] (Fig. 15.4B).

If there is resistance to catheter advancement, the catheter is most likely outside the vessel and the blood flow or flash is from the stylet. If the catheter and stylet have been separated, do not attempt to put them back together. If rejoined, the stylet may amputate the distal portion of the catheter. If amputated the free portion of the catheter is subcutaneous, it can be easily removed. If the free portion of the catheter is amputated and is free in the vessel, it may migrate to the right atrium. Once the catheter is seated, place an injection port or "prn" or "T" piece to occlude the catheter.

Securing the Catheter

There are several methods of securing IV catheters. Ensure that the skin surrounding the catheter is dry. The catheter may be sutured in place, securing the hub of the catheter with suture tightened in the groove of the catheter hub. A tape "butterfly" may be used to suture the catheter in place. Tissue glue is rarely needed to secure venous catheters but may be used in conjunction with tape to secure the hub. When using tape (Wet-Pruf Kendall; Tyco Healthcare UK LTD) to secure the catheter, 1-inch tape may be purchased and torn longitudinally. Half-inch tape may also be purchased. There is special tape (Cloth Adhesive tape; 3M, St. Paul MN 55144–1000) used for cats that may be easily removed without damaging the skin. The sticky part of the tape is used to encompass the hub of the catheter and the tape is adhered to itself prior to encircling the leg. Leaving a tab on the end of the tape used to secure the catheter will help the technician remove the catheter. A second piece of ½-inch tape is used to "pull" the catheter into the vessel. The second piece of tape is placed sticky-side down and is butted up against the hub and catheter junction. The remaining length of tape is used to encircle the leg and is taped over the hub being careful to leave a tab for easy removal. Try to pull the tape in the direction that is consistent with the course of the vessel (i.e., if placing a catheter in the left forelimb, the tape will encircle the leg clockwise). Finally, a 1-inch piece of tape may be placed under the injection port of the prn, encircling the leg in order to provide a clean space for injection of drugs or fluids. To avoid inadvertent catheter removal, be careful not to anchor the catheter with tape that crosses a joint (Fig. 15.5).

If the catheter is not needed immediately, a small piece of Vetwrap may be used to loosely cover the catheter after placement. After surgery, a similar wrap will help protect the catheter until recovery is complete. Adhesive remover (MS Adhesive Tape Remover; Miller-Stephenson) may be used to remove tape if the catheter is firmly adhered to the skin.

Cephalic Catheterization

The easiest venous access in dogs and cats is usually the cephalic vein, which courses down the craniodorsal surface of the foreleg, lateral to medial. Although more difficult to secure, the auxiliary

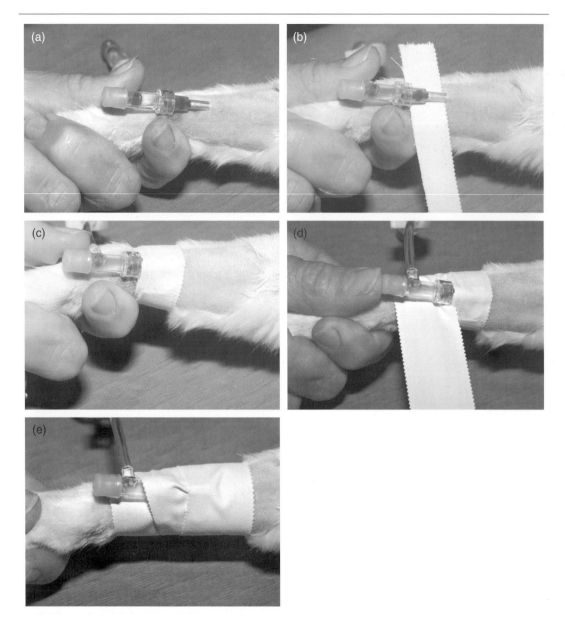

Figure 15.5. Securing the catheter: (*A*) catheter placed with T-port in place and leg dried. (*B*) The sticky part of ½-inch tape is used to encompass the hub of the catheter and the tape is adhered to itself prior to encircling the leg. (*C*) Leaving a tab on the end of the tape used to secure the catheter will help the technician remove the catheter. (*D*) A second piece of ½-inch (or 1-inch tape is used to "pull" the catheter into the vessel. The second piece of tape is placed sticky-side down and is butted up against the hub and catheter junction. (*E*) The remaining length of tape is used to encircle the leg and is taped over the hub being careful to leave a tab for easy removal. Avoid taping over a joint.

cephalic vein that branches off the cephalic vein at the metacarpus and proceeds medially is also available for catheterization. If the cephalic branch is catheterized, the carpus should be stabilized to prevent flexion during taping. The cephalic vein can accommodate a variety of sizes (gauges) of catheters depending on the size of the patient (i.e., 24 gauge to 18 gauge).

Routine, simple restraint for cephalic intravenous catheter placement requires a technician to support the patient in sternal recumbency and cradle the head to prevent the patient from biting the person inserting the catheter. The technician uses the other hand to hold off the vein and restrain ("pin") the patient between the technician's arm and body. The person placing the catheter may help stabilize the vessel by placing the thumb of the nondominant hand lateral or medial to the vein and keeping the skin taught (see Fig. 15.5).

Lateral Saphenous Catheterization in Dogs

The lateral saphenous vein (see Fig. 15.2C) is also routinely catheterized in dogs (Fig. 15.6). The patient should be restrained in lateral recumbency with the technician's arm across the neck grasping the front legs; the back legs are held with the other hand. In large dogs, it may be necessary to grasp only the down legs. Another technician or tourniquet is necessary to hold off the vein of the "up" leg by grasping the thigh. In large dogs, an additional technician may be required to help restrain the rear limbs as well.

Medial Saphenous Catheterization in Cats

In cats, the medial saphenous vein (see Fig. 15.2B) may be used for catheterization. The patient is restrained laterally with the medial aspect of the down rear limb exposed. The technician restrains the rear legs by pulling the up leg into the body and placing pressure on the down leg for restraint and to occlude the saphenous vein. Problems with placing catheters in the saphenous vein include difficulty in securing the catheter to the limb and increased tendencies for occlusion due to the patient positioning.

Lateral Tarsal Catheterization

The tarsal vein is an additional readily accessible vein that can be catheterized, especially in larger patients. The tarsal vein is located on the *dorsal* aspect of the tarsus and can be quite prominent. A smaller catheter is usually needed (24-gauge to 22-gauge), but a 20-gauge catheter may be safely placed in large dogs. Positioning of the foot as well as surgical ties placed above the catheter can contribute to inadvertent catheter occlusion.

Confirming Placement and Troubleshooting Catheters

There is some controversy over the withdrawal of blood through catheters. In short-term catheters, both being able to withdraw blood and easily flush the catheter is important. Typically, heparinized saline can be used to flush the catheter, withdraw blood, confirm placement, and flush blood back into the patient. Some of medications (e.g., thiopental, dopamine) are harmful if extravasated, so it is important to confirm appropriate placement of catheters. Adequate flow-through catheters are important if fluids need to be administered quickly.

There are several additional methods used to ensure proper catheter placement. Some anesthetists palpate the vessel while flushing the catheter. In so doing, the flush can be felt passing under fingers held lightly over the vein. Some people rely on the fluids flowing well to confirm placement. This is probably the least reliable and should be combined with another technique to ensure appropriate placement. When catheters are placed in small peripheral vessels, it may be difficult to withdraw blood because the negative pressure created by pulling on the syringe's plunger collapses the vessel. Connect the intravenous fluids to the catheter; fluid should run quickly if catheter is in place. Then lower the bag below the level of the heart. If the catheter is in the vein, blood will back up into the intravenous administration set.

Problems with catheter placement are best addressed before the patient is situated in the

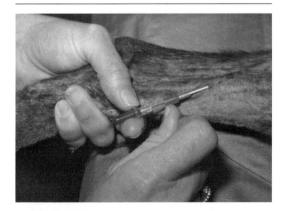

Figure 15.6. Catheterization of the lateral saphenous. Notice the technician is holding the stylet steady while feeding the catheter.

operating or technique room and draped. There are some common mishaps which occur with catheter placement. The common problems, diagnosis, and treatment are listed below:

1. A flash of blood is seen and the catheter is advanced easily for a small distance; then the catheter can no longer be advanced. Blood may continue to flow from the stylet.
   - The stylet is in the vessel, but the catheter is not. When trying to advance the catheter, it bumps against the vessel wall and is deformed.
   - The catheter is kinked or has penetrated the vessel and the stylet is still in the vessel.

The catheter should be replaced and a different vessel attempted.

2. With some resistance, the catheter flushes but blood cannot be withdrawn:
   - The catheter is kinked at the junction of the hub and catheter. Carefully, remove the tape encircling the limb and examine the connection. If possible, straighten the catheter and retape. Similarly, if the tape used to secure the catheter is too tight when it encircles the hub–catheter connection, passive flow may be occluded and retaping may be curative.
   - Catheter is kinked underneath the skin. The catheter may or may not be in the vein. The catheter should be replaced.
   - The length of the catheter may be important if the catheter tip terminates at the elbow or other joint, which may inadvertently occlude the catheter when the joint is flexed. Stabilizing the joint in extension should prevent occlusion.
3. Catheter flushes easily, there is no subcutaneous accumulation of fluids, and you feel fluid being flushed through the vessel, but you cannot withdraw blood.
   - The catheter is probably small and the pressure of withdrawal collapses the vessel. See above for confirming placement by lowering the bag of fluid.
4. All peripheral vessels are thrombosed, "blown," or unavailable (e.g., tied off during a catheterization procedure).

- If necessary, a jugular catheter may be used for induction and drug administration. Fluids often do not run well enough through a jugular catheter. If possible, once anesthetized, attempt another peripheral catheter.
- Some breeds (e.g., Bassett Hounds, Hound Dogs) have accessible ear veins. Avoid the central aural artery, unless it is needed for monitoring blood pressure rather than drug administration.
- If venous access is not available, intraosseous catheterization may be an option.

INTRAOSSEOUS CATHETERIZATION

Limited venous access in neonates and small exotics may necessitate intraosseous catheterization. Intraosseous catheterization is accomplished by placing a standard spinal needle (length and gauge should be determined by the patient's size) into the bone marrow cavity of the following locations: intertrochanteric fossa of the proximal femur, flat medial aspect of the proximal tibia distal to the tibial tuberosity and the proximal tibial growth plate, proximal shaft of the humerus, and cranial aspect of the mid-diaphyseal ulna. The location selected should be clipped and scrubbed aseptically. While wearing sterile gloves, the location should be palpated and the needle inserted while staying parallel to the long axis of the bone to prevent accidentally exiting through the cortex. It should be noted that the chosen bone should not have been fractured and the skin over the insertion site should be healthy. As the needle enters the cortex, pressure should be firm and steady. Once placed, the stylet of the spinal needle can be removed; the needle should be aspirated to confirm placement and then flushed with a heparinized saline. The following flow rates can be applied: not to exceed 11 ml/min with gravity flow or 24 ml/min with fluid pumps. Swelling in the surrounding soft tissues indicates that the needle has traversed the cortex and should be repositioned or withdrawn.

Like all catheterization techniques, the placement of an intraosseous catheter is not without its own risks. Complications may include osteomyelitis, damage to growth plates, subcutaneous or subperiosteal leakage of fluids, fat embolization, malposition of needle, partial or total occlusion of the needle, inability to enter the marrow cavity, damage to nerves, localized cellulitis, and subcutaneous abscesses associated with pre-existing infection of the skin.

Once an intraosseous catheter has been placed properly, most drugs and fluids that are labeled for intravenous administration can be administered through it.

Long-term Long Indwelling Catheters: Jugular Catheter Placement for Measuring Central Venous Pressure (Protocol Based on our Intensive Care Unit Procedures)

There are several reasons to place a long-term catheter. For our purposes, the primary reason anesthesia requires a long-term catheter (e.g., jugular or in very small patients, a lateral saphenous catheter) is for measuring central venous pressure (CVP). When placed in the external jugular vein for measurement of CVP, the end of the long indwelling catheter should lie between the thoracic inlet and cranial to the right atrium in the anterior vena cava.

In some instances, a central catheter is helpful if administering irritating drugs (e.g., etomidate). Other reasons applicable to emergency situations are not helpful in anesthesia. Due to surgical positioning, rapid fluid administration is difficult using a jugular catheter during anesthesia.

Supplies

The needed supplies include:

- Catheter: select the appropriate gauge, length, and number of lumens
- prn or T-port with male injection plug (flushed with heparinized saline)
- Suture material
- Antibiotic ointment and gauze pads
- Surgical scrub and alcohol or water based on manufacturer instructions
- Cast padding, soft rolled gauze (2 inch), Vetwrap, 1-inch adhesive tape
- Heparinized flush syringes
- Sterile gloves, fenestrated drape
- Clippers

Placing the Catheter

To begin, place the patient in a comfortable position, either in lateral or sternal recumbency. Clip the skin in the ventral region of the neck to facilitate a surgical scrub prior to placement of the catheter. Measure the external anatomy to estimate the length of catheter required. A small infusion of 2% lidocaine may be administered subcutaneously prior to making the initial placement of the introducer catheter/needle. Flush each lumen of the catheter and clamp or attach injection caps to the appropriate pigtails. Make sure to leave the distal pigtail available (uncapped) for guide wire placement. Insert the introducer catheter/needle into the jugular vein. Withdraw the needle from the introducer catheter and observe for free flow of blood. If no flow is seen, attach a syringe and gently aspirate until blood flow is established. Insert the tip of the spring-wire guide through the introducer catheter/needle into the vein. Hold the spring-wire guide in place and remove the introducer catheter/needle. Maintain a secure grip on the spring-wire guide at all times. After the removal of the introducer, thread the vessel dilator over the guide wire to gently enlarge the puncture site and open in the jugular vein. Do not leave the dilator in place as the possibility of vessel perforation exists. After removing the dilator, thread the catheter of the spring-wire guide. With a gentle twisting motion, advance the catheter through the skin. Advance the catheter to its final length of insertion by referring to the cm marks on the catheter. The length of insertion was previously measured externally and the correct length noted. While holding the catheter at the desired length, remove the spring-wire guide. The catheter should pass freely over the wire. If any resistance is met, retract the catheter 2 to 3 cm; again attempt to remove the spring-guide wire. Should resistance continue, remove the guide wire and catheter as a unit. Kinking of the spring-wire around the catheter tip has been reported and further attempts to force the removal of the spring-wire could cause breakage. Once the entire spring-wire has been removed, ensure that the wire is intact. Check the patency of the lumen of the catheter by attaching a syringe to each pigtail and aspirating until a free flow of blood is observed. Flush each with saline and connect all the pigtails to a T-port, intravenous extension line or male injection plug. Position the wings of the rubber clamp on the catheter and snap the rigid fastener onto the catheter clamp. Suture the catheter clamp and fastener together to the skin utilizing the side wings to prevent migration of the catheter. Apply skin dressing and cover the point of insertion with an impervious dressing. Then the entire neck may be wrapped with soft gauze, followed by a soft elastic bandage. It is recommended that a radiograph be taken to ensure the actual location of the catheter tip. The neck bandage should be changed immediately if it becomes soiled, or changed once daily and the point of insertion should be inspected for any signs of swelling or redness.

OROTRACHEAL INTUBATION

Prior to ET intubation, it is essential to gather all necessary supplies to prevent any delay in establishing a patent airway.

Supplies

Supplies needed include:
- Three checked[5] endotracheal (ET) tubes in a range of sizes
- A 12-ml syringe for cuff inflation ("cuff" syringe)
- Guide tube[6] or stylet[7]
- Laryngoscope
- Sterile water-soluble lubricant
- Lidocaine and a cotton swab (for swabbing arytenoids of cats)
- Tie to secure the ET tube in place (rolled gauze).

Choosing an Endotracheal Tube

The success of orotracheal intubation depends on the skill of the individual choosing and placing the ET tube. There are a variety of methods to select the appropriate diameter (internal diameter [I.D.], mm) and length (cm) ET tube. The most common method is based on the weight of the animal (Table 15.1). For example, generally a 20-kg dog can accommodate a 9.5-mm (I.D.) ET tube. This method overestimates the size required for large cats and brachycephalic dogs.

A less reliable method of estimating ET tube size is holding the distal tip of the ET tube between the nares. In theory, if the tip fits between the nares, the tube should fit in the trachea (Fig. 15.7). This method also underestimates the size of ET tube needed to create a sufficient seal. When in doubt, palpate the trachea and have a range of sizes of ET tubes checked and available for use (e.g., if a 5.5-mm tube is the anticipated size, also have a 5.0-mm and a 6.0-mm tube available).

The length of the ET tube is as important as the width. To measure the appropriate length, place the ET tube near the side of the patient from the nares to the point of shoulder; do not contaminate a clean tube by allowing it to come into contact with the patient's hair or fur. To prevent an endobronchial intubation, the ET tube should not extend past the point of the shoulder. To prevent excessive dead space ventilation (e.g., where two-way flow occurs), the length of the ET tube should not extend past the

Table 15.1. Estimated endotracheal tube size based on patient weight, except for brachycephalic dogs and cats.

Endotracheal tube size (ID) by weight		
kg	lb	ID
9.1	20	7
11.4	25	7.5
13.6	30	8
15.9	35	8.5
18.2	40	9
20.5	45	9.5
22.7	50	10
27.3	60	11
31.8	70	12

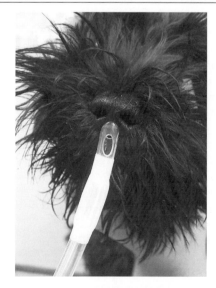

Figure 15.7. The tip of the endotracheal tube should fit between the nares in dogs.

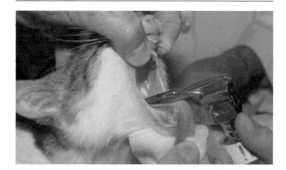

Figure 15.8. Proper positioning of a cat for endotracheal intubation.

nares. The machine (proximal) end of the ET tube may be shortened after temporarily removing the adapter-connector. Care should be taken not to cut the ET tube below the point of entry of the pilot line into the wall of the tube.

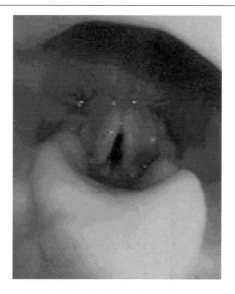

Figure 15.9. Visualization of the epiglottis and arytenoids of a cat.

Placing the Endotracheal Tube

Once the patient is induced, the technician should hold the patient's head up and out by grasping the maxilla caudal to the canine teeth. Then the anesthetist or the assistant should grasp the tongue with a dry gauze sponge, extending the tongue out of the mouth and over the incisors for visualization of the pharynx and larynx (epiglottis, glottis, and arytenoids) (Fig. 15.8).

The assistant should be careful not to grasp the throat; pressure exerted under the neck will cause distortion of the presented anatomy. When the patient is positioned correctly, the anesthetist should be able to visualize the larynx, including the glottis and arytenoid cartilages. If not, a laryngoscope may be needed. The tip of the laryngoscope blade should be placed at the base of the tongue ventral to the epiglottis. By placing downward pressure on the tip of the laryngoscope blade, the epiglottis should be revealed (Fig. 15.9).

If possible, avoid touching the epiglottis with the laryngoscope blade. If the tip of the epiglottis is not visible, the anesthetist may have to gently push the soft palate up to release the entrapped epiglottis. With the arytenoids visualized, gently slide the ET tube between the opened arytenoid cartilages. Do not use force. If too much resistance is encountered when introducing the ET tube or the ET tube is too small, choose the next size ET tube of appropriate

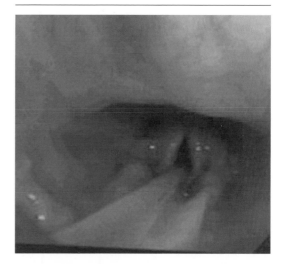

Figure 15.10. Placement of a guide tube through the arytenoids makes it possible to remove the laryngoscope. The endotracheal tube may be fed off the guide tube.

width and length. In cats and some small dogs, lidocaine may be required (swabbed on the arytenoid cartilages) to prevent laryngospasm. A guide tube may be needed in small patients, because visualization is difficult when a laryngoscope blade and an ET tube are both in place (Fig. 15.10).

The laryngoscope blade may be removed once the guide tube is appropriately placed through the laryngeal opening and into the trachea. The ET tube may then be advanced over the guide tube (Fig. 15.11). Generally, a stylet is used in larger patients when visualization is not an issue, but the ET tube is too pliable (Fig. 15.12). During intubation, a stylet should never extend past the distal (patient) end of the ET tube.

With an appropriate size ET tube in place, secure the ET tube around the maxilla or mandible in dogs and behind the head in cats and brachycephalic

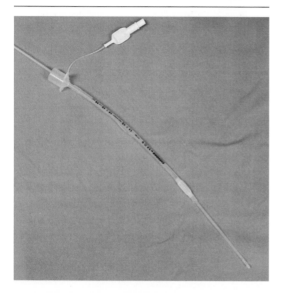

Figure 15.11. A typical guide tube and endotracheal tube for cats.

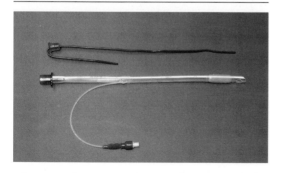

Figure 15.12. A stylet is used when the ET tube is too pliable.

dogs. A narrow gauze strip may be used to secure the ET tube, by placing one throw of a square knot securely over the ET tube (being careful not to occlude the lumen of a small ET tube). The throw should lay flat on the tube toward the maxilla or mandible, whichever will be used to secure the tube. The ET tube is then tied securely.

In patients at risk for regurgitation and aspiration, inflate the cuff of the ET tube to a light seal (by inflating the cuff with a syringe up to an inspiratory pressure of 20 cm H_2O while providing positive pressure ventilation (IPPV) prior to securing the ET tube. Otherwise, the ET tube is tied in place prior to inflating the cuff in order to avoid denuding the tracheal mucosa.

Once the ET tube has been secured, attach the breathing circuit to the ET tube connector and create a seal by inflating the cuff with a syringe up to an inspiratory pressure of 20 cm H_2O while providing positive-pressure ventilation (IPPV). If the cuff is inflated to an inspiratory pressure of 20 cm H_2O and the pop-off valve or overflow is inadvertently left closed, some of the excess gas in the respiratory system should move past the cuff before causing injury, providing a little extra time to diagnose the error. Overinflation of the cuff can cause tracheal irritation or necrosis. As the anesthetic plane deepens, a leak may be detected. This is most likely from the trachea relaxing and is remedied by providing IPPV to 20 cm H_2O and inflating the cuff until no leak can be detected at that pressure.

Special care should be taken when intubating cats. There are reports of tracheal rupture in cats after ET intubation (Hardie 1999; Mitchell 2000). Tracheal rupture is suspected to result from over inflation of the cuff. In cats, the cuff should be inflated in 0.5-ml increments to a light seal (as described above to an inspiratory pressure of 20 cm H_2O). Inappropriate use of a guide tube or stylet may also result in perforation of the trachea. When moving a patient or turning a patient from side to side, the ET tube should be disconnected from the breathing system to avoid denuding the tracheal mucosa or tearing the trachea.

To avoid damaging the trachea, always disconnect the patient's ET tube from the breathing system when moving the patient.

Special Circumstances

Special care should be taken during intubation in some instances. Techniques are available to decrease the risk when intubating patients with congenital anomalies, traumatic lesions, or esophageal abnormalities. If it is impossible to open the mouth normally, a guide tube should be available (Fig. 15.13). Other techniques such as retrograding a catheter from the mid-cervical trachea out of the mouth to serve as a guide have been described for pocket pets and can be adapted to dogs and cats. In some cases, pharyngeal intubation (see later in this chapter) will be necessary. In rare instances, a tracheotomy may be required.

RETROGRADE INTUBATION

By definition, retrograde means "directed backward" or "in the opposite of usual order." Therefore, retrograde intubation is the opposite of oral intubation. To facilitate this procedure, the ventral aspect of the patient's neck should be prepared aseptically. In exotics and small neonates, an over-the-needle catheter can be used as a stylet. Palpate and locate the trachea; pass the over-the-needle catheter between the tracheal rings as if you were planning

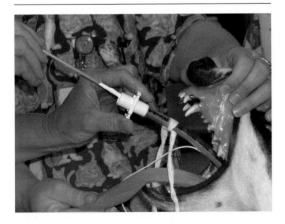

Figure 15.13. A guide tube is used to intubate a patient who may have difficult visualization due to mass or in case the patient's mouth cannot be opened very wide.

to do a tracheal wash. As the catheter with its guide wire enters the trachea, pass it cranially through the larynx and pharynx. Once the unit has been positioned correctly, the needle can be withdrawn from the trachea, leaving the catheter–guide wire complex in place. The catheter tip should be visible in the oral cavity and can now be used as a guide to facilitate intubation with an ET tube. As the ET tube is passed through the larynx, the catheter can be removed from the trachea and ventral neck. Secure the ET tube in the usual manner.

PHARYNGEAL INTUBATION

Occasionally, a patient will be presented in which normal ET intubation becomes a hindrance for the surgical team. These patients may present with fractured mandibles, masses that occlude the oropharyngeal airway, or other oropharyngeal procedures. In these circumstances, pharyngeal intubation may be necessary to facilitate surgery.

Just as in normal ET intubation, the ET tube is passed between the maxilla and mandible and through the glottis. Once the patient is at a surgical plane of anesthesia, a surgical approach is made near the angle of the mandible into the caudal aspect of the pharynx. At this time, the ET tube adapter can be removed and the machine end of the ET tube can be passed through the incision to the exterior (through the pharyngeal mucosa, subcutaneous tissues, and skin). Once the machine end of the ET tube is visible, the adapter can be reapplied to the tube and connected to the breathing circuit. For security measures, the ET tube should be sutured to the patient via a folded piece of water-proof tape ("butterfly") and the surgeon's choice of suture material.

MEGAESOPHAGUS OR FULL STOMACH

In a patient with megaesophagus or a full stomach, a rapid sequence induction should be performed and care should be taken to protect the airway. Patients should be intubated in sternal recumbency. In people, pressure is applied to the cricoid cartilage in order to prevent regurgitation (e.g., Sellick maneuver). If the patient has a full stomach or megaesophagus, there is an advantage to inflating the cuff immediately to protect against aspiration if regurgitation should occur. If the patient is fasted, it is appropriate to secure the ET tube prior to inflating the ET tube cuff to avoid denuding the tracheal mucosa by movement of the ET tube while it is being secured.

Cervical Trauma or Atlantoaxial Subluxation

Extreme care should be taken with patients with cervical trauma. After induction the neck muscles are relaxed and the patient can no longer guard (e.g., protect) its neck. In patients with cervical trauma or atlantoaxial subluxation and cervical instability, care should be taken not to overextend or flex the neck. Alternate techniques may be required for intubation to prevent further injury.

Increased Intracranial Pressure

For patients suspected to have brain disease, it is paramount to establish a patent airway quickly and provide modest hyperventilation. In patients with increased intracranial pressure, the effects of anesthesia and the resulting hypoventilation may promote vasodilation leading to increased intracranial pressure. Providing IPPV to produce modest hyperventilation (ETCO$_2$ 28 to 32 mm Hg), prevents a further increase in the intracranial pressure due to the inhalant anesthetic.

Placement Confirmation and Troubleshooting

The ability to quickly intubate patients orotracheally and to troubleshoot problems associated with improper intubation is very important. Troubleshooting problem intubations is a required skill. Before proceeding with any surgical stimulation, confirmation of proper placement of the ET tube is necessary. One method is to palpate the thoracic inlet for the ET tube in the trachea (e.g., the tracheal rings can be palpated as the ET tube passes the rings). To decrease the likelihood of mucosal damage, do not reposition the ET tube with the cuff inflated. Auscultation of bilateral lung sounds ensures that endobronchial intubation has not occurred. Observation of the movement of the rebreathing bag and condensation on the inside of the ET tube are other indicators that the tube is properly placed. An end-tidal carbon dioxide monitor may be used to rule out an esophageal intubation; gases exhaled from the respiratory system contain a significant amount of carbon dioxide. In smaller patients, plucking a small amount of hair and holding it in front of the adapter as the patient moves air through the tube and watching for any hair movement may indicates a patent airway; however, this method is not reliable and should not be used to replace auscultation of both lungs and the trachea to assure gas movement with each breath.

In an esophageal intubation, the following clinical signs may be present. The anesthetist may be unable to maintain a level plane of anesthesia, oxygenation of hemoglobin as indicated by SpO$_2$ values may be reduced, and an inflated ET tube cuff may not create a seal. There will be no movement of the rebreathing bag, gastric distention may occur, and ETCO$_2$ values may be very low. Deflating the cuff, extubating the esophagus, and re-intubating the trachea is corrective.

Aspiration pneumonia is most often caused by a misplaced ET tube (esophagus or bronchus) or a leaky cuff. Under anesthesia, the aspirate is usually regurgitated stomach contents, saliva, blood, or another fluid substance used during the procedure. The throat should be swabbed or suctioned before extubation of the trachea. Fasting patients before anesthesia will decrease the likelihood of regurgitation. Silent regurgitation may occur. If IPPV is used after regurgitation, the particles and fluid may be pushed farther into the lower airways.

If a bronchus is accidentally intubated, SpO$_2$ will be greatly decreased, lung sounds can only be auscultated unilaterally, and usually the patient will not stay anesthetized. Atelectasis of the unventilated lung may occur. Endobronchial intubation is readily remedied by deflating the cuff, gently withdrawing the tube until the lung sounds can be heard bilaterally and the SpO$_2$ improves to 95% or better. The ET tube is then secured in the new position and the cuff inflated.

With a tracheal rupture from intubation, subcutaneous emphysema may result. Radiographs and auscultation of decreased breath sounds will confirm improper ET tube placement. If possible, deflate the cuff and move the ET tube past the tear to create a seal and prevent further escape of gases into the surrounding tissues. Surgical correction will be required for large tracheal tears.

In the event of a pneumothorax, the intrathoracic pressure is relieved by a percutaneous needle insertion. This is done by inserting an over the needle catheter or large bore butterfly catheter in intercostal space 7 or 8 dorsolaterally with an attached stopcock and syringe. Air is aspirated from the thorax into the syringe and then emptied into the room by turning the stopcock off to the patient. Care should be taken to insert the needle properly to avoid the vessels and nerves which lay caudal to each rib in the intercostals space.

Once properly intubated, the patient can be repositioned for surgery. It is of utmost importance to disconnect the ET tube from the breathing circuit when repositioning the patient to prevent damage to the trachea, occlusion of the ET tube, or accidental extubation.

Extubation

A patient should be extubated only if it has a vigorous swallowing reflex and can protect its airway. There are several golden rules of extubation to prevent aspiration or loss of a patent airway. If regurgitation or hemorrhage has occurred in the airway during anesthesia, the oropharynx should be suctioned or swabbed to prevent aspiration; all liquid and particulate matter should be removed before extubation of the trachea. If there is any potential of foreign material to be in the airway proximal to the cuff, the tube should be removed with a partially inflated cuff. In brachycephalic breeds, basing extubation on the swallowing reflex is insufficient due to the risk of a long soft palate blocking the airway. Wait until the patient begins to chew the tube and cough before extubating the animal. Keep the ET tube between the incisors to avoid severing the ET tube; potential exists for aspiration or swallowing of the distal piece of the tube if the tube is completely sheared. In patients with megaesophagus or a full stomach, extubation should also be postponed as long as reasonably possible. If the patient is brachycephalic or has a megaesophagus or a full stomach, extubate with the cuff slightly inflated. Once extubated, a patient may still need assistance to keep the SpO_2 values in the normal range (see later in this chapter for oxygen supplementation).

> Keep the ET tube between the incisors to avoid shearing the ET tube when the patient begins to chew during recovery.

OXYGEN SUPPLEMENTATION

Oxygen enrichment can be accomplished by flow–by technique or tracheal administration via an ET tube; humidified oxygen is important. Oxygen is needed for delivery of inhalant anesthetics and proper enrichment of inspired gases.

The most reliable method of oxygen delivery to the patient is through the ET tube. This is especially helpful post inhalant as the patient exhales anesthetic. It has been noted that 5 to 10 minutes of oxygen insufflation immediately following inhalant anesthesia contributes to high SpO_2 values in the patient.

Oxygen can be delivered via a nasal cannula attached to an oxygen source (nasal insufflation). If needed chronically, the oxygen should be humidified as it is delivered or the patient should be placed in a humidified oxygen cage. If a patient is placed into an oxygen cage, the temperature and the oxygen concentration of the environment should be monitored closely to prevent excessive temperatures and oxygen toxicity.

Oxygen enrichment via an anesthesia mask can be a valuable tool to provide an environment with an elevated concentration of oxygen without the cost of an equipped oxygen cage. Care should be taken not to induce any more stress on a patient by application of the mask. Some patients may react violently to a mask or restraint. The anesthesia mask is especially helpful during preoxygenation of certain breeds and patients with specific surgical conditions. Brachycephalic patients may benefit from oxygen delivery before anesthetic induction due to their inherited breathing problems; however, the mask should be applied properly to avoid impairment of breathing. Patients with surgical conditions, such as pregnant patients for cesarean section, may gain from preanesthetic oxygen delivery to enhance oxygenation during intubation; both the dam and the neonates may benefit if even a short period of hypoxemia is avoided.

INTRA-ARTERIAL CATHETERS

Being able to palpate pulses is useful not only for obtaining pulse rates and evaluating the character of the pulse but also in identifying possible locations for placing an intra-arterial catheter. Locations for obtaining arterial blood samples or placing arterial catheters include the following: the ventral aspect of the tongue (lingual arteries), the dorsal pedal artery, the medial carpus, the brachial and femoral arteries, and the auricular arteries in dogs with large ears. Indications for arterial catheterization include measurement of direct blood pressures and obtaining blood samples for evaluation of the patient's acid-base and blood-gas status—metabolic and respiratory function, respectively. Contraindications and concerns related to arterial punctures and catheterization include patients with clotting disorders, the possibility of developing hematomas at the site of the arterial puncture, and thrombosis of an artery. Sites for access to arteries during surgical procedures include the dorsal pedal, auricular, carpal, and lingual arteries. A 24-gauge to 20-gauge over-the-needle catheter is generally used. The approach and puncture through the skin are at a steeper angle and more aggressive than with a venous catheter. Once a flashback is seen, lower the angle, hold the stylet steady, and thread the catheter into the artery. Place an injection cap on the catheter and secure the catheter in place with waterproof adhesive tape.

URETHRAL CATHETERIZATION

For critically ill animals (i.e., bradycardic cats with urethral obstruction, etc.), see Chapter 11. Most dogs (male and female) do not require sedation for urethral catheterization, although analgesia should be considered for female dogs. Most cats do require sedation and some require anesthesia.

Materials Needed

Collect the needed equipment prior to preparation of the vulva or tip of the penis:

- Sterile urinary catheter (appropriate sizes [Table 15.2]; see Procedure)
- Sterile gloves, sterile lubricant
- Dilute surgical scrub, sterile saline rinse
- Clippers
- Sterile saline-filled syringes
- Sterile syringe for urine collection
- For indwelling urinary catheters, also need sterile urinary collection system, 3–0 nylon suture, 1-inch tape.

Preparation of Site

Male dogs are usually placed in lateral recumbency, while female dogs are placed in sternal recumbency with the rear limbs extended off the edge of the table. In female dogs, the area around the vulva should be clipped and gently cleaned with a dilute

Table 15.2. Selection of urinary catheter size for canine and feline.

Canine		Size Fr red rubber	
Wt (kg)	Wt (lb)	Male	Female
<9	<20	3.5	6
9–23	20–50	5–8	8–10
>23	>50	20–12	10–12
Feline	Size Fr tomcat	Size Fr red rubber	
Any weight	Blocked 3.5	Indwelling 3.5–5	

disinfectant followed by a sterile saline rinse. In male dogs, the tip of the penis is rinsed in the same way.

Procedure: Selection of Urinary Catheter

Procedure

Prior to placement of a Foley catheter, the balloon should be inflated with sterile saline to ensure the integrity of the balloon. Deflate before placement.

Male dogs should be placed in lateral recumbency and an assistant should have the penis extruded from the prepuce. Premeasuring from the tip of the penis to the level of the urinary bladder assists with placement. While wearing sterile gloves, the tip of the urinary catheter is covered with sterile lubricant. The catheter should be advanced into the urethra until urine is visualized. If no urine is obtained after the catheter is advanced appropriately attach a syringe and aspirate for urine. Remove a diagnostic sample and either suture the catheter in place (indwelling) or remove the catheter. If the animal was obstructed, remove all urine and flush the urinary bladder with sterile saline until the urine is clear. Indwelling urinary catheters are attached to a sterile closed collection system.

Female dogs should be placed in sternal recumbency with an assistant holding the tail dorsally. While wearing sterile gloves, lubricant is placed on the tip of the urinary catheter. The lubricated gloved finger of one hand is inserted and the urethral orifice is palpated on the ventral vagina approximately 2 to 3 cm from the opening. With the other hand, the catheter is slowly inserted under the finger of the first hand while the finger guides the catheter ventrally and into the urethral opening. The catheter is advanced until urine is visualized. Alternatively, the urethral papilla can be visualized with a speculum or a sterile otoscope cone and then the catheter advanced into the urethral orifice. Once urine is obtained, the balloon is inflated if using a Foley catheter. Indwelling urinary catheters are attached to a closed urinary collection system. Suturing is not necessary with Foley catheters. A section of the collection tubing can be affixed to the tail to decrease tension on the catheter. Elizabethan collars should be considered in patients with indwelling urinary catheter.

THORACOCENTESIS

In the case of a traumatic pneumothorax or bullae (e.g., hit-by-car), anesthesia is often postponed until the thoracic pathology resolves. If it is impossible to delay anesthesia and surgery, the appropriate side of the thorax should be prepared prior to surgery and care should be used during IPPV (see Chapter 3). An emergency procedure is described above (discussion on placement confirmation and troubleshooting).

If fluid or air is compromising ventilation, it should be removed before anesthesia. The pleural cavity requires drainage in those disease states where it is no longer a potential space. Either air or fluid may become interposed between the visceral and parietal pleura in such volumes as to compromise respiratory function significantly. Accumulation of pleural air or fluid can be indicated by tachypnea, increased inspiratory effort, short/choppy breaths with increased abdominal component, and a decrease in breath sounds.

The need to drain the pleural cavity in small animals is not an everyday occurrence; in many situations, the ideal equipment is not close at hand and compromises have to be made. The result is that the sort of drain chosen and the manner in which it is maintained may depend largely on available equipment and personnel, on the perceived need, and, to a certain extent, on personal preference. Three forms of drainage may be considered: single-episode drainage, temporary drainage, and persistent drainage.

Different types of chest drains are available: wide-bore needle, large plastic intravenous catheter, proprietary trochar chest cannula, and intravenous tubing. All need some form of connecter such a three-way stopcock, Heimlich valve, or multiple-bore tube connecter, and a means of suction, such as a 60-ml syringe with intravenous extension tubing or suction pump.

Supplies Needed

Ensure that all materials are gathered before the thoracocentesis is performed to prevent the possibility of introduction of air into the pleural space. Supplies needed include:

- Clippers
- Surgical scrub and rinse as described by manufacturer
- Sterile gloves
- A 1- to 1.5-inch, 18- to 20-gauge needle, butterfly catheter, or indwelling intravenous catheter
- Three-way stop-cock, intravenous extension tubing
- A 35- or 60-ml syringe
- With or without sample collection tubes

Procedure

Clip and prepare a 4-inch window on either side of the thorax between the seventh and tenth rib space. If air is suspected, the prepped area should be dorsal to mid-thorax, and if fluid accumulation is suspected, the area should be ventral to mid-thorax approximately 3 inches above the sternum. The intravenous extension tubing should be preattached to a three-way stop-cock with the stop-cock in a closed position to the patient.

Insert the needle (catheter) at a 45-degree angle just anterior to the eighth rib space. Avoidance of the caudal aspect of the rib will ensure that the blood vessel in that location will not be penetrated. Once the needle (catheter) has been advanced about 1 inch into the pleural space, it should be placed parallel to the thoracic wall to prevent penetration of the lung tissue. Intravenous extension tubing is placed on the needle (catheter), and a 35- to 60-ml syringe is attached. Apply gentle suction, as vigorous suction may result in lung laceration when the pleural space collapses and the lung reinflates. If free air is encountered, when the syringe is full, use the three-way stop-cock and expel air from the syringe; repeat the aspiration until negative pressure is obtained.

ENDNOTES

1 Flushing venous catheters with heparinized saline prior to placement appears to decrease clotting during catheter placement.
2 Comments regarding catheters, like many clinical impressions, reflect bias and may not be true for everyone. Because the Sovereign catheter is so stiff, it is often easier to place if the technician does not have any help and must use a tourniquet.
3 When the stylet enters the vessel, a "flash" of blood is seen; the catheter is not necessarily in the vessel when the flash is seen.
4 Beginners tend to back the stylet out rather than keeping the stylet still and feeding the catheter.
5 The ET tubes should be checked to see if the cuff leaks after inflation.
6 A guide tube is used to direct the ET tube between the arytenoids into the trachea. It is generally 1.5 to 2 times the length of the ET tube. When visualization is difficult, the use of a guide tube allows the laryngoscope to be removed once the guide tube is placed through the arytenoids.
7 A stylet is generally used when ET tube is too compliant for accurate placement. The stylet does not extend past the end of the ET tub and makes the ET tube stiff. The stylet usually has a rubber stopper that occludes the top of the ET tube and keeps the stylet in place. When using a stylet, it should be removed once the ET tube is in place to avoid occlusion of the airway.

REFERENCES

Hardie, E.M. 1999. Tracheal rupture in cats: 16 Cases (1983–1998). *J Am Vet Med Assoc* 214: 508–512.
Mitchell, S.L. 2000. Tracheal rupture associated with intubation in cats: 20 Cases (1996–1998). *J Am Vet Med Assoc* 216:1592–1595.

ADDITIONAL READING

McCurnin, D.M., and Poffenbarger, E.M. 1991. *Small Animal Physical Diagnosis and Clinical Procedures.* Philadelphia: W.B. Saunders.
McMichael, M., and DeBiasio, J. 2005. *Veterinary Emergency Protocols.* College Station: Texas A&M University.

Appendix 1
Recommended Resources

Gwendolyn L. Canoll

ANESTHESIA/ANALGESIA

American College of Veterinary Anesthesiologists (ACVA) position statements: http://www.acva.org/professional/Position/pstn.asp

- Position statement on Pain Management
  www.acva.org/professional/Position/pain.htm
  Publication: Treatment of pain in animals. 1998.
  J Am Vet Med Assoc 213(5):628–630.
- Position statement on Waste Gas
  www.acva.org/professional/Position/waste.htm
  Publication: Commentary and recommendations on control of waste anesthetic gases in the workplace. 1996. *J Am Vet Med Assoc* 209(1):75–77.
- Position statement on Monitoring
  www.acva.org/professional/Position/monitor.htm
  Publication: Suggestions for monitoring anesthetized veterinary patients. 1995. *J Am Vet Med Assoc* 206(7):936–937.

EUTHANSIA

Website for 2000 Report of the AVMA Panel on Euthanasia: www.avma.org/resources/euthanasia.pdf

AVMA Grief Counseling Websites: http://www.avma.org/careforanimals/animatedjourneys/goodbyefriend/plhotlines.asp

PET LOSS HOTLINES FROM AVMA

- (530) 752–3602, or toll free (800) 565–1526 Staffed by University of California-Davis veterinary students; weekdays, 6:30 pm to 9:30 pm Pacific Time (PT); http://www.vetmed.ucdavis.edu/petloss/index.htm
- (352) 392–4700; then dial 1 and 4080, staffed by Florida community volunteers; weekdays, 7 pm to 9 pm Eastern Time (ET); or call (352) 392–4700 X4744 (Joy Diaz) at the University; http://www.vetmed.ufl.edu/vmth/companions.htm
- (517) 432–2696 Staffed by Michigan State University veterinary students; Tuesday to Thursday, 6:30 pm to 9:30 pm ET; http://cvm.msu.edu/petloss/index.htm
- (630) 325–1600 Staffed by Chicago VMA veterinarians and staffs. Leave voice-mail message; calls will be returned 7 pm to 9 pm CT (Long-distance calls will be returned collect)
- (540) 231–8038 Staffed by Virginia-Maryland Regional College of Veterinary Medicine; Tuesday, Thursday 6 pm to 9 pm, ET
- (614) 292–1823 Staffed by The Ohio State University veterinary students; Monday, Wednesday, Friday, 6:30 pm to 9:30 pm ET; voice-mail messages will be returned, collect, during operating hours
- (508) 839–7966 Staffed by Tufts University veterinary students; Monday through Friday, 6 pm to 9 pm ET; voice-mail messages will be returned daily, collect outside Massachusetts; http://www.tufts.edu/vet/petloss/
- (888) ISU-PLSH (888-478-7574) Pet Loss Support Hotline hosted by the Iowa State University College of Veterinary Medicine; http://www.vetmed.iastate.edu/animals/petloss/; operational seven days a week, 6 pm to 9 pm (CST) from Sept-April; Monday, Wednesday, Friday from 6:00 to 9:00 pm (CST) from May–August
- (607) 253–3932 Cornell University Pet Loss Support Hotline staffed by Cornell University Veterinary Students Tuesday–Thursday 6 pm to 9 pm ET, messages will be returned; http://web.vet.cornell.edu/public/petloss/

- (217) 244–2273 or toll-free (877) 394–2273(CARE) Staffed by University of Illinois veterinary students. Sunday, Tuesday and Thursday evenings 7 pm to 9 pm CT; http://www.cvm.uiuc.edu/CARE/
- Argus Institute: Grief Resources, Colorado State University. For the Argus Institute office, call (970) 491–4143
- (509) 335–5704, Pet Loss Hotline, Washington State University, College of Veterinary Medicine http://www.vetmed.wsu.edu/plhl/index.htm; staffed during the semester on Monday, Tuesday, Wednesday, and Thursday 6:30–9:00 PM, and Saturday 1:00 pm to 3:00 pm PT.

RESOURCES FROM AMERICAN ANIMAL HOSPITAL ASSOCIATION STORE FOR CLIENT EDUCATION

Downing, R. 2000. *Pets Living with Cancer: a Pet Owner's Resource*. Lakewood, AAHA Press.

Montgomery, M., and Montgomery, H. 1993. *Final Act of Caring: Ending the Life of an Animal Friend*. Montgomery Press.

Montgomery, M., and Montgomery, H. 2000. *Forever in My Heart: Remembering My Pet's Life*. Montgomery Press.

Montgomery, M., and Montgomery, H. 1991. *Goodbye My Friend*. Montgomery Press.

Loss of Your Pet (brochure). 2002. Lakewood: AAHA Press.

Loss of Your Pet (DVD and brochure). 1989. Lakewood: AAHA Press.

Moorehead, D. 1996. *Special Place for Charlee: A Child's Companion Through Pet Loss*. Partners in Publishing, LLC.

Appendix 2
Blood Transfusions

Maureen McMichael

CANINE BLOOD TYPES

Dog erythrocyte antigen (DEA) is the major antigen on canine red blood cells (RBCs). We currently type for six of these, including DEA 1.1, 1.2, 3, 4, 5, and 7. Because 98% dogs are positive for DEA 4 and 42% are positive for DEA 1.1, the universal blood donor is DEA 1.1 negative and DEA 4 positive. Dogs do not have naturally occurring antibodies against different RBC antigens.

FELINE BLOOD TYPES

There are three feline blood types: A, B, and AB. Type A is most common (~99% of cats in the United States). Type B is not common (higher percentage in Abyssinian, Birman, Persian, Somali, Scottish Fold, Exotic and British Shorthair, Cornish and Devon Rex). Be cautious, however, because some DSH cats are type B! Type AB is very rare.

Cats, unlike dogs, have naturally occurring antibodies against other blood types. Type B cats have very strong, naturally occurring antibodies against type A antigen. A transfusion of type A blood into a type B cat causes a rapid, severe hemolytic reaction and can cause death. All cats should be typed before transfusing. The average RBC life span after a transfusion in a cat is as follows:

Type A blood into type A cat—RBC life span ~36 days

Type B blood into type A cat—RBC life span ~2.1 days

Type A blood into type B cat—RBC life span ~1.3 hours often ending in DEATH!

> There is no universal blood type for cats.

CROSSMATCHES

A crossmatch should be performed for all animals that have received a transfusion over 4 days earlier. Major crossmatch—mix recipient plasma with donor red blood cells. Minor crossmatch—mix recipient red cells with donor plasma.

FRESH WHOLE BLOOD

Considered "fresh" for up to 8 hours after collection. Fresh whole blood provides RBCs, WBCs, plasma proteins, viable platelets, and all clotting factors.

Stored whole blood provides RBCs, plasma proteins, and the stable coagulation factors (loss of platelets and factors 5 and 8 occur after ~24 hours of storage).

One unit = 450 ml (dog), 50–60 ml (cat)
Dose 20 ml/kg OR 2.2 ml/kg will raise PCV 1%
Rate 5–10 ml/kg/hr OR in emergency can go as high as 20–25 ml/kg/hr

PACKED RED CELLS

Provides just the red blood cell part of whole blood. Packed cells do not contain plasma, coagulation factors, or platelets.

One unit = 250–300 ml (dog), 25–30 ml (cat)
Dose = 10 ml/kg or 1 ml/kg will raise PCV 1%

FRESH FROZEN PLASMA

Fresh frozen plasma contains all coagulation factors (including factors 5 and 8 and the labile factors).

One unit = 250 ml (dog), 25 ml (cat)
Dose 10 ml/kg

271

Shelf-life is 1 year (after that time, it can still be kept frozen and considered frozen plasma or stored plasma.)

FROZEN PLASMA (OR STORED PLASMA)

Contains stabile coagulation factors (all vitamin K–dependent factors); contains albumin, does not contain the labile factors (factors 5 and 8).

Dose 10 ml/kg
Shelf-life = 5 years

CRYOPRECIPITATE

This is the precipitate that forms at the top of a unit of fresh frozen plasma as it is slowly thawed. It allows a higher concentration of specific coagulation factors in a smaller volume. This is advantageous when you have an animal with normal volume that needs prophylactic protection (i.e., a dental in a dog with von Willebrand's disease) or in an animal that cannot handle excess volume (i.e., a Doberman with dilated cardiomyopathy and von Willebrand's disease). Cryoprecipitate does not contain anything more than fresh frozen plasma; it is just a concentrated form. In other words, if you have an animal with hemophilia A or von Willebrand's disease and do not have cryoprecipitate, use fresh frozen plasma. Cryoprecipitate is especially important for small-breed dogs with concurrent cardiac issues that could not handle the full plasma load. It contains factors 8, fibrinogen, fibronectin, and von Willebrand's factor. It is especially suited for animals with von Willebrands disease and hemophilia A.

Dose 1 unit per 10 kg
Shelf-life = 1 year

Administration

All blood products, including plasma, should be administered through a blood filter. A 170-μm filter should be used. Plasma may contain microthrombi, which will be filtered with standard blood transfusion filters.

OXYGLOBIN

Oxyglobin is a hemoglobin-based oxygen-carrying substance that increases colloid oncotic pressure and increases oxygen-carrying capacity. Oxyglobin is unique in that it is the only oxygen-carrying substance that will increase colloid oncotic pressure. It does not contain coagulation factors, albumin, alpha macroglobulins, or 2,3-DPG (because cows use chloride for this purpose). A major downfall is that Oxyglobin interferes with several chemistry analyzers and some values may be erroneous after administration of Oxyglobin. This is clearly marked on the package insert, so you will know what values you will lose before you administer it. The dose is based on the half-life of the oxyglobin molecule, which is very different from other forms of blood. Availability is limited at this time.

Dose for dogs; 15 ml/kg (lasts ~24 hours), 30 ml/kg (lasts ~72 hours); do not exceed 10 ml/kg/hr
Dose for cats; do not exceed 5–10 ml/kg; do not exceed 1–3 ml/kg/hr

RISK OF BACTERIAL CONTAMINATION

The risk of bacterial contamination increases exponentially after 4 hours at room temperature. All blood transfusions should be completed within 4 hours!

TRANSFUSION COMPLICATIONS

Signs of a transfusion reaction can include fever, tachycardia, tachypnea, vomiting, agitation, hypotension, and shock. Transfusion reactions can be separated into mild, moderate, and serious.

Mild Reaction

A mild reaction can be characterized by just a fever or can proceed to urticaria and angioedema. A transfusion fever is a temperature increase of 1°C over the pretransfusion temperature. The transfusion should be stopped, the bag checked for discoloration, the blood being transfused and the animal should be checked for hemolysis, and in most instances, the transfusion can be continued at a slower rate. An injection of diphenhydramine can be considered before restarting the transfusion.

Moderate Reaction

A moderate reaction can be characterized by fever, urticaria, angioedema, vomiting, restlessness, tachycardia, tachypnea, and hypotension. The transfusion should be stopped, the bag and the patient should be checked for hemolysis, and the bag checked for discoloration. Oxygen should be administered and intravenous fluid diuresis should be started (ideally after a baseline BUN/creatinine).

The animal should be monitored for signs of acute renal failure if there was hemolysis present. If agglutination is present and the animal still needs oxygen carrying capacity, Oxyglobin should be considered.

Severe Reaction

A severe reaction can be characterized by acute collapse, vomiting, tachycardia, tachypnea, fever, restlessness, hypotension, and shock. First, obtain an airway, intubate, and ventilate if necessary. Start shock doses of crystalloids (LRS, 0.9% NaCl), and administer a low dose of epinephrine (at 0.01 mg/kg IV) if the animal is collapsed, severely hypotensive, or in shock. If the animal is ventilating on its own, administer oxygen. Check a PCV for hemolysis, check the urine for hemoglobinuria, and check the blood bag for hemolysis or any other abnormalities. Take a sample of the transfused blood for culture and sensitivity and refrigerate the bag (mark "DO NOT USE" on it). Get a baseline chemistry panel for BUN/creatinine. If there is not already a CBC and urinalysis, get baseline data for these now. Continue intravenous fluid diuresis, consider bactericidal antibiotics if sepsis or infection is suspected, and monitor for acute renal failure and other complications. If oxygen-carrying capacity is still needed, consider Oxyglobin.

Index

DATE DUE

GAYLORD			PRINTED IN U.S.A.